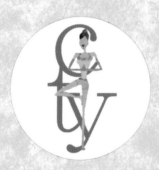

STRUCTURAL YOGA THERAPY™

structural YOGA therapy™

ADAPTING
TO THE
INDIVIDUAL

MUKUNDA STILES

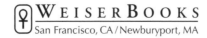

WEISER BOOKS
San Francisco, CA / Newburyport, MA

First published in 2000 by
Red Wheel/Weiser, LLC
with offices at:
665 Third Street, Suite 400
San Francisco, CA 94107
www.redwheelweiser.com

This hardcover edition, 2013

ISBN: 978-1-57863-177-3

Library of Congress Cataloging-in Publication Data

Stiles, Mukunda
  Structural yoga therapy™ : adapting to the individual /
  Mukunda Stiles
        p. cm.
  Includes bibliographical references and index.
  ISBN 1-57863-177-7 (hardcover : alk. paper)
  ISBN 157863-209-9 (pbk. : alk. paper)
    1. Yoga, Hatha—Therapeutic use.   I. Title.
  RM727.Y64 S75 2000
  613.7'046—dc21   00-033471

Typeset in 11/13 Adobe Garamond
Cover and book design by Kathryn Sky-Peck
Illustration of Patanjali on part title pages used by permission of B. K. S. Iyengar.
Cover photography © 2000 Photodisc, Inc.

PRINTED IN THE UNITED STATES OF AMERICA
MV
15 14 13 12 11 10

The paper used in this publication meets the minimum requirements of the American National
Standard for Information Sciences—Permanence of Paper for
Printed Library Materials Z39.48-1992 (R1997).

A Yogi's Prayer

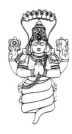

May all who are mean return to good;
    May all who are good obtain true peace.
May all who are peaceful be freed from bonds;
    May all who are free set others free.

Blessings upon all the earth;
    May all the world's rulers uphold righteousness.
May only good fortune reach everyone;
    May all the world's creatures be happy.

May rain fall when the earth is thirsty;
    May all the storehouses be filled.
May everyone here be free from injury;
    May all who are good be free from fear.

May everyone know a life of joy;
    May everyone live a life of health.
May everyone see only good in the world;
    May everyone soon be released from pain.

May everyone overcome all their woes;
    May everyone see only good in the world.
May everyone realize all their desires;
    May everyone everywhere be glad.

May our mother and father be blessed;
    Blessings upon every creature on earth.
May our works flourish and aid everyone,
    And long may our eyes see the sun.

    Om shanti, shanti, shanti (peace).

Contents

Part One
Origins and Theory of Yoga Practice, 1

Part Two
Preparation for Practice, 25

Part Three
The Benefits of Yoga Practice, 69

Part Four
Anatomy and Yoga, 107

PART FIVE
THE PRACTICE OF YOGA ASANAS, 191

PART SIX
YOGA FOR SPECIFIC GOALS, 261

List of Figures

List of Tables

Acknowledgments

I am most indebted to my spiritual teacher, Baba Muktananda, whose guidance led me to a life-style as a yogi. Through his constant presence in spite of his physical death in 1982, I have been directed to the work that is the focus of my life. With his assistance, I have found access to insight and higher wisdom in my constant inquiry into who I am through my studies of anatomy and Classical Yoga.

I thank B. K. S. Iyengar for his invaluable insight into Hatha Yoga and the functioning of the physical body. I have drawn largely from his work with yoga asana to create this series. From training in his method during the period of 1975 to 1976, the inspiration for this Structural Yoga Therapy™ method arose.

Many other Hatha Yoga teachers and colleagues have contributed to my life and shared my path to yoga. They include: Rama Jyoti Vernon, my dear friend and first teacher of Iyengar Yoga; Mataji Indra Devi, the most loving yogini I've ever met, whose persistent encouragement to "send love and light to everyone" is the highest teaching of yoga; Sri T. Krishnamacharya, whom I never met, yet whose motto, "adapt to the individual," has been a constant source of guidance in the development of my personalized approach to yoga therapy; T. K. V. Desikacharya, whose reminder to adapt yoga to the individual helped me to see beauty in the variety; Paul Copeland, M.D., who introduced me to Krishnamacharya's vinyasas and inspired my interest in yoga physiology; Judith Lasater, whose knowledge of anatomy and kinesiology inspired me to study those subjects for over twenty years; and Jean Couch, whose friendship and personal drive to help people in pain, through her development of balance, I cherish.

My principal teachers of the Classical Raja Yoga method of Patanjali's *Yoga Sutras* have been Swami Shyam of Kulu, and Swami Muktananda Paramahansa. Both gave me invaluable insight into the living, eating, breathing, and walking of this ancient Yoga. Special thanks to Dr. David Frawley, whose scholarly insight into Patanjali as a Bhakti—a lover of God—influenced my poetic rendering of the *Yoga Sutras*.

I have had tremendous assistance in the writing of this book over a twenty-year period. I want to thank my ex-wife, Yogini Tara Stiles, whose consistent love has helped me to find stability during challenging periods. I am grateful to Dr. William Beer for taking the time to review the anatomy and physiology material for accuracy. I especially want to thank the many wordsmiths who contributed much to revisions, editing, and making the information accessible to a wider range of yoga students. Among them are Geralyn Gendron, Barbananda Baccei, and my dear friend, Yogini Shar Lee.

I am especially indebted to those yoga students whose curiosity and suffering propelled me to seek an innovative approach to yoga therapy. I offer my Namaskar to you, with great respect and love.

The quoted material on the Part Title pages comes from the following sources: Parts One and Two: *Yoga Sutras of Patanjali*, to be published by Samuel Weiser in 2001; Part Three: Richard Lannoy, *Anandamayi: Her Life and Wisdom* (Boston: Element, 1996), p. 139; Part Four: Swami Prakashananda in Titus Foster, *Agaram Bagaram Baba: Life, Teachings, and Parables: A Spiritual Biography of Swami Prakashananda* (Berkeley, CA:

North Atlantic, 1999), pp. 79–80; Part Five: B. K. S. Iyengar, *Body the Shrine, Yoga Thy Light* (Bombay: D. B. Taraporevala, 1978), pp. 234, 245; Part Six: T. K. V. Desikachar, with R. H. Cravens, *Health, Healing & Beyond: Yoga and the Living Tradition of Krishnamacharya* (New York: Aperture, 1998), pp. 99, 121.

The original illustrations are by Jesse Tarantino. The anatomical illustrations were adapted from the following sources: Carmine D. Clemente, *Anatomy: A Regional Atlas of the Human Body* (Baltimore: Urban & Schwarzenberg, 1987); Lucille Daniels and Catherine Worthingham. *Therapeutic Exercise for Body Alignment and Function* (Philadelphia: W. B. Saunders, 1977); Louise Gordon, *Anatomy and Figure Drawing* (London: B. T. Batsford, 1979); Helen Hislop and Jacqueline Montgomery, *Daniels and Worthingham's Muscle Testing, Techniques of Manual Examination* (Philadelphia: W. B. Saunders, 1971); Frank H. Netter, *Atlas of Human Anatomy* (Summit, NJ: CIBA-GEIGY Corporation, 1989); and Clem Thompson, *Manual of Structural Kinesiology* (St. Louis: Times Mirror/Mosby, 1989). The models for the illustrations are Laurie Hastie and Mukunda Stiles.

Introduction:
The Evolution of Structural Yoga Therapy™

Asanasthah sukham hride nimajjati
One who is established in a comfortable posture
while concentrating on the inner Self,
naturally becomes immersed in
the Heart's ocean of bliss.[1]

—*Siva Sutras* III, 16

This text of the teachings of Kashmir Shaivism declares that the nature of our True Self is bliss. When I first studied with Baba Muktananda, my first spiritual teacher, I was given experiences of a place in myself that was this True Self. The language was unfamiliar, the trappings were strange, and even the smells were exotic. The experience, however, was one of coming home in the most profound sense. I had been a teacher of Hatha Yoga before meeting Baba in 1974. At that first meeting, Baba gave me initiation in Siddha Yoga, his term for the modern version of the devotional tantrik kundalini yoga tradition. This consisted of a personal transmission of the presence of yoga given through the life-force of his breath. Upon receiving this, my life began to change spontaneously for the better. Although I had no contact with him or his teachings for a year, this Presence grew inside me, until my motivation for life changed to follow its inner guidance. Over the course of time with Baba, a growing desire inflamed me to translate the process of knowing this Presence, which he called the inner Self, through the hatha/physical Yoga discipline.

I had been introduced to the *Yoga Sutras* of Patanjali by an inspiring teacher of Indian philosophy, Dr. Epstein, while pursuing a degree in economics at the University of California at Davis in 1973. In some mysterious way, my pursuit of a CPA license and the wealth to afford a Jaguar XKE lost their captivating quality after connecting with Baba. The *Sutras*, however, began to glow like an inner flame that I was irresistibly attracted to study. I changed my major to Religious Studies and was given free rein to write my own program because I was the first student to pursue this program. I chose to write my senior thesis on Patanjali's *Yoga Sutras* and, through interlibrary loan, obtained all the translations of this ancient text, which contained the secret to define, clarify, and share the experience of yoga as Self-knowledge. I knew it was in there, and yet my studies of the translations were unable to satisfy my desire for a direct experience of this Truth. I could sense a literal step-by-step understanding of a path that offered an intellectual comprehension coupled with the immediacy of personal experience of this secret teaching.

A year later, when Baba returned to California, the Presence guided me to pursue a career in yoga and to move to the San Francisco Bay area for studies with Rama Jyoti

---

[1] Jaideva Singh, *Siva Sutras: The Yoga of Supreme Identity* (Delhi, India: Motilal Banarsidass, 1979), p. 163. Paraphrase by author.

Vernon and her staff at the Institute for Yoga Teacher Education (now the Iyengar Yoga Institute). Toward the end of my studies, the inspiration for the program, B. K. S. Iyengar, came to stay in our home for an intensive week-long program of Hatha Yoga classes. I had been having much trouble with my hyperextended knees, due to their increased mobility and sensitivity, and could never find a placement for them that felt right despite having some of the best advisors teaching me—Judith Lasater, P. T., Ramanand Patel, and Rama. In the teaching of the first class, in fact the first pose, Mr. Iyengar came to adjust me in the basic standing pose, Tadasana. As one whose desire to learn is strong, I have always placed myself directly in front of my teachers in order to watch them closely. He immediately recognized my instability in simply standing still. He placed his hands lightly on my shoulders, looked me straight in the eyes and swiftly drew his bent knee up between the insides of my knees.

Immediately, I experienced the essence of the *Siva Sutras* stanza quoted at the beginning of this chapter. My mind emptied as if a giant drain had been opened and a profound stillness of absorption in samadhi ensued. I had no interest in anything outside of myself and I was caught without any desire to escape. When the mind returned (and I did sense it then as *the* mind, not *my* mind), I knew that this was what I wanted to know. I desired to find this experience myself and, by an intimate knowledge of this presence, to share it with others. I sought nothing more from Mr. Iyengar; he had given me what I wanted in one initial contact. He had a tremendous amount to offer in terms of understanding the physical body, though being the independent person that I am, I had to make my own way.

Soon afterward, I began to explore my own way of comprehending this experience. I knew instinctively that there must be some physical training necessary to gain this knowledge, and yet, I knew that by pursuing only physical training, I would be lost. My intuition urged me to learn more about the doorways to this multidimensional Presence of my Self. Clearly, however, there was something to be learned from Mr. Iyengar's swift motion bringing about physical stability. My next step was to learn all I could about anatomy and kinesiology to gain an understanding of the body mechanics of Hatha Yoga. At the same time, I continued to see Baba on a daily basis at his Oakland ashram, just a mile away from Rama's home where I lived.

Over the years, I have been given insights into how adjustments through Hatha Yoga to relieve subtle postural tensions can sometimes bring people into an immediate experience of their own innate Presence of Yoga. The insights first expressed themselves during the early 80s when I was a staff yoga teacher at Muktananda's ashrams in California, New York, Massachusetts, and India. During that period, Baba began to encourage Hatha Yoga training in addition to meditation training. He was quite specific about how the practices must be given, even going so far as to demonstrate the practice of bellows breathing (bastrika) himself in public. It was remarkable to watch him remain absorbed in his inner experience, unchanged by this profound physical pranayama. His stillness and devotion touched me deeply.

Another student of Baba Muktananda, Dr. Gabriel Cousens, sought me out for personalized instruction to help him rebuild his athletic body into the suppleness of a meditating yogi. When I applied what I had been given to bring the body into the pose of the Presence, Gabriel went into a meditative state. He was not interested in achieving this through Hatha Yoga, however, and insisted on using my knowledge of anatomy to change his physical body to have less density in his muscular and skeletal structures.

Through Dr. Cousens, I was introduced to some of Baba's American Swamis (monks) who were suffering from back pain. The ashram schedule required about six hours daily of sitting on hard floors. The Swamis had been doing a Hatha Yoga practice, although it was usually minimal compared to the hours spent daily in chanting or sitting for meditation. One of them, Baba's secretary, had been doing the Extended Triangle (Utthita Trikonasana) pose, which I thought should be helpful for his back. When I asked him to show me how he did it, I saw that he was not following the basic principles that Iyengar stressed for body alignment. Once I adjusted him in the pose according to these standards, he swooned into an all-encompassing bliss state of absorption into samadhi. He left his physical body to enter this bliss and crumpled like an infant in my arms. Tears of joy streamed from his eyes and he was, of course, quite free of back pain.

Another Swami with whom I worked was an accomplished hatha yogi before he met Baba. He had a beautiful practice for many years, and yet he experienced persistent back pain. Rather than diagnose him and give my prescription, I asked him to show me his practice. His poses were all effective for his overall health, though I could see that they were not therapeutic to his back condition. When I had made some minor adjustments and explained the deep anatomy of the spine, he began to feel within himself how to use his body more exactly. He learned quickly and saw how to go through the layers of his multidimensionality (explained in chapter 6) using his physical and energetic bodies, and his mind and spirit to integrate them. His experiences of "getting it right" were comprehensive—he stayed in his body and also accessed his bliss of samadhi.

From these few moments with these highly trained yoga meditators, I learned a great deal about integrating the process of Hatha into Raja Yoga that Patanjali had so beautifully described two thousand years earlier. The magnificence of the true teachings is that they are timeless and apply to the mind/body regardless of culture, sex, age, or time period. Yoga is the most profound practice I have found. It affords its disciplined practitioners all they could ever want to know or experience about themselves.

My intention in putting forth yet another name for a form of Hatha Yoga is to create a living understanding of anatomy and movement based on deep reverence for the integrity of the human body and Spirit. The body can and does adapt itself to injuries—physical as well as emotional and mental. This adaptive force, which is referred to in yoga as prana shakti kundalini, is the root inspiration for structural yoga therapy. Through in-depth study of the gross physical body, the subtle body can be appreciated more—as can Albert Einstein's words, "God is subtle." To know the subtle workings of the body is to appreciate and respect the indwelling Being that remains changeless as our appearance changes from infancy to childhood to adulthood to old age.

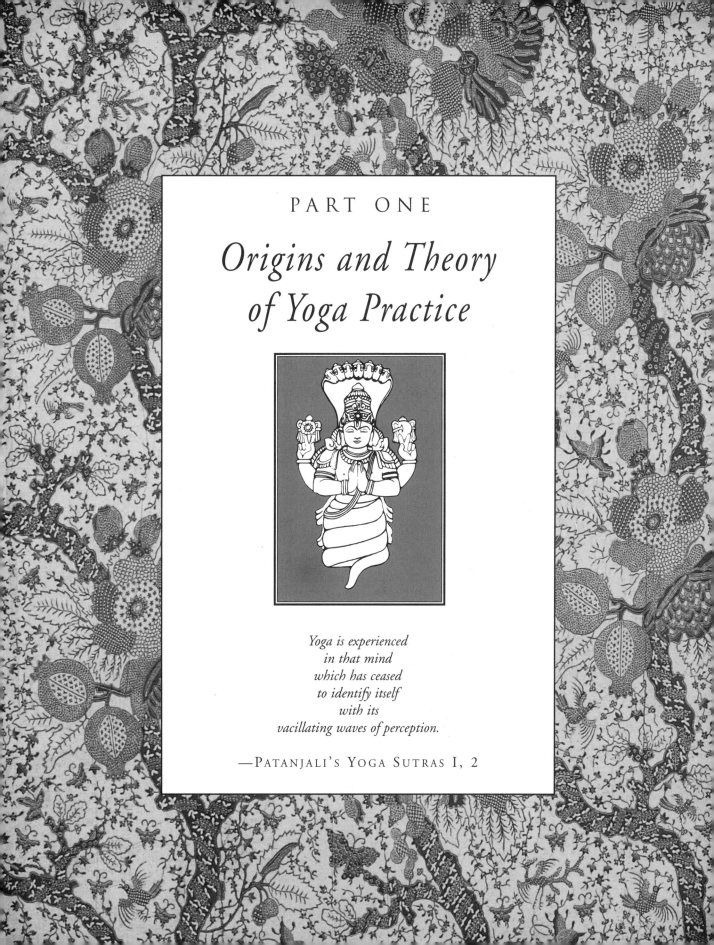

PART ONE

Origins and Theory
of Yoga Practice

*Yoga is experienced
in that mind
which has ceased
to identify itself
with its
vacillating waves of perception.*

—PATANJALI'S YOGA SUTRAS I, 2

INTRODUCTION

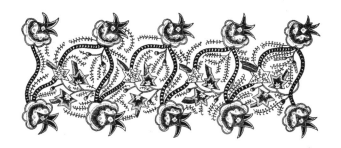

In the beginning, according to Indian mythology, the world was filled with a vast ocean and a few small islands. In this primordial sea, Matsya, a fish, was swimming near the shore of an island. He happened upon a conversation between Lord Siva and his consort, Parvati. Seeking instruction in the practice of Yoga, Parvati inquired: "I want to attain union with you. You are so attractive, so beautiful to me, and yet when I feel myself close to you, something holds me back, something keeps me from merging totally into you. My love is so strong for you, and yet something within me—what could it be?—is holding me back. I want to lose myself in you. I know you would keep me safe and respect me as your own Self. Please help me to merge more fully into you."

So Siva began a great teaching dialogue with Parvati, saying, "Your love is so strong, so genuine. That which you seek, union with me, is not an attainment. There is nothing to do, for I am your own True Self. I am not separate from you. The way to me is through knowing your own True Self. Out of your love for me, I will reveal the secret that is Yoga—the experience of communion. Yoga is the process by which you lose all identity of yourself as a separate being and become united with your nature as both Shakti and Siva—expansive, creative energy, as well as stillness, eternal bliss. Both these qualities are within you."

"The path to yoga is threefold," Siva continued, "but the goal is the same. The first path is purifying the ego through loving selfless service to others, known as *Karma Yoga.* The second is the study of sacred texts and reflecting upon their underlying question, Who am I? This is known as *Jnana Yoga,* the path of wisdom. The third path is the dedication of all actions to the Divine Presence, known as *Bhakti Yoga,* the path of devotion."

Hearing this teaching, Matsya the fish became more and more absorbed, and then more still. Through the stillness and these comforting words, he attained perfect posture (asana). He became light, was raised up to the surface and arched his back in the Matsyasana Fish Pose so that he could hear more clearly. Through the inspiration, he began to feel his heart open. The process of the pose began to transform him. He began to extend himself out of the water. A sublime force began to awaken within him through this spontaneous motion and he found himself effortlessly floating on the surface. As he became more still, his breathing was steadied and regulated; he became motionless in the water. He felt a transcendent life-force absorbing his mind, and yet he was not breathing. He was experiencing perfect Pranayama, in which the life-force hidden within his breath became suspended. An attraction to the inner experience held him, his steadiness increased. His mind turned within, as his senses detached from the outside world (a process called pratyahara), and he became totally absorbed, experiencing unity with everything and everyone.

As the experience deepened within him, he began to imbibe the state of samadhi, the state of absorption, and he lost all awareness of his fish nature. He experienced all objects as being composed of pure consciousness. Siva felt him merging into the same consciousness that was his essence. Feeling this oneness, he touched the fish, giving him his blessing, his initiation. The blessing of the lord instantly transformed Matsya from a fish into a human being. Siva gave him a new name—Matsyendra—Lord of the Fishes. Matsyendra came onto the land, sat, and listened to the discourse between Siva and Parvati until the instruction was full and he felt complete. As he listened to the teachings of yoga, he sat in a particular posture that twisted his spine and enabled him to remain free of physical distractions while listening attentively. This posture has been handed down in yogic lore as Matsyendrasana, the spinal twist.

From this story we learn that the essence of yoga is transformation. The great master, Sri Aurobindo, said:

> The true and full object and utility of Yoga can only be accomplished when the conscious Yoga in man becomes, like the subconscious Yoga in Nature, outwardly conterminous with life itself and we can once more, looking out both on the path and the achievement, say in a more perfect and luminous sense: "All life is Yoga."[1]

Through this transformation process, the fish Matsya became the first yoga teacher, Matsyendra. This myth is corroborated in the *Hatha Yoga Pradipika*, a 14th-century textbook on Hatha Yoga, which acknowledges that Matsyendra was the first to teach Classical Yoga practices.

---

[1] Sri Aurobindo, *The Synthesis of Yoga* (Pondicherry, India: Sri Aurobindo Ashram, 1984), p. 4.

Chapter 1

WHAT IS YOGA?

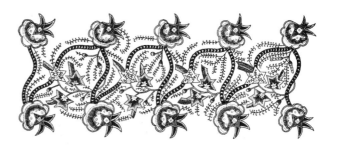

Everything has two fundamental aspects: the superficial—which is obvious, clear, and revealed—and the unknown—which is secret, unclear, and hidden. For example, a tree has a trunk, branches, and leaves above the ground. These draw nourishment from the light, while unseen roots draw strength in the darkness from the soil and water. In yogic philosophy, the obvious, that which is in constant motion, is called Shakti. The opposite pole of the unrevealed, that which is eternal and unchanging, is called Siva. In Chinese philosophy, the latent, dark, unexposed aspect is called yin, while yang is the patent, the bright, the exposed. The Shakti, or yang, aspect is the public part, generally called the exoteric aspect. The Siva, or yin, aspect—the inner, hidden part—is called the esoteric. Similarly, in describing human nature on the superficial psychological level, psychologist C. G. Jung noted that we have a public side that we reveal, and a private side that we keep hidden. On the transpersonal psychological level, we share common traits in our personalities. We also share transcendental traits, in that we have limited qualities of the Eternal One, omniscience, omnipotence, and omnipresence.

C. G. Jung said, "There is good reason for yoga to have many adherents. It offers not only the much-sought way, but also a philosophy of unrivalled profundity. Yoga practice is unthinkable, and would also be ineffectual, without the ideas on which it is based. It works the physical and the spiritual into one another in an extraordinarily complete way."[1]

---

[1] C. G. Jung, "Yoga and the West," in *Psychology and the East,* R. F. C. Hull, trans. (Princeton, NJ: Princeton University Press, 1978), p. 81.

The word *yoga* literally means "yoking," in the sense of the coming together of a harmonious relationship between our separate aspects. Different aspects of our perception make yoga either exoteric or esoteric. The yoga teachings regarding bringing the body, mind, and emotions into harmony, such as Hatha Yoga, are exoteric. Those teachings focused upon the outer self in harmony with the Inner Self, such as Classical Yoga, are esoteric. In exoteric-based Hatha Yoga, the practices focus on developing health to optimal physiological and psychological levels. In esoteric-based Classical Yoga, the practices focus on developing insight to know the hidden truth about one's nature.

In the yogic view of human anatomy, there are five bodies. Exoteric yoga practices strengthen the physical body (the first body), while at the same time purifying the hidden bodies. The second body is the subtle body, which makes up the emotional sense of vitality and energy. The third body is the mind, the embodied perception of thoughts and feelings. The fourth body is called the body of wisdom, the higher mind. The fifth body is composed of great joy that arises from "dispassionate nonattachment" to the experiences of the other bodies. (For more details see chapter 6.)

In the story of Matsyendra, Matsya, the fish, traveled through the five bodies as he grasped the teachings of Siva. The result was absolute one-pointedness that transformed him from a fish into a human. This allegory points to the hidden transformation available to yoga students through devoted practice. The lower nature, the fish, refers to that consciousness concerned with moving in a school, following the lead of others, as one who is held by water (emotions) and living a life based upon avoiding pain while pursuing pleasure.

Classical Yoga

Classical Yoga was first described as a systematic approach to Self-realization by Maharishi Patanjali about 200 B.C. His classical text, the *Yoga Sutras*, describes the nature of the mind and ways to control its restlessness. Unlike the five other classical Indian philosophical systems, Yoga is based on a process of physical and mental training culminating in the direct experience of realizing the universal Self within everyone.

Yogas chitta vritti nirodhah
tada drastuh svarupe avasthanam

Yoga
is experienced
in that *mind*
which has *ceased*
to identify itself
with its
vacillating waves of perception.

When this happens,
then the Seer is revealed
resting in *its own essential nature,*

6

and one realizes
the true
Self.[2]

Patanjali defines guideposts to keep the student of yoga progressing along the path. While there are numerous paths to yoga, they have a common thread that has been delineated in the *Yoga Sutras*. In fact, the *Sutras* can be taken as a guide for anyone undergoing any discipline of body, breath, emotions, mind, and spirit. The goal of yoga is to merge the mind into the True Self, and thus to be true to your Self in all thoughts, words, and deeds. Anyone proceeding any distance along this path cannot help but experience more joy and health.

Yoga is not a religion. People of all faiths practice yoga. From a yogi's point of view, everyone is doing yoga—everyone is seeking the joy found in the experience of the Self as our innate spirituality. Yet, most of the time, we do not realize that the joy we seek is experienced within, in the discovery of the Self. We erroneously believe our joy comes from objects of sensual pleasure. In completing activities, there is a momentary experience of stilling the mind, and thus we feel peace. This state of fulfillment is what the yoga practitioner seeks to gain more consistently, more permanently.

Yoga, then, is a continuous process. For serious students, it is a life's work. Yoga—as the stilling of the mind—occurs momentarily in many people without training. Often, following periods of concentration, people will report that they were performing a task (such as reading) and became perfectly still. Their breathing became nearly unnoticeable and they lost all sense of time. During these periods of active meditation, access to intuitive insights is available. We will intuitively understand how to manage ourselves in situations that formerly produced difficulties. This natural process is what Patanjali defined as yoga. It is through the study of yoga, in the context of the guidelines laid out in the *Yoga Sutras,* that these momentary experiences become part of daily living.

Patanjali's practical means of knowing the inner Self is known as Ashtanga Yoga, the yoga of "eight limbs." It is also called Raja, "royal," Yoga, the yoga of the royal path to self-realization. Raja, which also means "to radiate," is the practice of radiating the royal light of the true Self. The mysticism of Raja Yoga, simply put, means to be radiantly happy and share that compassionate affection for all creation. The eight component limbs, found in his *Yoga Sutras* II, 29–III, 3, are:

1. Yama—external attitudes for guiding conduct within society
   - Nonviolence (*ahimsa*): when mastered, one creates an atmosphere in which violence ceases;
   - Truthfulness (*satya*): when perfected, one's words and deeds exist in service to that Truth;
   - Abstaining from stealing (*asteya*): when mastered, that which you consider precious is drawn to you;

---

[2] Mukunda Stiles, *Yoga Sutras of Patanjali,* chap. I, sutras 2–3 (this book is a forthcoming publication from Samuel Weiser, York Beach, ME).

- Behavior that moves one toward the Truth (*brahmacharya*): when perfected, vitality is gained;
- Noncoveting (*aparigraha*): when mastered, knowledge of the hidden lessons of the repetitive cycle of birth and death is gained.

2. Niyama—internal attitudes for personal discipline

- Purity (*sauca*): when established, one desires to protect the physical body and has no interest in contact with others of an adverse nature;
- Contentment (*santosa*): when perfected, one gains supreme happiness;
- Perseverance in selfless service (*tapas*): when mastered, leads to a dwindling of all impurities and a perfection of the body, mind, and sense organs;
- Study of the Self (*svadhaya*): when mastered, leads to communion with your personal chosen ideals or deity;
- Devotion to God (*Ishvara pranidhana*): when mastered, leads to absolute absorption into the Divine Presence.

3. Asana—yoga posture. When regularly practiced, all movements end in a "steady and comfortable" pose that is performed by relaxation of effort and results in no longer being disturbed by duality, praise, and/or criticism.

4. Pranayama—regulation of the in- and out-flow of breath/prana. When perfected, one feels the life-force (prana) permeating everywhere, transcending the attention given to either external or internal objects.

5. Pratyahara—withdrawal of the senses from their objects. When the senses become detached from external objects of the mind's desire, the mind sees its source as pure consciousness.

6. Dharana—contemplation of one's true nature. When mastered, the mind is confined to one place of attention.

7. Dhyana—meditation. When mastered, a continuous flow of awareness to a single point of attention is maintained.

8. Samadhi—absorption in the Self. When achieved, it is the meditation that results in only the essential light of the object remaining. The object loses its concrete form. The Spiritual Light prevails and is experienced as the essence of all of creation.

This eightfold process is exactly what happened in the transformation of the fish Matsya into the yogi Matsyendra. Through a strong interest in the subject (yama and niyama), his body became still. In losing all awareness of his body, those sensations common to willful movement ceased (asana). His breath became subtle and steady (pranayama). Then his prana and senses withdrew their awareness of the distinction between outside and inside (pratyahara). Next, his mind focused upon listening intently to the teachings (dharana and dhyana). Finally, he lost the sense of himself and was left with only the awareness of himself as Pure Consciousness without an object to pull it (samadhi).

Chapter 2

WHAT IS HATHA YOGA?

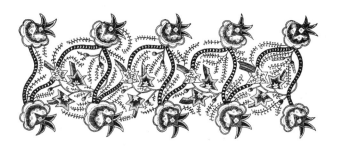

The word "yoga" is usually preceded by a descriptive adjective that connotes a particular method. In general, most yogas in America today are variations of Hatha Yoga. Hatha Yoga is the physical discipline of Classical Yoga, comprising stages three and four of the eight stages (Ashtanga Yoga) of Patanjali's *Yoga Sutras*. Hence most yoga methods—the exceptions being Classical and Kriya Yoga—delete training about yoga life-style, ethics, philosophy, preparation for spirituality, and meditation. Hatha Yoga emphasizes methods of doing yoga poses (asanas) and energetic breathing exercises (pranayamas) for physical health and well-being. Proponents of Classical Yoga utilize these techniques for the purpose of preliminary training in meditation, then proceed to give instruction in meditation and yoga life-style.

There are many types of yoga available for study today. New methods are brought out each year. Yoga is extremely popular these days, with an estimated ten to twelve million practitioners in America alone. For more information, see *Yoga International* magazine's Yoga Teacher Directory published in the January–February issue each year. This features a comprehensive description of the major methods of yoga. For information about yoga organizations on the Internet, go to www.sportscenter.com.ar/yogaorganizations.html.

Methods of Hatha Yoga

There are a number of major styles of Hatha Yoga in America. The following are summaries of methodologies of the most common lineages of yoga.

ASHTANGA YOGA

Ashtanga Yoga is the name applied by Indian master Pattabhi Jois, now in his 80s, to his system of yoga poses. Pattabhi Jois developed the system while being mentored by Prof. T. Krishnamacharya of Madras, South India. There are three levels, the first challenging enough to meet the requirements of even the most athletic student for several years. It is a system that was given to him in his youth to meet the high energy level of his developing body. In America, it is presented in modified formats, sometimes milder in form, as hot yoga, or power yoga. While the series does end with a pranayama series, it deletes the practices of meditation. Ashtanga Yoga, while named for the "eight limbs" of Patanjali's Classical Yoga, rarely presents the eight limbs or Patanjali's text.

The benefits of this method are its tremendous challenge to physical strength and flexibility. It is enjoying a period of popularity and so it is easy to find a teacher of this method.

CLASSICAL YOGA

Classical Yoga appears in two major forms, as the Ashtanga Yoga of Baba Hari Das, or as Viniyoga, originating from the teachings of Prof. Krishnamacharya and his son/successor, T. K. V. Desikachar.[1] This yoga is presented in the context of Patanjali's *Yoga Sutras* and hence incorporates study of the text, the source of the teachings, and adapts to the individual with many varieties of practices beyond the commonplace asanas. These may include pranayamas, kriyas, mudras, and bandhas.

Its benefits include thoroughness and well-rounded study of yoga as a life-style and the ability to receive individually tailored practices for your situation.

INTEGRAL YOGA

The Integral Yoga of Swami Satchidananda of Yogaville, Virginia is also a gentler spiritual-based yoga that is clearly leading to devotion and meditation practice. Swamiji, a disciple of the renowned Dr. Swami Sivananda of Rishikesh, came to America in the 1960s and is responsible for converting many hippies from a life-style of sex, drugs, and rock 'n' roll to family life, yoga, and chanting. His appearance is one often associated with yoga. He is a tall mild-mannered man, soft-spoken, who wears long white robes and has long flowing white hair and beard. His brand of yoga emphasizes poses taken to the extremes of flexibility as a way to awaken the kundalini spiritual energy, numerous traditional pranayama breathing exercises, chanting, candle-gazing, and meditating on the chakra energy centers. (For details see his book *Integral Yoga Hatha*.[2]) This yoga is not to be confused with the integral yoga of Sri Aurobindo, a spiritual yet practical meditation technique.

The benefits of this method are that it is a well-rounded program supervised by an Indian adept who has lived in America for over thirty years.

---

[1] See Baba Hari Das, *Ashtanga Yoga Primer* (Santa Cruz, CA: Sri Rama Publishing/Hanuman Fellowship, 1981); and Gary Kraftsow, *Yoga for Wellness: Healing with the Timeless Teachings of Viniyoga* (New York: Penguin/Arkana, 1999).
[2] Swami Satchidananda, *Integral Yoga Hatha* (New York: Henry Holt and Company, 1970).

The Sivananda Hatha Yoga method of Swami Vishnu-Devananda is essentially the same as Integral Yoga, as the same master trained both teachers. Swami Vishnu-Devananda also has a valuable book referencing all the aspects of yoga practice, the *Complete Illustrated Book of Yoga*.[3] The benefits of this method are a thorough practice in all the aspects of yoga to meditation. This method is popular, with over 7,000 teachers trained in a style that focused on twelve principal asanas.

IYENGAR YOGA

Iyengar Yoga is named for its creator B. K. S. Iyengar of Poona, Maharasthra (West-central) India. Iyengar, also a student of Prof. Krishnamacharya, has become the trademark of popular yoga in the West. His book, *Light on Yoga*,[4] has become an authoritative standard for thoroughness in asana. America's most popular yoga magazine, *Yoga Journal*, was founded by his students and remains a format of his teachings more than any other line of yoga. His yoga focuses on asanas done with precision, maintaining anatomical alignment, often with the use of props that he designed. The practice is physically challenging, and is often disrupted by the teacher giving adjustments and explaining the corrections to the students. Some teachers are known for giving only 3 or 4 poses in a 90-minute class.

The benefits of this method include heightened body awareness, improved carriage, improved respiration, and health. These benefits are refined and developed by many Iyengar-trained teachers such as Jean Couch, whose work to re-establish "balance" brings remarkable results in six sessions.[5]

KRIPALU YOGA

This Hatha Yoga style is named for the Indian master, Swami Kripalvananda, yet was created by Yogi Amrit Desai, former head of the Kripalu Yoga Association in western Massachusetts. It is generally known as a gentler, kinder yoga, placing emphasis upon the spiritual traditions of humility, devotion, and meditation. There are three stages of practice. In stage one, called willful practice, students learn the basics of asana details, alignment, and coordinating breath with motion. Stage two emphasizes will and surrender, begins the process of controlling the senses, and poses are held longer. Stage three surrenders to the wisdom of the body and allows for spontaneous movements to occur.

The benefits of this method include excellent community spirit, a nondogmatic approach, and practice that is done in a joyful manner.[6]

---

[3] Swami Vishnu-Devananda, *Complete Illustrated Book of Yoga* (New York: Three Rivers Press, 1988). See also The Sivananda Yoga Center, *The Sivananda Companion to Yoga* (New York: Fireside, 2000).

[4] B. K. S. Iyengar, *Light on Yoga* (New York: Schocken Books, 1979).

[5] Jean Couch, "Balance," in *Yoga International*, August/September (1998), pp. 26–30.

[6] See Christopher Baxter, *Kripalu Hatha Yoga* (Lenox, MA: Kripalu Center for Yoga and Health, 1998).

KUNDALINI YOGA

Kundalini Yoga, as popularized by Yogi Bhajan of the American Sikh tradition, utilizes Hatha and Tantra Yoga methods to willfully awaken the latent spiritual energy called kundalini. The procedure involves the use of yoga postures done rapidly in and out of the poses, often flexing, then alternately arching, the spine while breathing forcibly through the nostrils in a technique called "breath of fire." This breathing method is identical to the Hatha Yoga practice of bastrika, or bellows breath, well-known for awakening kundalini energy. Mantras are used to stimulate the seven chakras, and sometimes, white tantra (nonsexual, as contrasted with red tantra, which focuses on elevating sexuality) energy-awakening practices are used to receive the evolved energy of the teacher.

The benefits of this method are that this is a highly organized group with many adherents. Its practices are intense and, when followed, will increase your energy level and self-confidence. The practices may also be too intense for those whose mental state or nervous system is unstable. I do not recommend this practice for people who are taking psycho-therapeutic medications or are under the care of a psychiatrist.

Goals and Methodology of Hatha Yoga

Hatha Yoga represents asana and pranayama—steps three and four of Patanjali's eight limbs. *Ha* means "Sun" and *tha* means "Moon." The Sun represents the energies of the solar plexus, while the Moon represents the energies of the emotions located in the limbic region of the brain. The Bible's concluding book, Revelation, describes in its 12th chapter the radiance of the Sun that shines on the being who has mastered their Moon and thus stands upon it. By this is bestowed the crown of 12 stars, representing the attainment of fullness of all the zodiac signs. Thus, Hatha Yoga seeks to balance the body with the mind, gut instincts with intuition. Hatha Yoga is not an end unto itself; rather, it is a means to direct the mind by removing the obstacles of unsteadiness and discomfort that are experienced in the body, breath, and sensory awareness.

While the practices of yoga predate the Buddha (who practiced yoga in the fifth century B.C.), the surviving texts of Hatha Yoga are dated not earlier than the ninth century A.D. The *Hatha Yoga Pradipika*—the earliest major writing from the 14th century—states:

> *Hatha wisdom is offered solely and exclusively*
> *as a preparation for Raja Yoga.*[7]

Thus, in the tradition of Classical Yoga training, the disciplines of the body and breath were aimed at freeing the student from body consciousness. This transcending of the body leads to an awareness of one's life-force energy as transcendent. In the same manner, those who practice Raja Yoga are trained to become free of mental and emotional consciousness. This leads to an awareness of oneself as a spiritual being both immanent and transcendent.

---

[7] Swami Muktibodhananda, *Hatha Yoga Pradipika* (Munger, India: Bihar School of Yoga, 1985), chap. 1, sutra 2.

Patanjali's *Yoga Sutras* (chapter 2, sutras 46-49) state the process of asana and pranayama disciplines and the experiences that will arise when yoga is practiced in this systematic all-inclusive approach.

Yoga *pose*
is a *steady*
and comfortable position.

Yoga pose is mastered
by relaxation of *effort,*
to create a lessening
of the natural tendency
for restlessness,
and *identification*
of oneself as living
within
the *infinite* stream of life.

From that
perfection of yoga posture,
duality,
such as praise and criticism,
ceases
to be a disturbance.

When this is acquired
then naturally follows
a *cessation*
of the *movements*
of *inspiration and expiration;*
this is called
regulation of breath.[8]

Benefits of Yogasanas

The benefits of yoga practice manifest on two levels. The central benefit is produced from following the guidelines of Patanjali's classic *Yoga Sutras*, (II, 46). When this relaxation of effort and steadiness of body is created, the resulting pleasurable sensations of being in the stillness and contentment of the final posture pervades all levels of psychology, physiology, and consciousness. It is this benefit that makes yoga unique. The multidimensional being is put into a state of re-integration that organically creates the

---

[8] Stiles, *Yoga Sutras of Patanjali,* chap. 2, sutras 46–49.

feelings of wholeness. This benefit is common to all asanas utilized with concentrated, steady glottal breathing (ujjaye pranayama). The particular asana has little to do with this level of benefit. The general benefits create mental equilibrium, emotional health, calmness, sensitivity to yourself and others, and prepare the mind for meditative introspection. It was with this understanding that the early writers of yoga advocated the mastery of one asana. This can be seen in the *Hatha Yoga Pradipika, Gheranda Samhita* and *Siva Samhita.* In these medieval texts, the best postures were considered to be the sitting poses. In the *Hatha Yoga Pradipika,* the Perfect Pose (Siddhasana), a seated pose used principally for pranayama and meditation, is considered to be the best posture of the entire curriculum.[9]

The secondary benefit is from the practice of asanas that relate to specific movements of the body and how they positively affect the physiology. The secondary benefits are important from a health and curative point of view. They form the basis of yoga therapy. While much of this knowledge is subjective and lacking in objective research, the benefits are strongly supported by the experience of millions of practitioners over several thousand years. The variety of motions of yogasanas produces changes to cardiovascular functions, as well as benefits to musculo-skeletal structures. From this perspective, forward bending is known to be sedative, compared with backbends, which are stimulative. Standing postures and forward bends lower blood pressure, while backbends and inverted poses tend to elevate it. Some poses put pressure on the abdominal organs and may be directed to increase or diminish blood flow from the upper abdominal organs, such as the liver or stomach. Others increase blood flow to organs, like the shoulderstand, which promotes circulation to the neck region and is well-known for its beneficial effects for thyroid conditions.

Without receiving the general benefits of Classical Yoga, the specific benefits to health and physiology are short-lived. The general benefits are necessary to support the perceptual and life-style changes necessary for prolonged improvements in health.

The sign of mastery of yoga poses or asanas is clearly stated in sutra 48, that duality ceases to be a disturbance. An indifference to pleasure and pain, hot and cold, praise and criticism, flexibility and stiffness is the resulting mental state from perfection of yoga asana practice as Patanjali delineates it. This attainment is quite rare. There are millions of people practicing yoga asanas. There are but a handful who know this experience directly. For everyone else, the practice of asanas results in feeling well, improved health, better posture, or increased self-esteem. Although these are wonderful attainments, they are not cited in the text, which infers that they are not significant attainments in Classical Yoga.

The process of yogasana leads directly to those experiences described in sutras 49 through 52 for the practices of pranayama. There are a multitude of variations of how to breathe. Unless they lead to a subtle and prolonged breathing pattern and ultimately to a stillness of breath, however, the practitioner is not receiving optimal benefits

---

[9] Swami Muktibodhananda, *Hatha Yoga Pradipika*, chap. 1, sutras 39–43.

from the practice. These sutras further explain that the combined practices lead to a complete readiness for contemplation and meditation. Without this training, the benefits of meditation may arise, but will not be retained. Patanjali is interested in the process of sustained practice done over a full lifetime. These goals may not be what the reader seeks, so reflection is necessary to see where you are starting and where you will want to proceed.

By setting a clear concise goal, your mind will be able to achieve it, provided you remain positive, have good guidance, and are persistent in your discipline. Any really good yoga teacher can help you attain these physical goals from your Hatha Yoga practice. This is true regardless of which method of yoga you choose.

This book is written to assist you in attaining these goals, and also to remind you that there is a much greater goal—knowing yourself and realizing your multidimensional nature. The goal of asana is indeed freedom from duality. The attainment of this goal reveals something more of you than body consciousness.

Chapter 3

SIGNS OF PROGRESS
IN YOGA PRACTICES

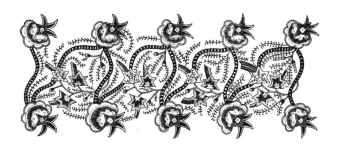

The sequence for a complete practice of all the techniques in Classical Yoga is breathing exercises (ujjaye pranayama), joint-freeing series (pavanmuktasana), spine-freeing series, yoga poses (asanas), yoga posture flows (vinyasas), respiratory locks (bandhas), hand gestures (mudras), cleansing practices (kriyas), contemplation exercises (dharanas), and meditation (dhyana). Every practice builds upon the previous technique and the attainment of fundamentals of the procedure to follow. Thus, step one leads to step two, and so on. Unlike linear learning, however, practicing step three with awareness and devotion enhances the capacity of the practices of steps one and two. This, in turn, leads to greater insights and attainment from step three. A self-generating and self-enhancing cycle is created

By beginning with learning how to breathe properly and slowly progressing into pranayama, you can find the hidden power of the breath. The breath is the string that ties all the other practices together into a cohesive whole.

The practice of the Joint-Freeing Series will teach you how to move steadily and rhythmically, in harmony with breath without forcing toward a goal. This will improve the circulation of blood and eventually of prana to enable muscles to be better prepared for change. It will also bring an increased energy level. The joint-freeing series also improves the flow of lymph fluids through the thoracic duct, located anterior to the lumbar spinal column. This strengthens the immune system and improves the practice of asanas that focus upon the spinal column. It will develop your capacity to isolate muscles, thus bringing definition to the Joint-Freeing Series. Through this practice, the Shoulderstand, Bridge, and Spinal Twist become more effective—their benefits can be more readily perceived.

Yoga asanas develop the capacity of sensitivity and self-restraint, so that the messages of the body can be heard and followed. The differences between stretch, strength, strain, and pain are slowly revealed and made distinct. You will learn how to pace your motions, adapt your effort level, and handle pain with discriminative awareness.

Yoga posture flows, vinyasas, strengthen your mind by developing a continuity of awareness of breath. This, in turn, develops your capacity to sustain effort without producing stress. Vinyasas integrate the yoga motions into daily life activities so that you can carry the practice with you wherever you go. They may be specific as in the Sun Salutation or personally designed for you by your teacher.

Bandhas powerfully enhance the respiratory function. They change breathing into an internal exercise that restores lost energy and elevates energy productivity. They prolong the practice of pranayama and allow the asana practice to quiet the mind.

Mudras are gestures, especially of the hands, though they may involve the entire body, as in Maha Mudra (a variation of Head-to-Knee Pose—Janu Sirsasana) or Viparita Karani Mudra (a variation of the Shoulderstand—Salamba Sarvangasana). Their intention is fully realized when applied to meditation practice. They indeed are the techniques of pratyahara, sensory focus, the fifth stage of Classical Yoga.

The most common mudra is to place your hands together at your heart in a prayer gesture. This is called Anjali Mudra. Laying your hands flat on your heart is called Hridaya Mudra, seal of the Spiritual Heart. Placing your palms down against your torso with thumbs and forefingers joined creates a triangle shape called Devi Mudra, seal of the Goddess of Radiant Light.

Kriyas purify the physical body and restore a balance from the stresses of illness and injury. They are especially recommended during the changes of seasons, or as a supplement to deepen the benefits of cleansing diets or fasting. They can also be used as an adjunct to Ayurveda's Pancha Karma, five cleansing practices, to promote rejuvenation.

Contemplation practices are most useful for training and directing the mind to understand and appreciate the reward of leading a spiritual life. They are meant to be interwoven with meditation practices so that the subtler aspects of anatomy may weave their benefits into the grosser aspects of the body and mind.

The disciplines of yoga must be practiced with joy, reverence, and happiness in order to receive the fullest benefits possible. Otherwise, yoga is just hard work, just another way to discipline an unruly body and mind.

Types of Yoga Poses

Very commonly, yoga asanas are classified into three levels of difficulty—beginner (up to six months of practice), intermediate (6 to 24 months of practice), and advanced (over two years of continuous practice in the same method or with the same teacher). As you progress, greater joint flexibility, muscular control, stability, concentration, and an increasing commitment to practice on your own is required. It is assumed that more advanced students have achieved their level as a result of stability and confidence in the teachings and the teacher. Going from teacher to teacher, you can only gain a mediocre intermediate level of understanding, regardless of the level of performance achieved.

Another distinction is made between static asanas and dynamic sequences in which asanas are linked into posture flows called vinyasas. Vinyasas are especially suitable for enhanced vascular circulation and general health. Static poses are known for their ability to focus circulatory benefits to specific organs or systems. By holding a pose for several minutes with deep rhythmic breathing, you produce a calming effect on the mind through the reversal of the "stress response" and the induction of the "relaxation response."

In this book, groupings of yoga exercises and postures have been created according to the various functions they serve. Rather than follow classification according to difficulty of performance, I have created categories according to the following themes:

1. Pavanmuktasana—"joint-freeing," a dynamic series for the purpose of limbering the joints, evaluating for normal range of motion, learning musculo-skeletal anatomy, and, with regular practice, freeing subtle energy flows called nadis (literally "tubes") to permit access to the experience of meditation.

2. Spine-freeing movements—dynamic motions that teach students to isolate strength into commonly weak muscles and, at the same time, release overworked stressed muscles.

3. Structural yoga asanas—a series of 24 static postures that develop a full range of motion and muscular stamina. They can be used therapeutically to improve posture, to develop individual muscle tone, to eliminate pain, or to balance strength with joint freedom.

The Signs of Progress in Yoga Poses

Each of the phrases of the *Yoga Sutras* on asana and pranayama reveals an attainment, a step along the path of Hatha Yoga. By walking the same path every day, you become familiar with it and can move steadily deeper, provided you stay alert and remember where you are going.

The first phrase of sutra 46 reveals that, by doing yoga poses, you can remove the causes of discomfort and instability. In order to root out these causes, you must take a close and fearless look at your bodily experience. Performing the joint-freeing series and the spine-freeing isolation series develops awareness by concentrating on one region and one specific motion at a time. By coordinating these exercises with rhythmic breathing, the habitual aches and irregular motions of the body are revealed. Practicing with diligence and attentiveness begins to lessen physically based distractions.

I have often seen how students with pain have gone through these simple joint-freeing motions, not realizing until the end of a 90-minute class that their chronic aches and pains were gone. My usual habit in teaching yoga classes is to ask at the beginning of a series or workshop how your body is doing today. I want to know if there are any new aches, or if there has been a change to your body from previous classes.

A new student in her late twenties, Sara, came to class and was quiet when I asked for feedback on these questions. During the class, I noticed that her right shoulder was not as mobile as her left. When I asked her about it, she said she had had pain ever since a doctor injected her with cortisone for bursitis following an athletic injury. I decided to add more variations to the joint-freeing series, giving some unusual combinations of motions. I had the class do internal rotation on one shoulder and external rotation on the opposite shoulder. Then we practiced the Eagle (Garudasana) pose arm placement and went up and down with the elbows and forearms crossed in front of the face. All of a sudden, Sara's face lit up. She exclaimed, "My pain is gone. I don't know what happened, but it's gone." She then revealed that she had been plagued with constant pain since the incident 10 years earlier. Sara continued to come regularly for the next year with no return of the pain in her right shoulder. Her mobility had returned equally in both shoulders in all the directions of motion.

I have found that many students, especially those who have been practicing yoga asanas for some time, experience new awakenings from the simple preparatory exercises. They bring about new insights into the more complex asanas, and, more importantly, they reveal the daily tasks that one performs that unconsciously block comfort or stability. I call it a return to the life-force. The prana begins to flow in new and previously unfamiliar ways, bringing with it, not only bodily changes, but also new ways of perceiving the body/mind complex.

With this increased energy flow and awareness, the first phrase of the next sutra on asana (47) can shed new light on the practice of being in asana. By learning to relax and easing excessive effort, you stimulate neurons to find new awareness pathways. Proprioception is stimulated. This is an awareness of where the body is in space that does not rely on visual cues. Grace is the natural result of making the right use of effort and will. The body begins to move in a naturally gracious manner in all activities, for the training is not limited to the time spent on the yoga mat. The training affects all motions that the anatomy makes.

When grace begins to flow, there is a certain discomfort with this process. We naturally fidget, wiggle, and can't sit still. There's the anticipation of something about to happen and we don't know what it is. That "unknowingness" is quite unsettling. Patanjali understood this process well and wrote about the sequence of events associated with the attainment of each step of the eightfold path. Each phase builds upon the previous one. With the development of a certain level of steadiness and comfort in the body/mind, a new level of restlessness arises, albeit much subtler than the previous tensions. At this point, the tensions carried in the body may be unnoticeable, except by a highly trained or intuitive body reader.

Unless you are taught to relax and be still, the training stops before this level. You leave the pose feeling you have done it and that you know all there is to know about it. This may be true on a certain level. You know as much as you have learned. However, there is always more to learn about yourself. This is an infinite body. It contains hidden accesses to infinite knowledge and infinite awareness. By this, I do mean that we are omniscient—not in the way this concept is usually interpreted. I refer to someone being omniscient in the same way that I might refer to someone as being an omnivorous eater. They can and will eat everything, just not all at once. In the same way, this body/mind is infinite, one moment at a time. It is omniscient, one insight at a time.

After a certain amount of relaxation and acceptance of the insights that arise from this training in Classical Yoga, you begin to have glimpses into the last phase of this second sutra on asana. There is such a profound relaxation of tension—that in essence is expressed as a release of fear. The gracious actions of your body begin to open a new level of vitality and the experience of the oneness of life is given. The infinite stream of life is experienced in a uniquely personal and profound manner. It may be gentle, something previously known, or a life-transforming shattering of the ego's individuality.

A little-known aspect of physical Hatha Yoga is that the preliminary processes deepen the experience of the next level and the higher levels of practice deepen the experiences of the most basic processes. In simple practices, the mind gets to play at simplicity, at being a beginner. As a beginner, insights about energy or states of concentration will arise naturally with experience—insights that had been lost because, previously, you were learning. By no longer focusing upon the technique, you can more readily see yourself. This can often lead to insights about your anatomy, such as which muscles are involved? What are you feeling? Where do you feel the reaction? Or they can reveal emotional insights—how feeling the tightness of your hamstrings may reveal an underlying resistance to change, or how weakness in your buttocks also shows a diminished capacity to feel pleasure. Students for whom consciousness is the natural place of attention may be given other insights into how physical sensation creates vitality or how energy reveals a shift in consciousness. By staying a student of basic practices, you are more apt to gain insights into your basic human qualities.

The classic text on Hatha Yoga, the *Hatha Yoga Pradipika*, claims this is a truth for the larger scheme, and I also find its validity in the step-by-step process.

> *There can be no perfection if Hatha Yoga is without Raja Yoga*
> *or Raja Yoga without Hatha Yoga.*
> *Therefore, through practice of both,*
> *perfection is attained.*[1]

The Signs of Progress in Pranayama

The *Yoga Sutras* state another sign of the mastery of asana practice:

> *When this is acquired*
> then naturally follows
> a *cessation*
> of the *movements*
> of *inspiration and expiration;*
> this is called
> *regulation of breath.*[2]

---

[1] Swami Muktibodhananda, *Hatha Yoga Pradipika* (Munger, India: Bihar School of Yoga, 1985), chap. II, sutra 76.
[2] Stiles, *Yoga Sutras of Patanjali,* chap. II, sutra 49.

Hence, there is a continuum of asana into pranayama when the intense focus on the breath dissolves the sense of solidarity of the yoga pose. This process is sometimes delayed by unknowing yoga teachers encouraging their students to "keep breathing." While this may be appropriate in the beginning due to lack of heightened awareness from shallow breathing, it is not appropriate for students of Classical Yoga and meditation. A pause in the rhythm of breathing is a natural outcome of concentration and a lessening of fear. A distinction is made between holding the breath, which is symptomatic of fear, and pause, where fear is not present.

For those who do not experience this spontaneous cessation of breath during their asana practice, Patanjali offers the training of the breath through three major methods.

> *The motions* of breath
> are either *external,*
> *internal,* or *stationary,*
> they may be *regulated*
> three ways:
> *by location, time, or number;*
> then they will become
> *prolonged and subtle.*[3]

By pranayama training of the three phases of breath—external and internal motions, and natural pauses—the breath becomes slower and subtler, yet more profound in its ability to deepen concentration. Its sensations, and with it the awareness that it promotes, increase and students may report experiencing other dimensions than those previously perceived of as being merely tissue. The training can be given in terms of where to direct the breath, its duration and the number of repetitions. This training is rarely given, because there are few competent masters available to train teachers. There are many variables in this process and it is not recommended except in direct teacher-to-student training.

> *Pranayama cannot be learned by toil,*
> *Try however many times one may.*
> *Strain, and pain, and surely weariness*
> *Are the most one can hope to gain.*[4]

The natural experience of breath stillness is considered the best form of pranayama, so I do not recommend practices other than those cited in this book. The *Yoga Sutras* (II, 51–53) are clear in their elucidation of the process of pranayama and the experiences that are signposts of following the Classical Yoga meditation path.

> In the *fourth* method
> one's breath is extended

---

[3] Stiles, *Yoga Sutras of Patanjali,* chap. II, sutra 50.
[4] Swami Muktananda Paramahansa, *The Nectar of Chanting* (Oakland, CA: S. Y. D. A. Foundation, 1975), *Guru Gita,* sutra 53.

into the Divine Life Force
and prana
is felt permeating everywhere,
transcending the attention
given to either
external or *interal* objects.

As a result
of this pran-ayama,
the veil obscuring the radiant
Supreme light of the inner Self
dissolves.

And as a result
the *mind becomes fit*
for the *process of contemplation.*[5]

The natural pranayama of Patanjali is often spoken of as prayer. It provides a unitive experience with wherever the mind is directed. It clears the mind of preconceptions and illusory impressions. Pranayama is the focus of the third chapter of the 13th-century text, *Vasistha Samhita,* a collection of verses attributed to the sage Vasistha. He states

Those who are purified by Pranayama,
Reach the supreme goal. . .

Pranayama is the savior for those
who are drowned in the
ocean of the transmigratory world.[6]

Reference to the process of breath ceasing is also given in the 14th-century *Hatha Yoga Pradipika:*

By stopping the prana through retention,
the mind becomes free from all modifications.
By thus practicing this yoga,
One achieves the stage of raja yoga (supreme union).[7]

---

[5] Stiles, *Yoga Sutras of Patanjali,* chap. II, sutras 51–53.
[6] Swami Kuvalayananda, Swami Digambarji, and P. R. G. Kokaje, eds., *Vasistha Samhita* (Lonaula, India: Kaivalyadhama, 1969), chap. III, sutras 20–21.
[7] Swami Muktibodhananda, *Hatha Yoga Pradipika,* chap. II, sutra 77.

PART TWO
Preparation for Practice

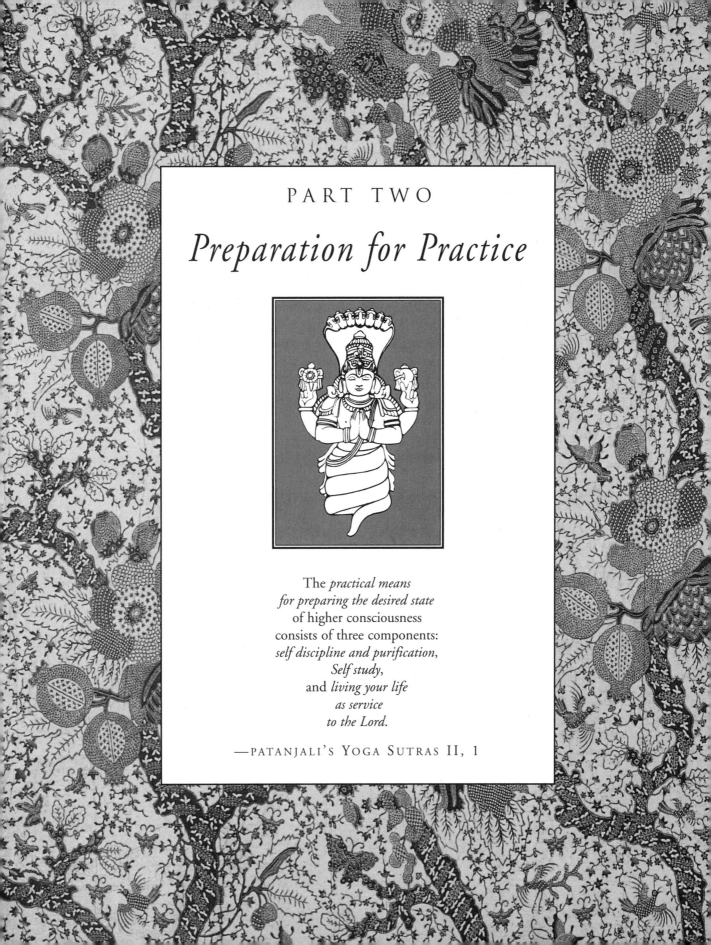

The *practical means*
for preparing the desired state
of higher consciousness
consists of three components:
self discipline and purification,
Self study,
and *living your life*
as service
to the Lord.

—PATANJALI'S YOGA SUTRAS II, 1

INTRODUCTION

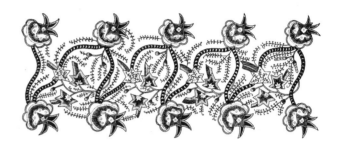

This book is best used as a supplement to class instruction. Nothing can take the place of personal guidance and class participation. The class will provide a direct living experience of yoga learned from a teacher who can share, not only the information of their years of practice, but also the transformation yoga has given them. This book is provided as a reminder of the processes you learn in yoga class.

Before beginning with practice, take a few minutes to read What is Yoga? in Part One and Guidelines to Practice, which follows, in Part Two. These sections are important in order to develop a consistent mindfulness in your practice. In practicing on your own, you should follow the same guidelines as your teacher uses in presenting the material to you. Here is a sample outline of a class:

1. Contemplation: focus on your goal and ask for guidance from your inner teacher or Higher Power;

2. Breath-awareness exercises;

3. Joint-freeing series (pavanmuktasana);

4. Strength-isolation exercises;

5. Structural yoga poses;

6. Deep relaxation (Savasana);

7. Energetic breathing (Pranayama);

8. Meditation;

9. Closing thanks to your inner teacher or Higher Power for guiding you.

When doing your own practice, follow these stages to produce a complete physical and mental workout. In the beginning, go especially slowly and read over the instructions to each part of the practice. Then do only that segment of practice before continuing on to the next phase. The best way to learn yoga is to go "step by step." That is the essence of vinyasa, a flowing posture sequence designed to master the nuances of a particular asana. Include each part in your practice each time. They will deepen, maturing with patience and regularity.

Chapter 4

GUIDELINES FOR PRACTICE

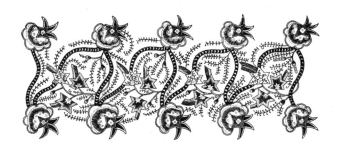

The most important guideline for the successful practice of yoga is the cultivation of a proper mental attitude. This awareness comes from patient, persistent practice, and from the contemplation of the unity of all life. First, you must learn not to cause yourself pain, injury, or unnecessary strain. Your body may be stiff when you begin, but with regular practice, it will become free and supple. The goal of yoga, however, is not increased flexibility. This achievement can be seen as merely a stepping-stone along your path to being at peace with yourself.

The practice of Hatha Yoga can lead you to a deep understanding of the unity underlying all forms of life. The asanas (poses) of Hatha Yoga are named after animals, plants, legendary heroes, sacred geometric figures, and deities.

As your body undertakes these various forms, you will come to realize the inherent life-force that exists in all creation. While this force moves all creatures in various ways, there is an inherent commonality in this force: it is universal.

A mental attitude based on unity is the ideal attitude for the Hatha Yoga practitioner. In the development of this ideal, your only competition is inside—that is, your only obstacles are within you. Comparing yourself to another is counterproductive. The inner struggle is to be rid of laziness, anger, delusion, and desire for being different or better than others. The constant struggles that characterize our outer lives become apparent through the practice of postures. By attempting to attain the classical ideal of "a steadfast, comfortable position" (*Yoga Sutras* II, 46) you will gain insights into all of your struggles.[1]

---

[1] Stiles, *Yoga Sutras of Patanjali*, chap. II, sutra 46.

How you approach asana is a metaphor for how you live your life. If it is your personality to approach your work as a struggle, you will approach asanas the same way—and ultimately find that it doesn't work. If it is your personality to be too relaxed, to give up too easily, you will approach asanas the same way—and find that it doesn't work either. Holding still in asana changes your inner chemistry. With persistent practice, sensitivity to your own mental and physical limits will result in an internal balance of your whole system—a change not limited to the yoga classroom.

Levels of Yoga Students

I recognize only three levels of yoga students. Level one consists of those people who are trying yoga out. Often, students stay at this phase for years without fully seeing the value in commitment. These people commonly enjoy the superficial study of the multitude of ways. They like to try out one teacher for a month and then another, one style for a season and then, next season, yet another. As a result, they never turn the soil over enough to plant a crop. They only scratch the surface of many styles of yoga and superficially test many teachers. Level two consists of those students who are consistent at coming to class and are exploring self-discipline. They alternate between wanting more and not wanting to commit to nurturing themselves in this way. Level three consists of those students who have committed themselves to a life-style that incorporates regular yoga practices under the guidance of one systematic approach. More about this development is described in chapter 33.

Where and When?

Ideally, yoga is practiced in the same place and time each day. The space should be well ventilated, so that air circulates freely. It should have natural light and also be able to be completely darkened for relaxation. There should be a carpet or mat large enough to stretch out on fully. If a padded mat is used, it should be used only for floor exercises. Standing poses are best done on a bare wooden floor or a thin, "sticky mat." The room should be kept clean and neat. Animals, smoke, perfume, and other distracting odors are best left out, because your sense of smell is greatly heightened as a result of yoga practices.

The room should also be quiet and free from distractions. Tell your household members when you're practicing, so that they can join you or leave you alone. Put on your answering machine or take the phone off the hook. Privacy is necessary to create concentration. Keep your practice to yourself.

A yoga studio will have all of these qualities, plus the benefit of providing space that is used only for yoga. After a while, such a space takes on the quality of yoga. The room feels relaxing and inviting to enter. It is a comfortable place to be. You'll find you want to sit for meditation or lie down and rest upon entering. If you can find a yoga center with such a feeling, you will have found a great asset.

You can create this feeling at home by setting aside a room or a section of a room just for practice. Over time, the energy will collect there, until it is clearly recognizable, even by people unfamiliar with yoga. To retain energy, I don't recommend you do yoga in public or outdoors, especially not in the Sun. Hatha Yoga can increase energy. With too much heat, you can become exhausted and unable to sit quietly for meditation after practice.

To increase your aesthetic or spiritual inclination, create a focal point with a display of flowers or soothing pictures. Keep the display simple enough so that it is naturally eye-catching for those exercises that involve fixed gazing.

At What Time and for How Long?

Yoga exercises are most beneficial if completed about an hour before meals. In this way, the stomach is empty and less likely to create digestive problems. In the morning, the body is stiffer, so morning practice should be gentle and slower in pace and vigor than evening practice. Morning practice can give energy to working hours when it is most needed. This is a prevention-oriented practice, and for this reason it is generally the best time.

If your life-style is not accustomed to early morning activity, try practicing yoga when you get home from work—it can relieve the fatigue of the day. This is a treatment-oriented approach to practice.

Practice in the late evening is beneficial for inducing a deeper sleep. Night yoga should be similar to early morning practice, yet with an even gentler attitude, so that movements gradually progress into full postures. This time is excellent for absorbing the benefits of days that have been challenging, or for preparing for early morning demands.

Whatever time you choose, it is important that it be a time that is least likely to be disrupted with schedule changes. The amount of time spent per week in home practice should be equal to time spent in classes. If you are attending a 90-minute class twice a week, a good minimum time for practice is every day for 20 to 30 minutes.

In the beginning, spending more than 30 minutes daily is not advisable, at least until after completing your first eight-week course in Hatha. This is because your body chemistry is subject to a tremendous amount of change. It needs time to reach a plateau and stabilize, so that the chemical and energetic changes can become integrated. This cycle of change, integration, and leveling off is more obvious when attending classes. The energetic changes in others, plus the teacher's chemistry, create a great opportunity for growth. Sometimes, this growth is too much, too fast, so practice at home may produce more changes at first than you are capable of integrating into your life-style.

It is a good idea to have a private session with your teacher at regular intervals, ideally once a month or at the beginning of each new series of classes. This practice can tremendously deepen your benefits from class.

What Should I Wear?

This is probably the most difficult question you'll face in a serious yoga practice. It is a challenge even for the best of yogis to keep up with what one should wear to the yoga studio. Personally, I avoid the fashion parade, so I lighten up on what is the latest rage in yoga attire. My feeling is that the best clothing to wear is that which conforms to your body shape without being too revealing and without restricting your movements. For women, a cotton leotard is ideal. For men, cotton T-shirts and gym trunks are good. This will allow a complete view of legs, hips, and midriff. This visual awareness is especially important when doing standing poses in which proper placement of these regions can prevent strain and pain. Natural fabrics that allow the skin to breathe and perspire freely are ideal, since yoga enhances the respiratory process throughout the body, including the skin. Remember to keep your feet bare to breathe.

What Should I Eat?

Your stomach should be empty when practicing Hatha. The best guide is to eat *after* yoga practices. If you must eat before class, allow at least 90 minutes for digestion. Certain practices, like the extremes of spinal twisting and of forward and backward bending, have the strongest effects on the digestive tract and can produce nausea or dizziness if you practice too soon after eating.

A vegetarian diet is optimal for receiving the most benefit from a committed yoga practice. However, it is not a pre-requisite for beginning yoga practice. If you do want to change your diet, it is advisable to wean yourself from a flesh-eating life-style. A major benefit in this area is that yoga can provide heightened sensitivity to your bodily responses to diet. Americans have been taught to dissociate from the truth of their reality. The truth is that, when we eat meat, fish, or fowl, we are eating animals. The Supreme Court Justice Oliver Wendell Holmes put it bluntly when asked why he did not eat flesh. He replied, "I do not want to make my body into a graveyard for dead animals." Words worth contemplating.

One of my teachers, B. K. S. Iyengar, said little about diet. But when pressed he said, "If the food doesn't make you salivate, don't eat it." This is great advice, as it will point out your true body's hunger, which sometimes is different from what you want to eat.

Remember that food choices often reflect our attitude and mood. Just as yogis do not recommend that you exercise if you are sad, hungry, angry, or irritable, they also recommend that you not eat if you are moody. The exception, of course, is if you have hypoglycemia—then, eat. If emotions are strong at mealtime, it is best to fast on liquids until you feel yourself more centered. Sit alone for some time in a quiet space, even if your only privacy is in the bathroom. Take full-body wave breaths until your emotions clear and give you insight into the message they wanted to deliver to you.

> Food is that which you eat,
> as well as that which eats you.[2]

Just as the consciousness of yoga class is largely created by the teacher, so also "the consciousness of food depends mostly on the consciousness of the cook. It is true that food itself has its own consciousness, but since the cook is a human being, he has a more evolved consciousness than the food. So the cook can transform the consciousness of the food if it is necessary and he wants to do so. He can add to the consciousness of the food

---

[2] Anonymous.

or he can even bring the consciousness of the food into his own consciousness for enlightenment."[3]

DIETARY GUIDELINES

1. Eat in a settled and quiet atmosphere. Do not work, read, or watch TV during meals. Always sit to eat. Avoid talking while you are chewing your food.

2. Dine either alone or with people you genuinely like. Negative emotions, whether yours, the cook's, or those of the people around you, have a harmful effect on digestion.

3. Eat at the same times every day. This will promote a digestive rhythm that will enable your body to receive the optimal benefit from a vital diet. Unless you are hypoglycemic, it is best not to snack, and avoid eating after 9 P.M. Snacking and late meals disturb your digestive rhythms and promote toxins from the lingering presence of undigested food.

4. Don't eat too quickly or too slowly. Leave one-third to one-quarter of your stomach empty to aid digestion. Start with a portion that would approximately fill your two cupped hands. If you are still hungry when you have finished that, wait about five minutes. This will help you determine if you are really still hungry, or if you are just experiencing the memory of previous hunger. If you are still hungry, take more. It is ideal not to leave the table either hungry or overly full.

5. Avoid taking a meal until the previous meal has been digested. Allow approximately three to six hours between meals. Have your largest meal at lunch, when digestion is strongest. Dinner should be a modest meal that can be digested before bedtime. Ideal foods for breakfast are fruits. This meal should be your smallest meal of the day.

6. Take a few minutes to sit quietly after eating before returning to your activity.

7. Water served at room temperature is fine to sip during meals. A good idea is to make water your beverage of choice. The benefits of water are vastly underestimated because many people are chronically dehydrated.[4] Better yet is to sip hot water slowly. This can help to digest any remaining food from the previous meal. It may also uncover false hunger and restore your true sense of appetite. Drink milk separate from meals, either alone or with other sweet foods. Milk may be taken with toast, cereals, or sweet-tasting foods, or separated from a meal by at least 20 minutes.

8. In general, it is best to include all six tastes—sweet, sour, salty, pungent, bitter, and astringent—every day.

9. Search out foods that have the most vitality; those that are alive with the breath of life, prana. Eat fresh food suitable to the season and your geographical area. The best foods are fruits, vegetables, and dairy products raised in your area. These foods have thrived on the same air, water, nutrients, and sunlight that you grow on.

---

[3] Sri Chinmoy, *The Body—Humanity's Fortress* (New York: Aum Publications, 1978), p. 14.
[4] F. Batmanghellidji, M. D., *Your Body's Many Cries for Water* (Falls Church, VA: Global Health Solutions, 1997).

10. Minimize raw foods. Lightly cooked food (stir-fried or sautéed) is much easier to digest.

11. It is best not to heat or cook with honey, as it becomes undigestible when hot.

12. Avoid iced beverages or food as they interfere with digestion.

13. Yogurt, cheese, cottage cheese, and cultured buttermilk should be avoided at night.

My favorite advice about food is that, *if I cannot bless what I am eating, I don't eat it*. If my blessings of the food and its source feel genuine, then it will be nutritious and uplifting.

Devotee: *Will not Bhagavan give me some blessed food (Prasad) from his own leaf plate as a mark of His Grace?*

Ramana Maharshi: *Eat without thinking of the ego. Then what you eat becomes God's Blessing.*[5]

Concerns about Health

A wide variety of health problems can be improved, if not entirely eliminated, with proper exercise, diet, and common sense. If you are sick, however, it is generally recommended that you do only limited practice, unless specifically instructed by your yoga teacher. If you have a cold, do only the Joint-Freeing Series (pavanmuktasana), gently. This will improve circulation, while enhancing your immune system's ability to adjust to your cold. If you have a more serious health complaint that may require the attention of a medical practitioner, let your yoga teacher know whether or not you choose to seek medical assistance. The teacher will advise you as to what practices are appropriate at this time.

Remember that very few yoga teachers are trained as yoga therapists. It is not within the normal scope of their training. Most teachers can give general advice, but do not expect specific health advice unless you are blessed with a yoga teacher who is also a certified health professional. Consult the International Association of Yoga Therapists for someone in your area. (See chapter 5 for details of yoga organizations.)

A wealth of information on yogic health comes from the companion science of Ayurveda. This holistic health system was born in India and raised on the consciousness of millennia of spiritual seekers and yogis. According to Ayurveda, the word for health in Sanskrit is *svs'tha*, which means literally "Self stay." In other words, to stay where the Self is produces health. The search for health is the search for the source of your own spiritual wealth.

A body-mind-spirit connection exists in many cultures. In the West it was championed by Aristotle who said, "Just as you ought not attempt to cure eyes without head or head without body, so you should not treat body without soul."[6]

---

[5] *Maharshi's Gospel, Books I and II*, T. N. Venkataram, ed. (Tiruvannamalai, India: Sri Ramanashram, 1994), p. 36.
[6] Donna Arbogast, "Massage, Yoga and Aromatherapy—Can They Help GI Conditions," *Digestive Health & Nutrition*, January/February 2000, p. 11.

Precautions

If any of the following conditions apply to you, be certain to let your yoga instructor know as soon as possible.

> Arthritis or questionable joint pain
> Asthma or shortness of breath
> Contact lenses
> Heart malfunctions (regardless of the date of the incident)
> High or low blood pressure
> Injury to the spine or nervous system
> Painful back or herniated or slipped spinal disc
> Persistent pain anywhere in your body
> Pregnancy
> Any recurring disease or injury
> Any unpleasant mental or physical reaction during or after yoga practice (at home or at class)

Whenever there is a change in your health, let your teacher know. If you have doubts about your physical or psychological health, please consult a physician or licensed health practitioner familiar with yoga (ideally, one who consults with your yoga teacher), so that, together, they can assist you in getting the maximum benefit from your yoga practice.

Your yoga instructor is trained to assist you and to adapt practices so that they will not aggravate health concerns. Your instructor can only be effective, however, if he or she is in contact with your reactions from both your subjective and an objective view. Yoga teachers are not trained as yoga therapists or physical therapists. They probably cannot give you practices to alleviate your symptoms. Do not expect them to cure you of your pain. Yoga is beneficial for many conditions, but it is not therapy for them. Training is available for yoga therapists who can assist in the alleviation of chronic pain and disease. Remember, however, that this is relatively new field, so there are few trained to work beyond the wellness level. Keep an open attitude about what is possible, but remember to temper it with common sense.

For Women Only

Fully 80 percent of the people coming to yoga classes are women. Hence, most yoga teachers are equipped to know the specific needs of women during their cycles of life. In general, it is not recommended that you do yoga asana or vinyasa sequences during the heaviest days of your menstrual cycle. The Joint-Freeing Series (pavanmuktasana), Energy-Freeing Pose (Apanasana), or Child Pose (Darnikasana) often provide relief from cramping. These poses can also help you eliminate excess energy and fluid during this time. They are particularly beneficial when you apply them gently and progressively. Go into and out of the poses twice as many times as normal and allow yourself to start with small motions that gradually get you to your complete range of motion after ten or twelve repetitions. These motions are beneficial during the pre- and post-menstrual days as well. No inversions—Shoulderstand (Sarvangasana) or Headstand (Sirsasana)—should be done during your period. If you're having your period, let your teacher know in order to avoid potentially harmful practices.

When you become pregnant, yoga takes on a wonderful new depth that allows the changes of your body's chemistry to occur more naturally. Exercises to strengthen and isolate the entire pelvic floor (Mula Bandha), the genital area (Vajroli Mudra), or the anal sphincter (Aswini Mudra) are especially beneficial. These practices are seldom taught. You will need to do some research to find a teacher who is familiar with them. Deep stretches, such as prolonged squatting (Utkatasana), open hip postures, such as the Warrior (Virabhadrasana II) and the Extended Triangle (Utthita Trikonasana), and stretches of the inner thigh adductor muscles, such as Spread-Leg Stretch (Upavistha Konasana) may help to prevent tearing or the need for an episiotomy to widen the vaginal opening during delivery. Stretches for the groin and hamstrings, such as Forward Bending (Paschimottanasana) coupled with low-back and gluteal strengthening poses like Cobra (Bhujangasana) and Bridge (Setubandhasana) can keep your body more relaxed as it changes.

As long as you begin yoga before your pregnancy, few changes in the ordinary yoga routine are needed until the end of the second trimester. I would not recommend that you begin yoga for the first time during your pregnancy. If you do, I highly recommend having private sessions with an experienced teacher who knows how to adapt to your situation. There are often changes that may need to be made sooner in your case—change that an established student would make only later in pregnancy. Such changes include eliminating balancing poses, twists, lying on the abdomen, and inversion poses. A teacher trained in prenatal yoga can give you more specific guidance. Enjoy this wonderful opportunity to share yoga with your child!

For Men Only

Congratulations on joining yoga. I'm pleased that you have made a commitment to your personal development and awareness through yoga. There are several precautions as you start that I'd like to impart to assist you in maintaining this commitment. I've noticed that the percentage of men who take yoga classes is inevitably smaller than that of women. Whatever your motivation for beginning yoga, keep with it. Pay more attention to yourself while in class. This guideline is given to everyone, but it is especially important for men to remember to avoid the pitfall of making this an athletic event or an opportunity for showing off. Surely you will be able to do strength postures that women cannot easily do. But take this as an opportunity to be humble and get free of your intimidation of women, whose bodies are naturally more flexible than men's. Yoga is not only for flexibility, but you will definitely become more limber from a sustained practice. Yoga can give you an opportunity to understand the blessing it is to be male.

Men have a mood cycle, which I sometimes refer to as the male menstrual cycle. Be especially cautious if you find yourself having reactions that you might be tempted to attribute to the lunar phase or pressures at work or home. Separate yourself from the outside influences and look to see what is really going on with you personally. Make yoga an opportunity for you to get to know yourself.

Women tend to be more in touch with their feelings. Often this enables them to be more sensitive to themselves and others. Yoga can provide an opportunity for you, as a man, to learn about body signals that are precursors to wanting something. You may not be able to verbalize what you want, but perhaps you may be irritable, making it difficult for others to be with you. Anger is a powerful emotion that especially arises in us when we have an unfulfilled desire. Use yoga not only as a tool to discover the sensual experiences your body feels, but also to reveal what your emotional self craves.

YOGA MAKES MEN BETTER LOVERS

You can learn, not only to be more responsive to your own feelings, but to observe your beloved's emotional state as well. Yoga is a vehicle that allows you to observe your feelings, and, thus, detach from them in order to focus on what your partner wants and is feeling. The flexibility to consciously choose between focusing on your own feelings or your beloved's feelings is a great enhancement to lovemaking. It enables you to become more sensitive to your mate's level of arousal, and allows lovemaking to become prolonged and sensual to the point of timelessness. The best loving takes place in a state of meditation. Yoga can take you there, without the challenge of meeting your own or your beloved's expectations.

The main factor for improved sexual and emotional intimacy is sensitivity to your self. It is also important to acknowledge there are a host of yoga exercises that strengthen the muscles necessary for sexual expression. A bumper sticker circulating in the yoga community says "Yogis do it everywhere." Regular practice of yogasanas will definitely increase your capacity to move beyond the missionary position. In general, many yoga asanas will improve your hip mobility, which in turn releases lower-back stiffness and pain. Before considering an application for the Sexual Olympics, your hips and lower back must be in great shape. In addition, all exercises cited earlier to strengthen the pelvic floor for women will also improve men's stamina, prostate tone, bladder control, and the ability to delay ejaculation. These include Root Lock (Mula Bandha), Pelvic Tilt and Bridge Pose (Setubandhasana). I especially recomment practice mastering the Rolling Bridge variation that produces wonderful self-control and stamina.

Chapter 5

HOW DO I FIND A YOGA TEACHER?

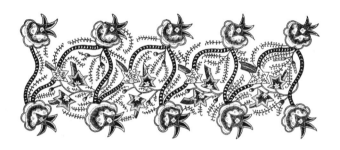

The importance of a teacher cannot be overemphasized. The teacher plays an important role in guiding the student. The teacher can share his or her experience and help you to avoid mistakes, pitfalls and dead ends. The teacher's presence conveys the "living experience of yoga," something rarely attained by simply reading about it. The consciousness of the teacher elevates the student. Using voice or hands, teachers can adjust you so that the stress and pain you carry may be alleviated. At the same time, they can facilitate you becoming more attuned to your true Self, increasing your sense of peace and contentment.

Yoga has become so popular that classes exist in even the most remote areas. Finding a class is usually not a problem, but finding a competent teacher is more difficult. To find a good teacher, it is safest to rely on word of mouth. Advertising can be deceptive in the "real world" and the yoga world is no exception.

Training in yoga is not standardized, either for students or for teachers. There is no board that certifies all yoga teachers. However, there is a national movement called the Yoga Alliance gaining support for elevating the standards of teacher training. In the meantime, be aware that a "certified teacher" may have trained in a weekend course or in courses lasting several years. When you search for a teacher, ask them about their background. A competent teacher will not be offended by your query. Consider asking the following questions:

1. *Do you have confidence and a rapport with the teacher?*

This is the most important question of all. If the teacher passes this test, the other questions are most likely irrelevant. They add credence to the teacher's capacity to establish trust and confidence in you. The teacher should, most of all, be able to inspire you to want to do yoga, to become disciplined. Discipline is both the responsibility of the student, and of the teacher. The teacher's own discipline and love of the practice will produce a contagious fire in the truly interested student.

The teacher should also be able to dispel your doubts. This does not mean that teachers are authorities on every aspect of yoga, life-style, and the spiritual realms. It means that their confidence in the tradition and ability to access guidance is strong enough that they trust where they are going, even when they don't see the next step of spiritual life (sadhana). This confidence in the tradition is contagious, and sincere students will be impelled to trust their own innate guidance while using the teacher as a sounding board to check out their own stability.

Your teacher should inspire you without forcing you. If a teacher has a reputation for forcing students to achieve poses, STAY AWAY. There are teachers who injure their students, not necessarily due to lack of anatomical training or safety guidelines, but because they are frustrated at not achieving their own goals. This leads to pent up anger, resentment, and may come out in the form of pushing students to do more than they are able. There are numerous instances of good, even great, teachers badly injuring committed students. Some of the students found these physical injuries beneficial in moving them on from stuck places in their life. As for me, I can see no benefit in causing injuries.

2. Does the teacher practice daily exercise and meditation?

Some teachers present their own practice to students; they do not practice on their own. In teaching, they are really giving themselves a workout. This may endanger you, if you are not as strong or flexible as the teacher in some motions. A competent teacher spends more time watching and correcting than demonstrating.

3. Is the teacher certified? By what organization? How long was the training?

Yoga is often taught by people who were not trained to teach, but merely taught how to practice. "Only he who obeys can command."[1]

A competent teacher-training program shows a prospective teacher, not only how to do the exercises, but also when and how to present them, how to adapt them for individual differences in sex, age, ability, and changes in health. A few certification courses offer more than basic training in anatomy, physiology, and kinesiology as it relates to Hatha Yoga. This important body information enables a teacher to better analyze your physical potential for reaching your goals through Hatha Yoga without injury.

4. Is yoga a part-time hobby or full-time profession?

Part-time teachers are in the majority and can provide guidance at the beginning levels to the average student. Students with special needs (due to changing health conditions and injuries) and committed, persistent students need the assistance of a teacher who has devoted his or her life to this work. Only such a teacher can adequately train other teachers.

---

[1] From The Rig Veda.

5. *Does the teacher continue to study with his or her own teacher?*

Yoga training influences all aspects of one's life-style. In recognizing this, the competent teacher continues to study with his or her teacher, as well as seeking out other competent teachers for consultation. The study of yoga implies the immersion to varying degrees in an entire (yogic) philosophy. Philosophy means the "love of knowledge." The love of yoga generates a desire for higher knowledge, more insight, and greater clarity of expression.

6. *Is the teacher a member of a group of certified teachers?*

Yoga teacher associations exist in most states. They exist so teachers can share with their peers and continue to grow without blinders. Keeping an open mind to the benefits of the variety of practices and being in contact with a variety of teachers is important to competent teaching.

These guidelines will assist you in finding the right teacher for you. A well-known yoga teacher, Alice Christensen, writes: "We believe that yoga teachers must be exceptionally conscientious and professional in their work of transmitting to others the exacting disciplines of yoga. These personal commitments ensure that teachers avoid any injury or misrepresentation in their classes."[2]

Are You Looking for a Yogi or a Certified Yoga Teacher?

The presence of a teacher can bring attention to qualities you cannot learn from a book—how to incorporate yoga into your life-style and how to be yourself and express joy, comfort, and relaxation of effort in living life. Yoga training can influence every aspect of life for the positive, if you reach for it.

There are not only a lot of styles of yoga in the world today; there is also a huge assortment of ways that different teachers present the material. One great distinction is the difference between a yogi and a yoga teacher. In general, if you're looking for a yoga teacher, make certain that they are certified to teach. They should have completed a teacher training course taught by someone authorized to teach teachers, and they, in turn, are then authorized to teach students. There are undisciplined people making a living from teaching yoga without being authorized to do so by their teacher. Some are "self-taught," and have had "spontaneous realizations from an ascended master." These types feel their skill as students qualifies them to be teachers. This is not true.

A certified yoga teacher has gone through the fire of his teacher's discipline and passed the requisite exams. Regardless of how lengthy or difficult the undertaking, this is a sign of commitment. Make certain that the person with whom you are studying is authorized to teach and continues to seek training for on-going education.

A yogi is altogether different. This is an individual who clearly knows and expresses that her or his path is a spiritual journey to God. While yoga teachers may know tech-

---

[2] Alice Christensen, *American Yoga Association Beginner's Manual* (New York: Simon and Schuster, 1987), p. 16.

41

niques for relieving pain and stress, creating health, increasing energy, or even therapy for psycho-physiological issues, a yogi is a yoga adept who lives a committed life-style of nothing but yoga and spiritual practices. Yogis pursue their spiritual path to God living anywhere among the full range of life-styles—from the life of a householder to that of a renunciate monk.

Yoga teachers earn their livelihood teaching yoga. They need students to support their life-style and, often, to make them feel good about their contribution to the world. Yogis usually don't depend upon student income for their livelihood. If they do receive compensation for their teachings, it's by voluntary donation. They have little or no ego-investment in receiving the praises of their students. Their work is done as a selfless service in honor of what their teachers gave them, or as a blessing to God.

While yoga teachers are committed and may appear to be devoted, yogis are constantly reverent and devotional. To tell them apart is often not easy. If you are looking for a yogi, my spiritual teacher used to say, test them. Don't make a commitment until you've tested potential candidates for at least six months. Follow their advice and faithfully practice their teachings, but do not take initiation until you see that they live what they teach and that your own life is better for having taken their advice.

The test of a great yoga teacher is that he or she will awaken your innate desire for spirituality and this, in turn, may take the form of a yogi being pulled to you.

Chapter 6

REMEMBERING
THE BIG PICTURE

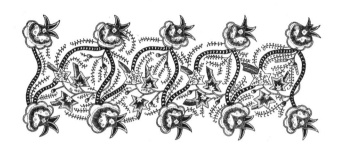

The yoga perspective of anatomy is quite different from that of Western anatomy. In the yogic view (darshan) we are composed of five bodies. The first body is the same in both yogic and Western views, but the other four bodies are unique to the yogic darshan. The names of these bodies reveal a radically different perception of reality. In the second part of the *Taittirya Upanishad*, it is said that our true nature is hidden from our perception because five sheaths enclose it.[1] Each of these sheaths has its own language and method of communicating across the layers of the personality.

The first yoga body (see figure 1 on page 44) is called the Annamaya Kosha, literally the "body sheath made of food, which is an illusion." This is our physical body. The physical body is created by and sustained by food. If the quality of the food is high, the illusory nature of the body is more readily perceived. This is one reason why live, fresh, seasonal food from vegetables and fruits is recommended as a yogic diet. Eating fresh food prepared immediately before eating results in an increase in live vitality available to nurture this "food body." When we eat overcooked, stale, or animal-based food, the food body becomes devitalized and has difficulty refining the food to a level of quality at which it can be converted into the needs of the second body.

The second body is hidden by a subtler sheath and is called the Pranamaya Kosha, the "body sheath made of prana, which is an illusion." This subtle body's anatomy is made of energy channels called nadis, which terminate in spinning energy centers called

---

[1] Swami Nikhilananda, *The Upanishads*, vol. IV (New York: Ramakrishna-Vivekananda, 1978), pp. 39–66.

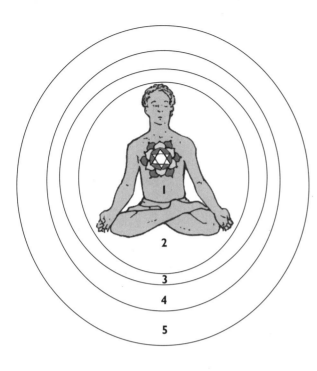

Figure 1. Yogic view of multidimensional anatomy.

chakras. The word *chakra* means wheel, implying an ever-spinning center of activity. The subtle body is composed of our senses and emotional states. The energy flowing through these channels is sensory input from the five gross senses and the subtler senses associated with the mind. Hence, these vortices and channels are always active during our waking state, seeking sensory and emotional stimulation. When we are fed beautiful sense impressions—art, nature, or live, vibrant, colorful, aromatic food—these are converted into the "prana" that keeps this subtle body healthy. From these stimuli, the chakras become open and functional. When we are not interested, repulsed, or fall asleep, the chakra activity slows down or stops. The energies withdraw from the outer world and we become replenished, provided we can assimilate the sensory input. With negative input—violent movies, stale odors, chemical food—there is less vitality available to be converted into prana.

The third body is called the Manomaya Kosha, the "body sheath made of thought, which is an illusion." This is the body of the mind. This body is made up of the refinements produced from the first two bodies, as well as its own capacity to generate positive uplifting thoughts. When thoughts are beneficial, the mind is content and at peace. From this, more positivity is generated and the mind refreshes itself. The nature of this body is thought. Mantra can transport the mind to a higher level of perception and cognition. Mantra literally means "the word which when contemplated transforms the mind." Mantras, given properly as a meal is lovingly prepared, will plug the mind into a higher and more creative mind, a mind that thinks of the welfare of others.

The fourth body is the Vijnanamaya Kosha, the "body sheath made of wisdom, which is an illusion." This body is made of transcendent thoughts. It is awareness free of self-centeredness. It is concerned for the welfare of all. This is generated by a naturally arising state of detachment from the grosser bodies. This body knows it is not the physical food body, therefore one established in this awareness is indifferent to what happens to the body. What happens to the physical body does not change the state of wisdom. Wisdom is the beginning of contact with transcendence. This state is accessed by meditation, reflection, and proper nourishment. Proper nourishment consists of good company, spiritual literature, and selfless service to others. Through a regular diet of these nutritious foods, the body of wisdom becomes more active and can fend off periods of unwholesome contact through dispassionate nonattachment.

The fifth body is the Anandamaya Kosha, the "body sheath of bliss, which is also an illusion." This body is said to be as small as a mustard seed, seated in the secret chamber of the interior heart to the right of the physical heart. This body is composed of happiness. It does not need anything to generate its happiness, as that is its natural state. The beneficial foods given to the four grosser bodies will be refined into the food that makes up this body. It is by nature joyful. Nor is that the end. According to the Yoga Philosophy, there is hidden beyond this body the truth of who you are.

Each of these bodies hides the next. Yet each also reveals something of the subtler body. The physical body appears to possess energy and vitality, yet it derives that substance from the subtler body of prana. In turn, when we have energy and emotional fulfillment, our mind appears healthy, yet it derives mind substance from an even subtler source.

The different paths of yoga focus upon re-establishing harmony between the koshas. Hatha Yoga is primarily concerned with the yoking of the first two koshas, making our energy and physical health strong and generating vitality. In one sense, when the first kosha is vital, it feeds the second, and so on.

This is how yogis perceive health. It proceeds from the grosser kosha being fulfilled; this, in turn, naturally produces a refined energy that becomes the material of the subtler kosha. Thus health of the body produces a by-product that is vitality and emotional health. This, in turn, creates a tendency for mental health. If the higher koshas are diseased by negative thinking or emotions they will block the efforts of the grosser koshas toward health. Hence, energy is wasted and the student's attainments are unstable. Classical Yoga is more concerned with the relationship of the third and fourth koshas bringing the mind into a receptive mode with the source of higher knowledge. All the yoga sadhanas (practices to establish a spiritual life-style) seek to promote health and the full receptivity of the being to the Creative Spirit.

For the yogi, health is not merely determined by the physical body, nor is it created by physical exercise alone. The Sanskrit word for health is *svastha*, which, literally translated, means "established in the self." To the yogis, true health is a coming home to your Self. In the condition of not being at home to your Self, there is dis-ease.

For most people, however, the bodies are separated, blocked from communicating with each other. Their energy is irregular, and perhaps dissipated in various directions. Many Eastern healing modalities, like acupuncture, jin shin jyitsu, reflexology, and polarity therapy, treat health problems by correcting the misdirected flow of energy patterns. Similarly, in yoga training, the proper practice of asana, pranayama, and contemplation returns the five bodies to a right relationship with themselves. Hence we are aligned again and re-established with ourselves. The experience of this is cited in the *Siva Sutras*:

> *One who is established in a comfortable posture*
> *while concentrating on the inner Self alone,*
> *naturally becomes immersed in the spontaneous*
> *arising of the Heart's ocean of bliss.*[2]

---

[2] Jaideva Singh, *The Siva Sutras* (Delhi, India: Motilal Banarsidass, 1979), chap. III, sutra 16.

Students of yoga cannot be reminded too often of the importance of detachment and constant practice. By detachment, in this context, I mean flexibility of mind. This is more important than rigid discipline enforced to create an iron will. The yogic attitude is to be flexible enough to respond to the needs of the moment—to be able and willing to assist others through deeds of loving kindness. This is the ideal culmination of yoga in action (karma yoga), and is more important than doing your yoga practices at the exact stroke of the clock.

Chapter 7

YOGA BREATHING

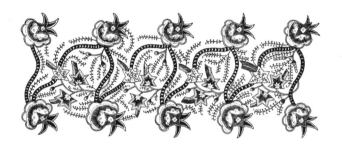

An important aspect of Classical Yoga is the strengthening and cultivation of the life-force energy called prana. While prana is not the breath, it is most readily discovered through the discipline of the respiratory function. This, together with the heightened sensitivity that is the hallmark of yoga training, reveals the hidden secret of the breath as prana. The word prana literally means "primary or vital air." Its prefix, *pra*, means forward, toward, or prior. The suffix, *na*, means to breathe or to energize.

In the second movie of the Star Wars trilogy, *The Empire Strikes Back*, Yoda spoke eloquently to Luke Skywalker about "the Force:"

> *You will know the Force when you are calm at peace. . . .*
> *The Force is my ally and a powerful ally it is.*
> *Life creates it, makes it grow.*
> *Its energy surrounds us and binds us.*
> *Luminous beings are we, not this crude matter.*[1]

His description is quite aligned with the yogic concept of "the force of prana." Indeed, it sounds like a modern interpretation of a Classical Yoga description of prana. For the yogi, the vital force is in the body, surrounds us, and interpenetrates all objects. Prana can be gotten from external objects, but this type is short-lived. The yogi seeks to refine his own breath into more prana, not unlike the alchemists who sought to transform base metals into gold. Yoga is indeed alchemy; the self become the Self.

---

[1] *The Empire Strikes Back*, George Lucas (London: Lucasfilm, Ltd., 1980), 128 minutes.

The practices of working with the breath to strengthen and extend respiration are the preliminary methods of yoga breathing culminating in pranayama. These exercises begin with simple breathing methods such as those a respiratory therapist might use for the alleviation of symptoms of shortness of breath or to develop a greater vital capacity in the lungs. These are quite powerful practices, given that most people breathe with as little as 25 percent of their respiratory capacity. Just to increase respiratory efficiency can give a tremendous relief to the vital organs, which have been starved for oxygen and pervaded with the waste gas carbon dioxide. It's no wonder that just learning how to take deeper fuller breaths efficiently and on a regular basis can have an uplifting effect on all the physiological systems.

The practice of asanas with a full breathing technique is central to the process of Classical Yoga. This is one of the hallmarks that distinguishes Classical Yoga from regular physical fitness or gymnastic exercise.

In Classical Yoga the poses are practiced in two ways: using rhythmic breathing to come into and out of poses practiced in a continuous flowing sequence called vinyasa, or practicing poses separately in a logical sequence, statically held, in a stable comfortable manner. According to Patanjali, the poses are perfected by a sequence of steps through which awareness of the life-force is cultivated.[2] To find this inner pose, which creates a stable, comfortable outer posture, smooth full breathing must be developed.

The breath is intimately connected to the mind. It is said, "If the breath is agitated, so is the mind." Therefore, to quiet the mind in order to direct its attention, we first learn to regulate the breath.

First Learn How to Breathe

To begin the process of breath awareness, lie down on the floor in the Corpse (Savasana) Pose, relax, and observe the motion of your breath. Let your hands rest at your sides, legs separated enough to relax your lower back. Begin by observing your natural breath pattern. Let your mindfulness training begin by noticing the air as it enters your nostrils. Watch where it expands as you inhale, where it releases as you exhale. Notice the rate/pace of your breath, and the contrast between inhalation and exhalation in terms of pace and effort. Your breathing pattern may vary at different points of the day. It may also change according to your mood, previous activity, and current thoughts. Many factors contribute to what you find as you simply relax and observe.

Feel the interior spaces as your breath enters your head and begins its interior journey down through your trachea into your lungs. Notice where you feel the natural motions of your breathing. Does it feel labored or effortless? Do you notice one target area receiving the breath more than some other regions? Can you distinguish a temperature difference between the inhalation and the exhalation as it moves through your nostrils?

---

2 Stiles, *Yoga Sutras of Patanjali,* chap. II, sutras 47–49.

Let your awareness now focus on your abdominal region and allow a gentle expansion there as you inhale. Now let the area contract and sink inward as you exhale. If this is different from your normal breath, place your hands on your lower abdomen and gently compress your abdominal muscles as you exhale. This breath awareness is for the purpose of concentrating your attention and toning your abdominal muscles. While the effort is mild, over time it will definitely tone your abdominals with its wave-like motions.

When you sustain this directing of the breath while lying down, it naturally stimulates a relaxation reflex. In reaction to this normal parasympathetic reflex, your respiratory rate will diminish, your heart rate will lower, and elevated blood pressure will begin to normalize. This comes about through a neurological sensor called the baroreceptor located on the wall of the descending aorta. This reflex is activated when pressure is applied to the middle abdomen during exhalation. The pressure change is sensed by the baroreceptor, which in turn signals the hypothalamus in the mid-brain. The hypothalamus is responsible for regulating heart rate and blood pressure. The tension of the arterial wall tells the system that less pressure is needed in the system, which causes the blood pressure and heart rate to be lowered. Once you can create these abdominal waves at will, you will find this to be an effective method to relax, regardless of what activity you may be engaged in.

To begin the process of breath awareness, observe the nature of your breathing pattern while visualizing your respiratory system (see figure 3, page 52).

Inhale: Your diaphragm goes down as air rushes into your lungs. The action of the diaphragm widens your rib cage and also pushes your abdominal contents downward and forward.

Exhale: Your diaphragm returns to its original position, and air is expelled from your lungs. Your abdomen draws in and up when you breathe out.

It is important to note that, for about half the population, this is not a normal event. The other half of the world breathes in reverse of this description. That is, they swell the belly during exhalation and expand the chest during inhalation. The belly contracts during inhalation and the chest relaxes during exhalation. This reverse breathing is due to the exaggerated use of the chest, neck, and shoulders. Accompanying this respiratory pattern are often chronic tension in the neck and shoulders and irregular biological rhythms—menstrual flow, constipation, frequent or evening urination, insomnia; elevated blood pressure, even tachycardia (irregular heart rhythms).

It has been my consistent experience that, when people regain this natural pattern, some of the most obvious symptoms of stress in their lives begin to fade away. So simple, yet so complex. This is the biological reflex of the life-force coming into and from the human body. To make this shift requires some patience and perseverance that are well worth the benefits you will experience.

Not convinced? Next time you are stressed out, check out your breathing and see how it is moving. I guarantee that the wave pattern is not present if you feel tense. Change your breath and allow any other change to follow from that.

In summary, the natural breathing pattern in yoga practice is wave-like, moving through the nostrils as follows:

To breathe in: expand your chest first and then let your breath descend like a wave to your lower abdomen.

To breathe out: allow your abdomen to go in, pulling in and up on your musculature, then let the wave return upward.

Anatomy of Natural Respiration

As you inhale, the large muscle of the diaphragm moves down, flattening out as it goes, causing the lower ribs to expand and the abdominal organs to move down and forward. Natural inhalation acts as a massage to the upper abdominal organs—liver, stomach, transverse large intestine, and pancreas. A full normal inhalation will massage even the mid-abdominal organs—the ascending and descending large intestine and the centrally located small intestines. The abdominal muscles must relax for this to occur. Thus, there is a slight swelling of the belly from top to bottom giving the appearance of a wave-like motion.

During normal exhalation, the abdominal muscles contract. With yoga training, the contractions will be felt like a reverse wave from the bottom of the abdomen toward the chest. This action is made possible by toning the centrally located rectus abdominis muscle. It is assisted in breathing by the tone of the lateral abdominals, the abdominus oblique internus and externus, and the abdominus lateralis. During full expiration, the diaphragm relaxes back to a dome shape, mildly compressing the lungs and heart, while narrowing the rib cage. The rib movements are caused by two sets of muscles between the ribs: the internal and external intercostals. These muscles depress and narrow the rib cage during exhalation, while in inhalation, they reverse the process to expand the rib cage's diameter, thereby increasing the internal cavity space to allow the lungs to open.

During normal breath training these sets of muscles—the diaphragm, rectus abdominis, and the two sets of intercostals—are strengthened and trained to move more air in and out. This increases the quantity of circulating air within the body (called the tidal volume) and diminishes the number of breaths per minute.

It requires both practice and heightened awareness to train your respiratory motions to reach your back. With persistence, the breath can stimulate circulation to the kidneys, spleen, and the adrenal glands located in the middle back. A good way to begin is to rest in a prone position—like the Crocodile (Makarasana) or the Fetal pose (Darnikasana)—and direct the breath to your lower back. In both these positions, the lower back is mildly stretched during inhalation. You will notice from the drawing of the diaphragm (see figure 2) that its posterior attachment is to the internal portions of the upper three lumbar vertebrae. By deepening your breath to your back, the diaphragm is encouraged to extend downward, which, in turn, can facilitate the opening of the lower lobes of the lung.

THE NOSTRILS AND WINDPIPE

Most yoga breathing exercises (pranayama) are done by drawing air in through the nostrils. The nostrils are lined with mucous membranes that serve to moisten the air and filter out any heavy particles that might become trapped and may be toxic to the internal organs. The nostrils are also lined with small hair follicles that act to change the direction of the airflow and heighten its speed. As the breath passes the nose, it enters a series of pathways called the superior, middle, and inferior meatus and the superior, middle, and inferior concha. These structures act like turbines to increase the speed and direct the flow of the breath toward the deeper lobes of the lungs. They also permit a warming of the air immediately before entering the pharynx en route to the trachea.

In contrast to this, with mouth breathing, the mucous membranes in the throat dry out, increasing the risk of irritation and infection. Notice the difference in yourself between mouth and nostril breathing. Which can you sustain? Which one feels most natural? Which gives you more air?

Breathing through the nose also stimulates the olfactory nerves, heightening sensations of aroma. Our sense of smell is connected to the earth element, according to Ayurveda. This element creates our sense of groundedness, a connection with gravity and the Earth.

THE LUNGS

The anatomy of the lungs is fascinating. They are pear shaped, with small upper lobes capable of containing only about ½ cup of air each. The lower lungs can contain about 1 ¼ quarts of air. The upper lobes extend above the collarbones and can be palpated by applying pressure at the sides of the neck where the neck joins the clavicles. The lower lungs are wider than the upper lungs when viewed from the front, and they fill the entire width of the middle rib cage. The bottoms of the lungs are concave, conforming to the shape of the diaphragm's dome.

THE DIAPHRAGM AND INTERCOSTALS

The major muscle of respiration is the diaphragm. This large flat muscle is shaped somewhat like a full parachute or a dome. It fills the entire inner circumference below the lungs and heart, attaching to the rib cage and lumbar spine. It serves to divide the vital organs resting above it, from the digestive organs that reside below it (see figure 2). The diaphragm's motion is similar to that of a piston, just as the lungs are similar to a combustion chamber. When the diaphragm contracts, it moves downward, pulling air inward with the inhaling motion. Its contraction transforms its shape from a lofty dome to something rather like a Frisbee saucer that has widened in its downward motion. During normal breathing, the motion is rather shallow, hence air does not enter the lungs' larger lower regions. With a full inhalation, air reaches into the lower lungs, where there is more space to receive the full capacity of respiration. "The blood supply to the lower lobes is gravity dependent, so that while we are upright there is far more blood available for oxygen exchange in the lower parts of the lungs. It is for this reason that diaphragmatic breathing, which draws air into those lower regions, is such an essen-

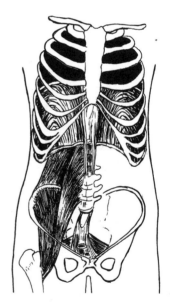

Figure 2. Cross section of the diaphragm and deep pelvic musculature. The pelvic diaphragm lies on the internal floor of the pelvis. It subtly moves with full respiration and is toned with yoga's Root Lock (Mula Banda).

51

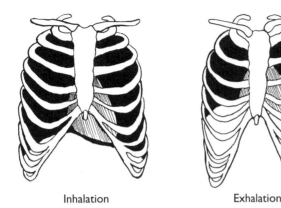

Inhalation   Exhalation

Figure 3. The action of the rib cage in the breath cycle. The diaphragm, shaped like a parachute, covers the entire inner rib cage, and extends down to attach to the anterior bodies of the first three lumbar vertebrae.

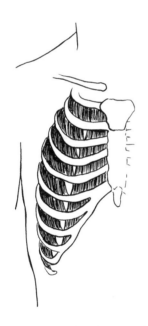

Figure 4. Internal and external intercostal muscles. Please note that this drawing does not show everything. The muscles overlap each other—they are a web permitting intercostal motions during full respiration.

tial component of optimal exercise breathing."[3]

In the yoga breathing practices, the diaphragm is contracted and lowered on the inhale, with the abdominal muscles controlled, so that the breath is drawn in slowly and consciously. "The combined action of the diaphragm and the abdominal muscles pulls up the lower part of the spinal column. . . . This pulling up of the vertebral column as a whole, gives exercise to the sympathetic and the roots of the spinal nerves."[4]

During exhalation, the diaphragm relaxes upward, which allows for the release of carbon dioxide and other metabolic waste gases. At this time, the diaphragm relaxes back to its dome shape, mildly compressing the lungs and heart while it also narrows the rib cage (see figure 3). The rib motions are caused by two sets of muscles located between the ribs called the internal and external intercostals. These muscles open and elevate the ribs to expand the circumference and increase the internal cavity for the lungs during inhalation (see figure 4). The muscles contract in reverse during the exhale.

With yoga breathing, these three sets of muscles, the diaphragm and the intercostals, are strengthened to such an extent that more air is moved in and out during a normal respiratory cycle. Thus, the effects of pranayama training last throughout the day. This increases the quantity of circulating air (called the tidal volume) and diminishes the number of breaths per minute. The net effect is a more efficient respiratory apparatus.

The piston engine of an automobile is similar in design to the respiratory system. When the piston goes down, it pulls air into the chamber above it. This action intensifies the pressure in the combustion chamber, located above the piston. When the piston rises, it forces air out, creating a strong burst of energy to be released to your car's drivetrain. The major difference in this anal-

---

[3] John Douillard, *Body, Mind, and Sport* (New York: Crown, 1994), p. 153.
[4] Swami Kuvalayananda, *Pranayama* (Philadelphia: The SKY Foundation, 1978), p. 113.

ogy is that, unlike a car's cylinder, your rib cage has the capacity to expand with the downward piston-like motion of the diaphragm. This additional dimension of motion allows for the possibility of tremendously increased power and vitality.

Diaphragmatic and Abdominal Breathing

Begin breath training by watching the breath as you inhale and exaggerating the expansion caused by the downward motion of your diaphragm. Place your hands on your abdomen at or below your navel. You will notice the lower abdomen gently swell during inhalation. A common misconception is that diaphragmatic breathing differs from abdominal. In yoga training, they flow one into the other. By emphasizing one, different benefits arise. Diaphragmatic breathing is more stimulative, and abdominal more relaxing, even to the point of being soothing or sedative. Some people are under the mistaken impression that this breathing motion will decrease abdominal muscle tone. Nothing could be farther from the truth. In yoga breath training, we emphasize relaxation during inhalation and controlled toning of the abdominals during exhalation. The control comes primarily from toning the large vertical central muscle, the rectus abdominis.

Breathing focused to just this region has a sedative effect if done for a 2 to 10 minute cycle. It can help you to relax as it lowers blood pressure and respiratory rate. If done regularly, it can be developed into a tool to help you fall asleep more rapidly. It is a vitally important breathing pattern to master, as it is a tool you will need for stressful periods of life. When you can accomplish it in an active standing position, you will be able to apply it during a stressful conversation to help relieve the physical tension accompanying your impatience or anxiety.

A variation is to breathe through your mouth with a sighing sound. By allowing an audible sound to escape, you can deepen the discharge of stress. You will probably note that you have done this in the past. Indeed, sighing is natural as you release a stressful event. By training the sigh to become prolonged and audible, you can make yourself more effective at putting the event into a discriminating perspective. This breathing is not recommended except for short periods of time. Your teacher may encourage you to use it more during a class situation should he or she feel it's warranted. Do not continue it more than five minutes, however, unless you are ready to sleep.

The Wave Motion

The second breathing exercise is the wave motion. This is a continuation of the diaphragmatic and abdominal breath in which a greater amount of air can be taken in when respiratory motions extend among three regions—the lower abdomen, solar plexus, and the chest.

During inhalation, your chest expands naturally first, then the expansion progresses to the lower ribs, and lastly into the abdomen. The inhalation is essentially a descending vertical motion. With this descent, the lower rib cage widens and the upper abdominal

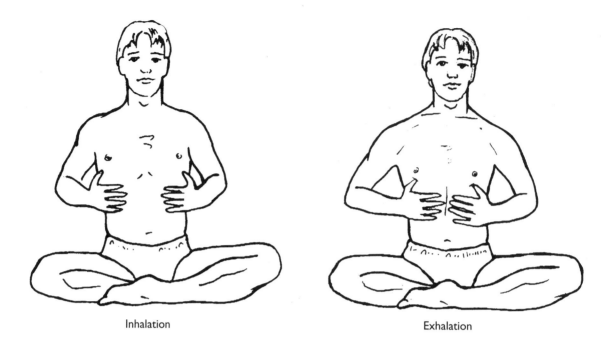

Inhalation   Exhalation

Figure 5. Intercostal breathing.

organs are displaced downward and forward. As in the abdominal breath, there is a mild expansion of the abdomen at the end of the inhalation.

The exhalation is the reverse of the inhalation. Its motion is an ascending vertical flow of breath. It begins with a mild contraction in the lower abdominal muscles to propel the exhaled air from the bottom of the lungs. During the mid range of exhalation, the lower rib cage narrows to promote the ascent of the diaphragm. This is the natural manner of breathing that coordinates the functioning of all the respiratory structures and musculature.

The desired effect is an evenness of motion in all three portions of the body—chest, rib cage, and abdomen. This exercise requires you to be motionless in order to feel the effect. Thus, it is best learned in a seated or supine position. The complete breath moves all of the respiratory muscles to full capacity in a passive manner, preventing stress to the heart and autonomic nervous system. If your breath expansion is too great in the upper region, this causes the clavicles (collarbones) to rise and stimulates your heart rate and blood pressure. This is the breath pattern predominant in people who have heart conditions or asthma. Changing their breathing pattern may lessen the underlying physical and emotional tensions.

Next, turn your attention inward and notice the quality of your breath. Allow your breath to become a natural wave that moves up and down your interior body. Ideally, it will become smooth and constant with no pause; an inhalation and exhalation of equal length. Maintain a consistent rhythm, full and deep, feeling more internal than external motion. The breathing cycle should be slowed to 8 to 10 breaths per minute, rather than the average 12 to 15 per minute. Breathing should be silent to others, making a nasal sound audible only to the practitioner. Your nostrils should not flare during the cycle. Your lower jaw should be relaxed, with your teeth slightly separated. In general, allow your face to be relaxed with a serene expression.

Once you understand—and feel—the anatomy of breathing, you will be able to move on to the subtler components of the breath. Unlike the abdominal breath, the complete wave breath is not sedative. Rather, it is an invigorating breath that brings your body to rest, while simultaneously promoting mental clarity.

VARIATION—INTERCOSTAL BREATHING

The middle component of the complete breath can become a more powerful tool for driving up your energy level. To expand your mid-range, place your hands in a curve around the shape of your lower rib cage (see figure 5, page 54). Exhale and press your fingertips together so that they meet just above your solar plexus. Inhale and expand the region beneath your hands. Continue and begin to press with your hands to emphasize the narrowing of your rib cage. Adjust the width of your hands to let your fingertips touch at the end of the exhalation. Inhale, expanding outward with the ribs to strengthen the intercostal muscles. Exhale, using the strength of your arms to narrow the ribs. Continue and notice how much expansion you can get with each inhalation. The ideal is to have two to three inches of expansion at your lower sternal region.

Ujjaye Pranayama

Your next breathing tool is *ujjaye* breathing. Ujjaye comes from two root words, *uj*, meaning "upward," and *jayi*, meaning "victorious." It is a breathing technique that helps the mind rise victoriously above its usually restless nature to experience the Self. The mind then becomes calm, and the stillness that is always there beneath your thoughts shines clear, giving an experience of your inner Self. An important technique for Hatha Yoga, ujjaye is a glottal breath in which the glottis at the back of the throat is partially closed to narrow the passage of air entering from the sinus cavities and nostrils to the trachea (windpipe).

Ujjaye is the basic pranayama technique from which most others derive. It is done best seated in a chair or a meditation pose, with your back erect and your head slightly down, as in bowing toward your heart. The chest/heart is raised to allow the lungs freedom to expand easily.

Place your hands, palm up, on your knees with the tips of your forefinger and thumbs joined in Jnana Mudra (Wisdom's Seal) and your arms straight. Place your attention on the breath sound. Maintain inhalation and exhalation at an even, steady pace. Create a constriction in the base of your throat that makes the sound more audible.

Begin by taking a deep breath and feel the soft juncture above and between your collarbones (clavicles) where the breastbone (sternum) sinks in. It is this contraction that creates the breath sound. The sound should be evenly made from the beginning to the end of each inhalation and each exhalation.

Don't pause while breathing, but maintain a smooth, steady in-out flowing cycle. When this has been stable for five minutes, you may begin the second phase of practice—extending the natural length of each breath. This follows with the second definition of pran-ayama.[5] Drawing out the breath deepens your ability to concentrate and maintain a still posture. Your breath becomes more subtle, the prana energy in the breath more apparent. The influence of the mind becomes more obvious.

The breath is said to create the natural mantra sound of *ham'sa*. *Ham* is the sound of the inhalation, *sa* the sound of exhalation. The mantra means, "I am that." "That" refers to pure awareness. In this way, breath can be used as a meditation device to attract your mind. You may become aware of *ham* on inhale and *sa* on exhale. By gently keeping your mind on this awareness, the process of meditation spontaneously arises from within. Deepen this process by practicing the guidance in chapter 31 on the inner process of asana as it leads you from Hatha Yoga to Raja Yoga.

VARIATIONS

There are numerous variations of this practice that alter the ratio of inhalation to exhalation, add breath pauses (Kumbhaka), or alternate the nostril through which you breathe. These practices are best learned directly from a teacher and hence will not be covered here.

BENEFIT

Ujjaye is excellent for respiratory patients, especially asthmatics. When regularly practiced, it is an excellent doorway into natural meditation.

Using Breath in Asana Practice

One of the hallmarks of Classical Yoga is the use of ujjaye pranayama (in the wave motion) consistently in asana practice. This feature, and the development of breathing exercises into pranayama, which enlivens the life-force, make Classical Yoga unique as a personal discipline. In asana practice, there are three general rules for the use of breath patterns.

1. *Inhalation occurs as you extend the spine, exhalation when you release tension and relax.*

Rhythmic breath is harmonized to be at the pace of the body motions. For example, if I am in an erect standing position (Tadasana) and I lift my arms up, I inhale during this motion. With practice, I can learn to pace the tempo of my arms' motions with the time required to fill my lungs. In this manner, the inhalation will be complete when the arms reach full shoulder flexion, fingertips aimed at the ceiling. Similarly, I can exhale to lower my arms to my sides and I run out of breath when my arms touch my sides.

---

5 Stiles, *Yoga Sutras of Patanjali*, chap. II, sutra 51.

2. Inhale when you move to center or become erect and exhale when moving away from centered position.

Bending forward is to be accompanied by an exhalation. Sitting up can accompany an inhalation. Twisting or side bending can be done with an exhalation; while returning to a centered erect posture can occur on an inhalation. If I move slowly into a forward-bending position, I extend myself, lengthening my spine with each inhalation, and moving forward with each exhalation.

3. Breath awareness is constant, even when your body is stationary.

If I hold an asana, my attention remains on the internal wavelike flow of ujjaye. If my intention is to deepen the physical pose by continually going into a wider range of motion, my breath can be used to release specific tension areas that restrict my breath or body sensations, wherever they may be. In this procedure, revert to the first rule and notice that your body continues to lengthen itself during inhalation. A keen concentration will uncover where the opening is taking place. On the next inhalation, gently move yourself in the pattern revealed by the openness of your breath. On the next exhalation, release the tension, observing carefully where and in what direction the release takes place. This will guide you to move on the next inhalation. Once you have reached the boundary of this openness, you can choose between staying at the new edge of your pose or inhaling on your way back to a centered position.

The qualities of the breath are intriguing to examine (see Table 1). Classical Yoga regulates all four parts of the breath—the two motions (inhalation and exhalation) and the two pauses that naturally follow the motions. The pauses are natural, provided there is no stress or fixed attention. During either of these events, the natural rhythm is altered and the breath will be shallower and the pauses longer. A major difference between stress and concentration is that the pause during stress is accompanied by effort and tension, and it increases internal pressure. With concentration, the pause is

Table 1. Qualities of the Breath.

INHALE (Puraka)	EXHALE (Rechaka)	PAUSE (Kumbhaka)
Warming	Cooling	Neutral
Openness	Defining boundary	Vulnerability
Extending motion	Grounding	Stillness
Spaciousness	Centeredness	Point of potentiality
Receive light	Release darkness	Harmony of light/dark
Ha—Sun	Tha—Moon	Hatha

a natural and effortless event. Upon closer examination, the breath is not held nor does it stop. Rather it persists with subtle, nearly imperceptible, waves.

Provided your concentration is genuine, do not encourage yourself to breath deeply during yoga asana practice. Only if you are exhibiting holding your breath should you be encouraged to breathe fully. Watching carefully for this distinction can permit you to move into a deeper connection with the process of Classical Yoga. It is often a missing link, a hidden secret, that practitioners disregard in learning how to transition from physical Hatha Yoga to mindful Raja Yoga practice.

HOW LONG TO HOLD A POSE

Based upon the breath patterns, there are different benefits for holding poses at varying lengths.

1. *Inhale into the pose; exhale to release the pose.*

This pattern is useful for the purpose of becoming familiar with the movement and how your body reacts. By repeated practice in this manner, sensitivity is heightened and your body will uncover its own homeostasis. When this method is repeated for up to six times, it is optimal for slowing down your mind, deepening your breath, and developing pranic energy. It is a form of pranayama that regulates the flow of prana into the areas of the body affected by the asana.

2. *Staying in the pose for 2 to 3 breaths.*

This pattern is useful for training concentration (dhyana) and integrating pranayama ratios into asana. It is particularly beneficial for improving memory, gently strengthening the lungs, and for students with scoliosis. At this level of concentration, two points of anatomical alignment may be maintained, but the practice is not for developing detailed body posturing. When this method is repeated, it heightens the body's ability to adapt, thus improving efficiency at eliminating stress and hypertension.

3. *Staying in the posture for 12 breaths.*

This is the level I recommend for optimizing the effects of muscular strength or flexibility for those students who are focusing upon eliminating specific muscular and postural imbalances. This develops optimal stamina in the shortest possible period of time. To proceed, begin by holding the pose with good alignment and steadiness at a lesser number of breaths, then increase the holding time by 2 to 3 breaths per week. When the posture can be held comfortably and steadily for 12 breaths for two weeks consistently, you can move on to the next level of challenge as indicated in The Kinesiology of Yogasanas (Table 6 in chapter 22, page 266).

Using Breath for Insight

As we grow older, we breathe less fully; some people use only one third of their lung capacity. Shallow breathing is an important factor in disorientation, loss of memory, and vitality. The brain requires three times as much oxygen as the rest of the body's tissue cells. Every tissue requires oxygen. An inadequate supply will impair organ function. By opening up your posture, you also open your respiratory muscles which in turn stimulates respiratory efficiency. Restricted breathing is known to correlate with depression and anxiety. Change your breath and you can change your mind.

The practice of yogasana is a wonderful opportunity to use your breath as a vehicle to feed your brain and access your higher mind. The mind contains all wisdom and knowledge. By this training, we can progressively increase our access to this abundant source of insight. Among the methods of inquiry that are available to yoga are questioning yourself during yogasana.

There is a method to systematically developing hidden regions. A series of questions can be asked during the exhalation—Where am I holding? During exhalation, request this region to release. Another question to ask during inhalation—Where am I opening/extending? While continuing to contemplate this question, have an intention of purposeful, willful extending. During the process, watch the inner sensations carefully to observe where the release or the extension is actually occurring. As long as the extension is occurring where your intention is, the yogasana is effective. When a point is reached where the extension halts or spontaneously takes on a new direction, then your mind is not merged with your body. By keeping mind and body united, you can begin to personalize the process of their energetic development to create personalized yogasana. This is the physical basis for spontaneous occurrence of asana, which develops naturally through spiritual awakening of the energy called Shakti Kundalini.

The Release of the Subconscious

After spending some time reflecting upon the force of the breath, it may become apparent that the breath is in a relatively constant state of change. Like our moods or emotions, it also varies. Who can say which comes first, a change in moods or a change in the breath? Just as our posture slumps when we are depressed, so also our breath becomes constricted, and vice versa. When we are elated, we tend to stand taller and breathe more fully. By watching ourselves, we can uncover these changes and have a choice to change what was previously subconscious. To see and feel all the emotional states, thoughts, and subtle energies that accompany our moods requires a commitment to courage and regularity in self-discipline.

Our emotions are a key element in self care because they allow us to enter into the body/mind's conversation. By getting in touch with our emotions, both by listening to them and by directing them through the psychosomatic network, we can gain access to the healing wisdom that is everyone's natural biological right. And how do we do this? First by acknowledging and claiming all our feelings, not just the so-called positive ones. Anger, grief, fear—these emotional experiences are not negative in themselves; in fact, they are vital for our survival. We need anger to define boundaries, grief to deal with our losses, and fear to protect ourselves from danger. It's only when these feelings are denied, so that they cannot be easily and rapidly processed through the system and released, that the situation becomes toxic. And the more we deny them, the more the ultimate toxicity, which often takes the form of an explosive release of pent-up emotion.[6]

The most potent of the endorphins is beta endorphin, which is most highly concentrated in the pituitary gland. By visualizing its release and secretion to the receptors throughout the body or to specific target sights, you can stimulate your immune system, control your emotions, or release the cravings of addictive substances. Endorphins can be seen as your own body's natural heroin. This goes back to the yogis idea that whatever we crave is already inside of us.

Simply uncovering the process of our change, however, is not enough. Just seeing your depression doesn't change it, any more than seeing that we are bound can contribute to liberation. Making a decision to change and consciously applying that decision while taking steps to change behavior can produce a result that will have durability. This process is known as contemplation, or dharana, in Classical Yoga. The process of being alert and insightful naturally follows a spectrum that leads to a heightening of intuition and higher knowledge (gnosis).

How Not to Breathe

A fascinating view of breathing is obtained by watching those who are healthy and contrasting your findings with those who are unhealthy. When you watch an infant sleeping, it is easy to determine that it breathes using primarily the diaphragm by watching the abdomen rise and fall. Two scientists, Alan Hymes, M.D. and Phil Nuernberger, Ph.D. were curious as to the respiratory patterns of heart-attack patients, so they instructed primary-care nurses in an intensive coronary unit of a large hospital in Minneapolis to determine how patients were breathing. They surveyed 153 patients divided into two categories—those who had suffered a heart attack or myocardial infarction (MI), documented by blood tests and cardiogram; and a second group suspected of having had heart attacks (NMI), but found to have no destruction of cardiac tissue. The results were as follows:

1. All patients (100 percent) were habitual thoracic breathers, no diaphragmatic motion was detectable;

2. Approximately 75 percent of all patients were chronic mouth breathers; 70 percent of these also exhibited open-mouthed snoring; 84 percent of the MI group who snored exhibited patterns of apnea, involuntary pauses of six seconds or more; and 48 percent of the NMI group who snored exhibited patterns of apnea.[7]

The authors suggested that "it may be that teaching the patient simple diaphragmatic breathing should be an integral pattern of the treatment process. Altering the thoracic

---

[6] Candace Pert, *Molecules of Emotion: Why You Feel the Way You Feel* (New York: Scribner, 1997), pp. 285–286.
[7] Alan Hymes and Phil Nuernberger, "Breathing Patterns Found in Heart Attack Patients," *Research Bulletin*, vol. 2, no. 2 (Honesdale, PA: Himalayan International Institute, 1980), pp. 8–10.

pattern to diaphragmatic breathing could increase the efficiency of ventilation/perfusion, resulting in a decrease in the amount of work required by the cardio-pulmonary system. This could help reduce the strain on the heart.[8] Their findings are consistent with earlier research, which found that "hypertension and heart disease are more common in heavy snorers than in normal subjects."[9]

Of particular interest is the relationship of apnea to health. During the survey "six patients who were part of the observed MI group died during the survey period. Every one of the six patients exhibited long, sustained periods of apnea lasting 30 seconds or longer, 24 to 48 hours prior to death. Again, it is not yet clear as to whether apnea is a contributing or a resultant factor."[10]

The Dangers of Holding Your Breath

"It is dangerous to hold your breath during any form of exercise," writes Michael O'Shea. "As you inhale and exhale, the pressure in your chest cavity increases and decreases. When you exercise and are breathing heavier, these pressure changes are even greater. When you hold your breath, you do not allow for the natural release of this pressure, and the stress on your heart and circulatory system can elevate blood pressure two to three times above normal. This can result in ruptured blood vessels, stroke or heart attack."[11]

In yoga practice, as in any unfamiliar activity, it is common to hold your breath due to the concentration involved. This should not be encouraged. For beginners, one major value of a teacher is to encourage full conscious respiration during all yoga activities. Once the student has spent about a year with the practice, there are exercises that can be given to allow for the natural pause between respiratory motions to be gently increased. This practice should be supervised and, in general, done only with the coordination of muscular locks to regulate blood pressure and heart rate. The side effects cited above can be alleviated with proper supervision. In general, however, it is advisable not to hold your breath during yoga practices of asana or pranayama. The muscular locks (bandhas) may appear easy to learn, but their proper development requires physical supervision by a teacher trained in their physical and energetic benefits.

---

8 Hymes and Nuernberger, "Breathing Patterns Found in Heart Attack Patients," p. 11.

9 E. Lugaresi, G. Coccagna, and F. Cirignotta, "Snoring and its Clinical Implications," in C. Guillemainault and W.C. Dement, eds., *The Sleep Apnea Syndromes* (New York: Krock Foundation Series, vol. II, Alan R. Liss, Inc., 1978), pp. 13–21.

10 Hymes and Nuernberger, "Breathing Patterns Found in Heart Attack Patients," p. 12.

11 Michael O'Shea, Ph.D., "Fitness," *Parade Magazine,* Sept. 5, 1993, p. 18.

Chapter 8

SUN SALUTATION: SURYA NAMASKAR

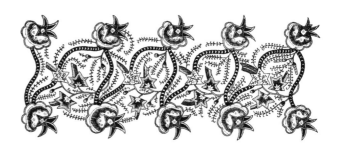

The Sun Salutation can become the great high point of your morning practice. While it has a definite heating benefit, I do not recommend that it be used as a warm-up, but rather as is sequenced in this book, after you are warmed up and have dealt with optimizing your strengths. Then you can use the Sun Salutation to enhance your respiration and cardiovascular functions. This is a beautiful sequence that can teach you to coordinate rhythmic breathing with body postures into a flowing routine. This suffices as a complete program when done for 15 to 20 minutes continuously.

Surya Namaskar, literally translated, means "beautiful light, you are my own Self." Surya is one of the twelve mantra names for the Sun. In the traditional practice of the Sun Salutation, the Sun is honored during the period of rising and setting, so that its energies can be taken in through the medium of mantra and pranayama—energetic breathing.

PRECAUTIONS

If you have a bad back, exercise caution during forward-bending poses by bending the knees. Cobra pose is safest if done without the use of your arm strength. If there is stiffness in your wrists, do not bear weight on your flat hands but rather use your fingertips or knuckles.

Instructions

1. Start in Mountain Pose (Tadasana), standing steady with your feet six inches apart, your palms together, centered before your chest in prayer pose, Namaskar (see figure 6,

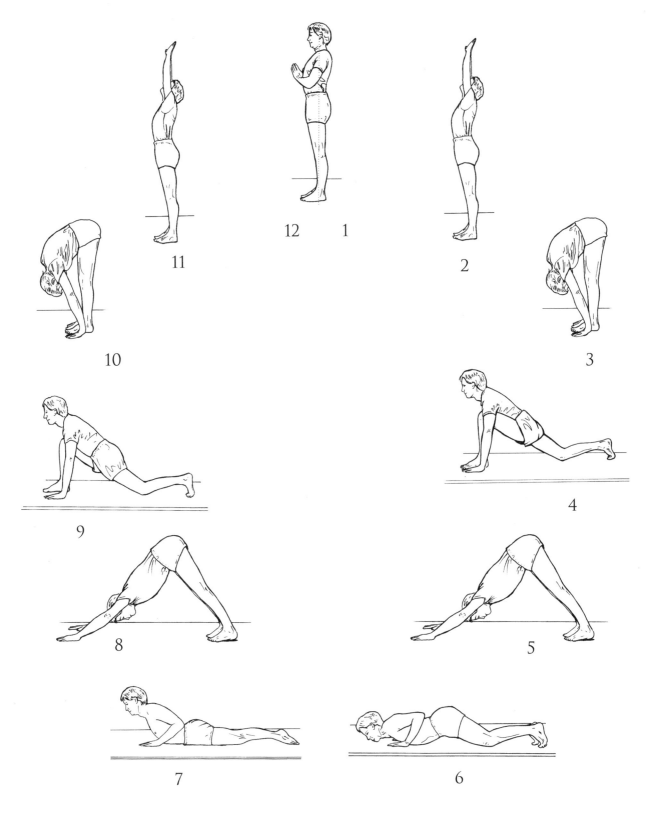

Figure 6. The Sun Salutation—Surya Namaskar.

page 64). Close your eyes, take a series of deep breaths so that the flow of your breath is centered in the region of your heart, the inner sun. Imagine your inner sun rising as you breathe, spreading its warmth throughout your body. Inwardly repeat this greeting to the Self in your heart:

I honor the divinity of my heart with all the warmth and cordiality of my mind.[1]

2. **Inhale**, arms extending forward and up, palms together in the Upward Salute (Urdhva Namaskar). Keep your buttocks firm as you look up at your hands.

3. **Exhale**, stretching forward in a sweeping forward bend that extends your spinal column. At the end of the Intensive Stretch (Uttanasana) forward bend, your arms are relaxed and your head is hanging close to your knees.

4. **Inhale**, bending your knees. Your palms are placed outside your feet, so that your fingers are in line with your toes. Stretch your right leg fully back, allowing your knee to drop to the floor in the runner pose. Your pelvis will be pushed down and forward to stretch your quadriceps. Lift your chest and head to create a mild backbend in the Runner Pose, also called the Equestrian Stretch (Ashwa Sanchalanasana).

5. **Exhale**, moving your left leg back, placing your left foot open, yet even with the right foot. Lift your hips high, slowly straightening your knees while pushing your chest toward your feet as you come into Downward Facing Dog Pose (Adho Mukha Svanasana). **Inhale**, lengthening your spine.

6. On the next **exhalation**, bend your knees, coming briefly into the Cat Pose. Let your chest lead you to the floor in the Cat Bow, also called Eight-Limbs Salutation (Ashtanganamaskar). Keep your elbows narrow at the end of the pose.

7. **Inhale** and squeeze your shoulderblades as you lift your chest, expanding it fully into the Cobra posture (Bhujangasana). Point your feet so that your thighs and legs are in one firm line.

8. **Exhale** and lower your chest. Then inhale into Cat Lift. Exhale, and lift your hips high up and back, coming to Dog Pose. (When you have developed sufficient strength and fluidity, move with one exhale into Dog Pose.)

9. **Inhale**, returning your right foot between your hands, with your toes placed even with your fingertips, returning to the Runner Pose with left leg now back.

10. **Exhale** and bend forward, your left leg coming forward, so that your upper body is in a forward-bending position, Uttanasana—the Intensive Stretch Pose.

11. **Inhale** and stretch your arms forward to initiate the lift. The upward pull of your arms will extend your middle back as you come up. Look up as you bend back, tensing your buttocks.

12. **Exhale**, bringing your palms to your heart position, Namaskar.

---

[1] Personal instruction to author from Paul Copeland, who received it from his teacher, Professor T. Krishnamacharya.

Repeat. On the next cycle, at position four, your left leg is brought back first, and again in position 9, your left leg is brought forward. Two repetitions, with the reversed leg position, creates one cycle of Surya Namaskar, the Sun Salutation.

COMMON PROBLEMS

Among the common problems in the Sun Salutation is that, when you establish the length of your extension of Runner Pose, that distance from hands to feet should be maintained throughout the sequence. Do not change your hand and foot positions to make other postures easier, as this will cause you to move backward over repeated sequences.

One helpful trick in making the transition to return to the Runner Pose (Number 9) from the Dog Pose is to reach your ankle and pull it up with a hopping motion to bring your toes level with your fingers. Another method is leave Dog Pose on your tip-toes, so that your hips are raised as high as possible. This will allow the maximum swing of a pendulum-like force of your leg being brought forward. Bring your knee up as close to your chest as possible. Slide your pelvis forward, maintaining your knee close to your torso, so that, in the final position, your shin is perpendicular to the floor when your hips are fully pressed forward.

BENEFITS

The Sun Salutation is the most beneficial of the traditional yoga sequences. It may be done slowly and gently for a meditative inner focus. It can also be done more vigorously over a 10 to 20 minute period for an aerobic effect to strengthen your cardiovascular system. The poses can also be sustained for developing muscular stamina. The Sun Salutation is the most widely known series of yoga poses. All yoga teachers present it in some variation. It is so highly regarded that there are entire booklets on this one practice.[2]

The Sun Salutation is a very powerful sequence of postures that both strengthens and extends the long muscles of the front and back of the body. It is a unique sequence, in that it can stand alone, without the need for other practice to maintain health. It can increase hip and spinal flexibility with practice. John Douillard describes the power of this practice as follows:

The coordination of the breath with the flexion and extension postures considerably enhances the effects of the Sun Salute. When the body is moving into extension during a backbend, the rib cage, spine, and muscles are all stretched or lengthened. With an inhalation coordinated with back-bending extensions, the diaphragm is moving in the opposite direction. During this inhalation the diaphragm must contract downward in order to pull oxygen into the lungs.

---

[2] Bhanawanvo Pant Pratinidhi (Raja of Aundh), *Surya Namaskara—An Ancient Indian Exercise* (Hyderabad: Orient Longman, 1989); and Swami Satyananda, *Surya Namaskara (A Technique of Solar Vitalization)* (Munger, India: Bihar School of Yoga, 1983).

During the contraction of the diaphragm (inhale) the Sun Salute posture is always one of extension. During this exercise, as the body extends upward, the diaphragm is contracted downward. This provides a deep internal massage, particularly for the diaphragm and the muscles of the rib cage. . . . The Sun Salute introduces a scissorlike motion, which can effectively breathe to hard-to-get-to muscle spasms in the rib cage that make breathing into the lower lobes of the lungs more difficult.

With continued practice of the Sun Salute, the rib cage will reestablish its normal range of motion and flexibility, making deep diaphragmatic nasal breathing—the preferred breathing technique both during exercise and at rest—easier to perform.

The best flexibility gains can be made when the muscles are warm, immediately after a workout. The Sun Salute because of its counterposing flexion and extension postures, is one of the most effective means of gaining flexibility. [3]

Initially, the Sun Salutation is practiced three or four times in sequence. For the first few days, concentrate on getting fullness in the movements. Later, develop your breathing rhythm and flow. The breathing should be slow and deep, in time with the flow of the poses. This may take a week or more of regular practice. Following that time, it can be increased to a total of six to ten repetitions, until your stamina is developed enough to maintain this flow without becoming winded. Gradually, in the second or third month, it can be increased to twenty or twenty-five repetitions. After that time, the effect on the heart and cardiovascular system will maintain health and vigor. Done regularly, twenty repetitions will tone your body and help to reduce weight. When done with full continuous breathing, each sequence should take approximately one minute for a half-cycle.

My first spiritual teacher taught a variation on the Sun Salutation. He recommended that it be practiced at gradually increasing speed. After you achieve twenty rounds slowly and rhythmically with the breath (which should take 20 minutes), this can safely be done. He recommended that teachers increase to one hundred times, or fifty rounds, doing them as fast as possible, so that the rhythm is not at breath rate (one inhalation or exhalation per movement), but rather the entire cycle is accomplished in 2 or 3 breaths. In this manner, the breath is steady and just as long as normal.

With regular practice, this can be done in about fifteen to twenty minutes. It has a tremendously strong aerobic effect on the cardiovascular system. It produces about the same effects on the cardiovascular system as running or swimming would, but without the jarring effects of running and without the need for a swimming pool. The Sun Salutation is a remarkable routine, because it energizes the body to the point that this is all you need to do to maintain optimal physical health.

---

[3] John Douillard, *Body, Mind, and Sport* (New York: Crown, 1994), pp. 182–183, 198.

PART THREE

The Benefits of Yoga Practice

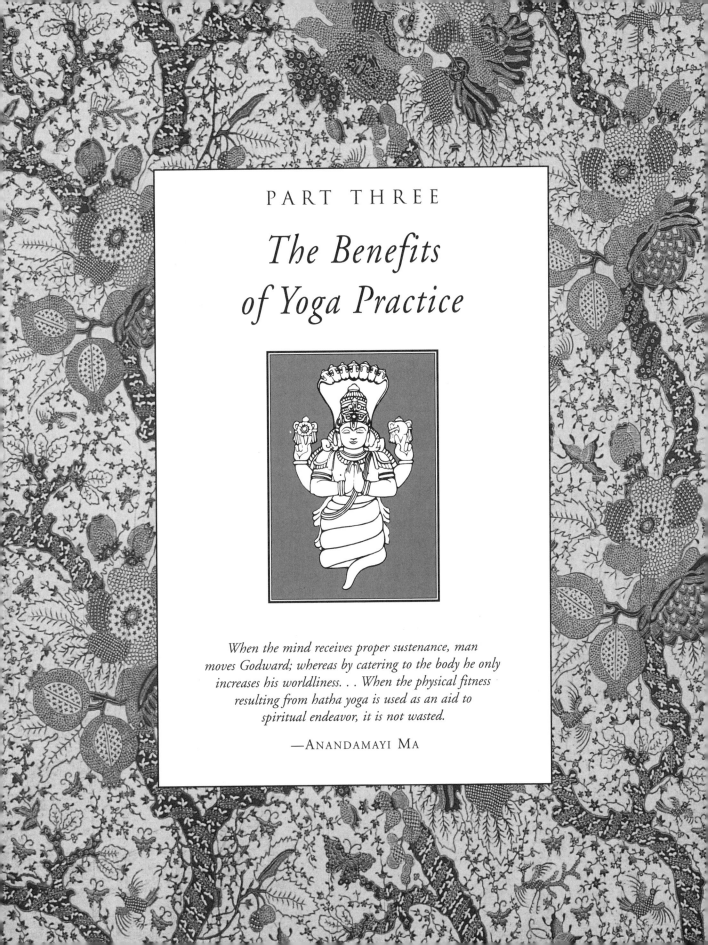

When the mind receives proper sustenance, man moves Godward; whereas by catering to the body he only increases his worldliness. . . When the physical fitness resulting from hatha yoga is used as an aid to spiritual endeavor, it is not wasted.

—ANANDAMAYI MA

INTRODUCTION

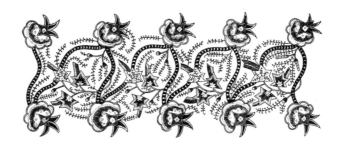

Sheik Nasrudin goes to market, or how not to ride a horse.[1]

Once upon a time, Sheik Nasrudin made his livelihood as a potter. All week long, he worked over the wheel, churning out pots of all sorts—pots for flowers, for cooking, for ornaments, even neti pots for yogis to douche their sinus cavities. Every day, he led a disciplined life of rising early and creating beautiful and utilitarian pots for his household and the community. Nasrudin's wife, Sarah, was a great contributor to his creative process. Often, she had unusual ideas come to her during her daily meditations or nightly insightful dreams. She described exotic shapes for common pots that Nasrudin used, and these frequently become his best selling-pots. On Saturdays, he loaded his pots carefully onto the back of his burro and slowly plodded off to the weekly market.

One day, his burro sprang loose from his coral and began to eat wild grasses in the neighbor's field. Among them were loco weeds. When Nasrudin went to fetch the burrow, he was unmanageable. *What to do?* In compensation for his difficulty, Nasrudin's neighbor offered his own horse to take the pots to market.

Nasrudin had never before ridden a horse and he was challenged by the task of getting all his pots on such a large animal. He was also delighted that he could load the horse with twice as many pots because of its great size. When it came time to mount the

---

1 Oral tradition received from Swami Muktananda, retold by author.

huge beast, he set his ladder to get onto the horse's back. Then he took his familiar cane stick to swat the beast as was his custom with his burro. As soon as he did so, the horse roared up onto its hind legs, leaving Nasrudin to grasp its mane with all his might in an effort to stay on. The horse bolted faster than Nasrudin believed possible. Nasrudin's legs and his pots were flying everywhere. He was pulled upside down and tried to hang on with his arms and legs encircling the horse's neck. When he passed the neighbor's home, the neighbor was shocked to see Nasrudin in such a state, so he shouted, "Where are you going in such a hurry?"

Nasrudin replied, "I don't know. Ask the horse."

. . .

Many of us will see ourselves in Nasrudin. We lack understanding of where we are going. So, like him, we are without understanding of our goals. The undisciplined body/mind is like the wild, terrified horse and Nasrudin—out of control, directionless, perhaps even recklessly so. Alternatively, we may move along slowly, deliberately. Our lives are predictable—until, that is, we get caught up in the speedy horse of our culture. This can happen through undisciplined, unquestioned, and attached reading of the newspaper, watching television, or just doing what our neighbors do. Who knows what's next? I don't know—ask the culture.

In another sense, the burro is like the untrained body/mind just living life and having the "freedom" to move outside the fence. We think that we are free because we can do what we want—we are free to drive anywhere we want, perhaps just to get ahead of our neighbors at the next intersection's red light. This is freedom without any awareness of the consequences. We are free to fall in love, and free to leave if the relationship gets too hot or if our partner wants their freedom. We are free to have our mood swings and to do what we like when we like, regardless of the impact on others. We may find, upon self-examination, that we are like the typical Boston drivers—in such a hurry to get ahead of the car next to us that we fail to notice the light ahead is red.

In the yoga sense, this is not freedom. Yoga is not a cultural phenomenon. It is not a "here today and gone tomorrow" marvel. Yoga is not a fad. Classical Yoga teachings are applicable to all cultures and religious faiths and are true for all situations. In Classical Yoga practice, we continuously strive to be free of fear, craving, and clinging by cultivating patience, enthusiasm, and equality of love for all of life. This type of freedom transcends all boundaries and sets us free to know the truth of life. This is what I believe we all seek, regardless of whether or not we are conscious of that search.

Exploring Yoga Research

Hatha Yoga limbers the joints and improves circulation through preparatory exercises (pavanmuktasana), develops muscular tone through postures (asanas), and develops powerful wind and heart muscles through breathing exercises (pranayamas). The benefits of Hatha Yoga are tremendous. Scientific research on the effects of yoga began as early as 1924 near Bombay, India, at Kaivalyadhama Yoga Institute, and at about the

Table 2. Summary of Research into the Benefits of Yoga Practice.

BEHAVIORAL	PHYSICAL	MENTAL	PHYSIOLOGICAL	PERSONALITY
Weight ⇓	Hand steadiness ⇑	Concentration ⇑	EEG Alpha ⇑	Anxiety ⇓
Nervousness ⇓	Reactivity to stressors ⇓	Memory ⇑	Respiratory efficiency and competence ⇑	Depression ⇓
Health complaints ⇓	Flexibility ⇑	Intelligence quotient ⇑	Oxygen consumption ⇓	Neuroticism ⇓
Clinical assessment of psychiatric patients ⇑	Relaxation ⇑	Mental fatigability ⇓	Respiratory rate ⇓	Conflict resolution ⇑
Psychological complaints ⇓	Muscular electrical activity (EMG) ⇓	Performance quotient ⇑	Chest expansion ⇑	Openness to experience ⇑
	Muscle tone ⇑	Shift in sequence of ideas ⇑	Lung capacity ⇑	Defensiveness ⇓
	Fitness ⇑		Breath-holding time ⇑	Guilt ⇓
			Tidal volume ⇑	Tension and instability ⇓
			Respiratory amplitude ⇑	Projective measures (number of responses) ⇑
			Cardiovascular efficiency and competence ⇑	Delay in responses ⇓
			Systolic and diastolic blood pressure ⇓	Hostility ⇓
			Heart rate ⇓	Submissiveness ⇓
			Peripheral blood flow ⇑	Self-criticism ⇓
			Oxygen transport system ⇑	Self-concept ⇑
			Adrenocortical efficiency and competence ⇑	Assertiveness and emotional stability in females ⇑
			Endocrine and metabolic competence ⇑	Body image ⇑
				Interpersonal relationships ⇑
				Self-esteem ⇑
				Spiritual orientation ⇑

73

same time at The Yoga Institute of Santa Cruz, Bombay. Since then, data has been accumulated by researchers around the world to show a remarkable variety of benefits. In 1981, Joan Harrington, Ph.D., published a summary of the outcome of Hatha Yoga practice in the Research Bulletin of the Himalayan Institute.[2] This summary of scientific studies revealed the scope and depth of Hatha Yoga's benefits. Although it was published nearly twenty years ago, this survey remains the most complete to date. (See Table 2 on page 73 for an overview of this report.) The report states:

> From this review of the literature surveying the effects of Hatha Yoga, it appears that physiological and psychological improvements do take place as a result of regular practice for four to six weeks. The longer the postures are regularly performed, the more definite the changes tend to be. Studies that show that the effective use of this physical intervention facilitates personality change lend credence to the body/mind approach to therapy. The influence the postures have on balancing the autonomic nervous system creates a calmer, less anxious physiological environment. Physiological indices, psychological tests and self-reports have measured the personality changes this may allow. There is also reason to assume that fewer psychosomatic complaints are manifest in regular yoga practitioners due to the direct manipulation of the muscles and viscera, the autonomic nerve system balance and the decreased anxiety.
>
> The studies in which somatic/behavioral measures are used as dependent variables demonstrate that the Hatha postures do in fact have significant effects on physiological, health and performance variables. Hatha Yoga seems to be highly effective in dealing with psychosomatic complaints and in enhancing feelings of well-being beyond the "not sick" level. Participants claim to enjoy the practice and note improvements in themselves after regular practice. Hatha could also be an important method of athletic training and of diminishing certain physical complaints so that higher-level personality concerns can be dealt with more effectively. Because it is a physical intervention, Hatha Yoga is especially useful in dealing with psychosomatic complaints.
>
> In summary, this review of the literature suggests that Hatha Yoga has potential as a useful intervention for improving physical well-being, reducing anxiety and enhancing personality development. . . . Hatha Yoga could be a helpful adjunct to medical and psychological treatment when practiced regularly by clients on their own to improve their feelings of physical health, reduce their anxiety, and enhance their self-concepts and emotional tone.[3]

You can see from this research summary that tremendous benefits are available from regular Hatha Yoga practice. This survey is meant to reveal the potential personal effects you

---

[2] Joan Harrington (Arpita), "Physiological and Psychological Effects of Hatha Yoga: A Review of the Literature," *Research Bulletin* (Honesdale, PA: Himalayan Institute, 1983), vol. 5, nos. I and II, p. 38–39.

[3] Joan Harrington (Arpita). From "Physiological and Psychological Effects of Hatha Yoga: A Review of the Literature," p. 41; used by permission.

can experience when you choose to pursue the practice toward these goals. Question yourself and discover what areas of your life you'd like to transform. I would highly encourage you to seek out a yoga teacher or yoga therapist to mentor you more completely toward fulfilling your goals, once defined.

While there are many benefits from Yoga practice, the benefits cited should not be the end, but, rather, the necessary means to facilitate the healthy pursuit of a high-quality life. Yoga, added to the practice of meditation, accelerates the inner work of personal and spiritual growth.

Chapter 9

PHYSICAL
TRANSFORMATION

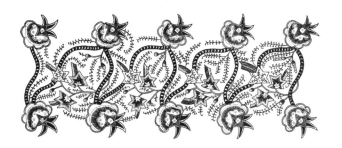

O ur bodies are living tissues in a state of constant change. The process of eating, digesting, and excreting is the process of being alive. Disrupt any phase of the process and we become ill. Maintain the proper balance and we experience physical health. All systems of the body interact with one another. Bones interact with muscles and, in turn, with physiological systems—nervous, digestive, respiratory, reproductive, excretory, and endocrine. To change any system is to change the whole. To promote improvement in any system is to promote improvement in the whole organism, and vice versa. This is the fundamental tenet of yoga and holistic health.

In yoga philosophy, the universe is composed of a trinity that has both masculine and feminine aspects. The masculine and feminine aspects of the forces are a creative force called Brahma or Sarasvati, a nurturing force called Vishnu or Lakshmi, and a transformative force called Shiva or Kali. These three primal forces interact with each other and, by that interaction, are transformed into any of the others. In the *Siva Samhita,* it is said the microcosm is the same as the macrocosm.

> Within this body dwells the mountain of Meru (the spinal column) . . . and there are rishis (all-knowing ones), munis (sages) and all the stars and planets, holy places of pilgrimage and temples. . . . (In this body) wander the sun and the moon—the cause of creation and destruction. . . . All creatures that exist in the three worlds (heaven, earth and hell) are also in this very body. . . . In this universe-patterned body, each of these objects is located in its own place.[1]

---

[1] Shyam Ghosh, ed. and trans., *The Original Yoga* (New Delhi, India: Munshiram Mancharlal, 1980), chap. II, sutras 1–6. Material in parentheses has been added.

What exists outside as the world also has a parallel component inside each individual universe. Hence, when we affect a positive change within ourselves, we are also positively affecting a change in the world around us.

Physiology and Kinesiology of Yoga

Clearly, Hatha Yoga practice generates change. There are some changes that even go beyond those cited in Dr. Harrington's research summary. Some may seem far-fetched, even mythical, to the uninitiated. Among the more unusual changes possible with yoga is the transformation of bone structure.

Bones are living tissue, composed of three types of cells—osteoblasts (that create new bone tissue), osteocytes (that maintain the strength of existing bones), and osteoclasts (that destroy weakened or unstressed bone cells that are not essential to the integrity of the bone). What is even more amazing, these three types of cells can be transformed into the others, depending upon the demands of stress or lack of it upon the bone tissue.

Thus the yogic trinity can be said to also exist within bone tissue. Brahma, the creator, correlates to the osteoblasts; Vishnu, the preserver, to osteocyte bone cells; Shiva, the destroyer/transformer, to osteoclast bone cells.

Studies have shown that bones respond to the stress of weight-lifting by becoming larger and denser. Conversely, we know that, without the stress of exercise, they become smaller and more porous, as is the case during extended hospital stays or long periods of weightlessness due to space travel.

I found that, when I was attending the Iyengar Yoga Institute in 1975 for my first yoga teacher certification, the ideas discussed about bone tissue piqued my interest to see what was possible with my knock-knees. I had been a long-distance runner for many years preceding yoga training. While stretching had always been a part of my warm-up routine, it had never changed the basic difficulty I had with my knees. I loved running through the pine forests surrounding my home in the Mt. Shasta area of Northern California. It was a tremendous high for me to just soar through the woods and breathe in the delicious pine-scented fresh air. I thought that I could run forever.

That is, until my knock-knees revealed their weakness and the inside of my knees began to scrape together. The curvature of my legs left me pre-disposed to weakness in my outer hips and a tightness in my groin. When I became fatigued, my knees would bang together. The situation was so severe that I often came back to the locker room with bloody scrapes on my knees and my wonderful natural high, erect posture degenerated into a depressed slumped posture.

The information in anatomy and physiology classes at the Yoga Institute made me wonder whether, if I changed the stress lines in the bones of my legs, I could actually sculpt the shape of the bones anew. This shattered the previously held concepts that my body's posture was genetically determined and hence outside my capacity to change. I had nothing to lose. At this time, I was practicing Iyengar Yoga vigorously for six to eight hours a day under the supervision of some of the best-trained teachers in America.

I decided to give it a good shot and calculated the poses that would stretch out the range of the group of five groin muscles, called the adductors, and strengthen the outer thigh and hip muscles, called the abductors. I especially focused on standing postures—Extended Triangle Pose (Utthita Trikonasana) and Warrior variation I and II (Virabhadrasana). I studied anatomy, not only in books but also as I experienced the shifting musculature's leverage increasing from the progressive improvement in these asanas.

I not only had knock-knees, but my knees were also quite hyperextended (see figure 15, page 101). The hyperextension was something I had developed during my formative years in high school and exaggerated by trying to look cool. In the mid-60s, I went to a high school that was about one-third African-American. The young men had all developed, to my eyes, cool and wonderfully unique ways of walking and standing. I, too, wanted to be cool, so I learned how to stand with my knees thrust way back beyond their normal shape and my arms folded across my puny chest. I even had my mother make me shiny black elastic stretch pants with the front crease line sewn in. One of my idols, a rippling hulk of a football player, commented, "Where did you get those pants?" I was elated, I had arrived—KOOL in 1966—Weed High School.

Later, at the Iyengar Yoga Institute, I had one pivotal session, working alone in my room while living in the household of the school founder, Rama Jyoti Vernon. I was extremely frustrated at not understanding her instructions on how to position myself during the Triangle and Warrior poses. Mostly, however, I focused on intensifying the heat of the poses into my thigh bones with the intention of commanding that my bones change their shape. I decided I was going to stand differently and change my legs no matter what. I was tired of the constant taps, slaps, or verbal commands to straighten my knees, bend my knees, pull the knee caps up, rotate the eyes of the knees, and so on. I had heard enough about knees. I just wanted them to go home where they belonged and not hear another thing about them. I was on fire with determination. I decided I would tackle Warrior II and stay there until my knees changed—not that I had any idea what I was doing. I just began to do the pose. I held it as long as I could on one side, then, when I couldn't stand it anymore, I changed my stance to the other side without straightening my legs. I did the same there, until I needed to change again to the first side. My legs began to tremble, my knees got red, my breathing was erratic and shaky. I could not hold my arms out parallel to the floor anymore. I put my hands down on my hips and pulled on the muscles telling them to exert their force into the knees to make them change. The trembling intensified; my outer hip muscles ached and felt as if they would spasm at any moment. Then I changed sides again and continued to pull the inner thigh muscles up and out. I pulled the outer thighs back and into the hip socket.

I was startled at the response of the tissue to my commands for change. My knees could not maintain the alignment that I was taught was crucial to keeping the knee joint safe. When I could stay in the pose no longer unaided, I pulled a chair over, placed it beneath my bent thigh, and worked to maintain a lift so the chair would not support much of my weight. In this manner, I could keep the bent knee aligned over the ankle and still struggle to stress the outer side of the knee by pulling my thighs, and thus my adductors, wide open. My knees literally became hot to the touch. After twenty-seven minutes in the pose, I could continue no more. I collapsed onto the chair and then onto the floor. Instinctively, I went into a fetal pose and sought to comfort myself. I lay there trembling, pulsating, throbbing in a fount of upheaval from the heat literally burning through my bones.

Somehow, I knew the pattern had been broken by this session. Six months from the start of the work, I discovered my knees had indeed been sculpted to a straight line. I found that I could not only change my body, I could transform it. The energy required was tremendous, yet I felt somehow invigorated and rejuvenated. I still find that, when I stand, my ankle and inner knees touch evenly, without the slightest suggestion that they had ever been otherwise.

Transforming Your Posture

I will explain how you, too, can transform your postural misalignments in this book. First, however, it is important to understand your body and its postural idiosyncrasies.

> In a worldwide survey of postural habits, Gordon Hewes showed that we sit, kneel, stand, and recline in ways that are socially determined. It's now clearly established that human posture, physique, motor habits and body image, as well as emotions and thought patterns, are culturally shaped.[2]

Jean Couch, an Iyengar Yoga teacher and author of the *Runner's Yoga Book*,[3] is passionate about her research discoveries along similar lines. She is studying a phenomenon she calls "balance." Her studies of American posture have revealed that "the past century has seen a radical change in the way we stand. Up until the 1920s most people in the United States stood with their support bones—the spine, pelvis, and legs—on the same axis . . . so the body weight is upright and balanced. . . . All children on Earth are balanced until around the age of three—after that they take on the posture of the adults around them."[4] "Balance" is based on Jean's study of people who have no back or joint pain. These people are from various countries all over the world, yet they all stand, bend, walk, sit, and recline the same way. By inquiring into the postural characteristics of "balance," Jean has devised a method of teaching people how to stand, sit, walk, and practice yoga in "balance." In my study with her, she claimed that this procedure of mimicking the actions of "balanced" individuals eliminates a range of musculo-skeletal pains, not merely pain due to bad backs or poor posture habits.

Perfect balanced posture—a relatively rare phenomenon in civilized societies—is the result of uniform balanced contraction and relaxation of opposing muscle forces around a joint. It is more commonly the case that, when we exercise, we continue to imbalance and exacerbate our poor postural conditions.

---

[2] George Leonard and Michael Murphy, *The Life We Are Given* (New York: J. P. Tarcher/Putnam Books, 1995), p. 188.
[3] Jean Couch, *The Runner's Yoga Book* (Berkeley, CA: Rodmell Press, 1991).
[4] Jean Couch, "Balance," in *Yoga International,* September, 1998, p. 26. For more details go to her website at www.balance-center.com.

Since muscles perform specific motions, an analysis of the functional knowledge of anatomy, called kinesiology, will reveal the individual muscles shortened that result in postural changes. Muscles work in opposition; that is, when one muscle contracts, its antagonist relaxes. The phenomenon we call a stretch is called relaxation by a physiologist. We can, therefore, conclude that a shortened muscle is paired with an overrelaxed (overstretched) muscle. A contraction of the biceps brachii and a relaxation/stretch of the triceps brachii create this motion, for instance, when we bend the elbow (see Table 3 in chapter 12, page 103).

From this perspective, we can recognize that an individual who begins yoga practice with knock-knees can be prescribed strengthening exercises in the gluteus medius and tensor fascia lata muscles. In addition, the student may need to stretch/relax the adductors, gracilis, and medial hamstring muscles. If, in practicing yoga exercises, these muscles are extremely weak or tight, the student will most likely avoid the motions that would be most beneficial to their muscle and joint balance, unless taught otherwise.

This tendency to avoid change reflects the fundamental biological principle of homeostasis, which views a system as tending to do whatever is necessary to maintain the status quo. In other words, the body/mind avoids change unless acted upon by an outside force. A person with knock-knees will tend to perform exercises in a manner that maintains the stress in their legs to reinforce the knock-knee posture. Homeostasis declares that what is, persists. Furthermore, this individual will tend to resist or ignore those movements that could alter the existing pattern. For any real change to occur, the body/mind must be clear and have enough vitality to manifest the intention to change. Even though change is desired, it may be accompanied by unfamiliar and, very likely, uncomfortable sensations. Without enough pain, discomfort, passion, or ego, no change will be made. There must be motivation for true transformation, not merely a desire to change superficially.

A structural change will affect, not only the way your body appears, but the way it functions. This is true for all tasks you may perform, but especially for the practice of asanas. For example, if you have a high right shoulder, when you sit to type you will be using your muscles in an uneven fashion. The shortened muscles will continue to be shortened and the weakened muscles will continue to be underutilized. The result is a predictable increase in tension on the upper right shoulder and neck. During practice of the Warrior II (Virabhadrasana), a student with a high right shoulder will continue to hold that posture with the entire arm being held higher. Good practice of this asana will bring awareness of the structural imbalance, thus aligning the shoulders and diminishing the chronic tension held in the right shoulder.

Self-awareness often improves the postural distortions that you bring into yoga practice. However, if you comprehend your structural changes and begin to correct them by consciously strengthening and stretching the specific muscles associated with the imbalances, your body will become more efficient in all its activities.

If, on the other hand, you simply align the body during the practice of asanas, the effect will not be complete, because it will not get to the root cause of the postural imbalance. For example, in the Warrior II example cited above, merely lowering the high right arm and shoulder will not necessarily strengthen the muscles causing the imbalance.

Lowering the high right arm will only serve to diminish the tension of the muscles that are too tight. Thus we are changing only half of the necessary forces causing the postural change. In this sense, postural alignment with asana makes the poses look better, but it is not yoga therapy.

Bringing attention to the strengthening needs as well as the relaxation needs around postural imbalance is required before sustainable change is possible. Attempts to compensate for physical tension alone, without understanding the basic dynamics of contraction and relaxation, will produce an unwanted change in some other part of your body. Simply lowering the high right shoulder will often move the pelvis to the left. This is especially true when the high shoulder is reflected in the common right thoracic scoliosis pattern.

Postural imbalances are best corrected in a gradual, systematic manner. Since we are not only biological, but also psychological and spiritual in nature, a change in our biology will affect our minds and enhance our spiritual awareness as well.

I have found the yoga of B. K. S. Iyengar to be particularly suited to the detailed practice needed to change postural alignment. In his yoga method, static asanas are held with attention to alignment from the ground up. In this manner, strengthening the muscles of the feet and ankles will promote strength and alignment of the calves and knees. In turn, this promotes balance in the thighs and hips, which, in turn, promotes balance of the abdomen with the lower back, and so on up the body. The asanas of the Structural Yoga Therapy™ model come from a kinesiological analysis of basic Iyengar Yoga poses. These 24 fundamental poses were chosen because they contain all the directions of joint motion and thus can be used to strengthen or relax/stretch the major skeletal muscles.

In terms of a structural therapy, more postures are not necessary and, in fact, can become a hindrance. Many advanced yoga poses exceed the normal range of motion and, when practiced, can result in increased postural misalignments. I have found that when the body is intentionally being re-aligned, the resulting asana practice is more likely to produce the results described by Patanjali in his Classical Yoga treatise.

Since many people begin yoga practice with an imbalance in their physical carriage, I have found it helpful to begin with the joint-freeing series as a way to analyze your body and free up the restrictive joints. The preparatory isolation exercises can then be performed more effectively to free the spine and strengthen commonly weakened muscles. After this, the body is ready to perform the yoga poses in a manner that naturally leads to heightened insight.

The Need for Stretching

In her article, "In Defense of Stretching," author Jean Couch cites a number of reasons for stretching in a manner that maintains normal joint mobility.

> 1. Muscle contraction stimulates its neurological brain—the muscle spindle—to define the muscle's resting length. Unless movements go through complete range of motion in an aligned manner, the muscle spindle resets the joint into a restricted position.

2. Stretching allows muscles to relax and receive increased blood flow and oxygen.

3. When injury or imbalanced physical activity hinders a joint's mobility, other joints make postural compensations.

4. Tight muscles on one side of a joint create weak opposing muscles (antagonists) on the other side of the joint.

5. These tight muscles pull the body out of alignment from the ideally balanced "anatomical position."

6. A muscle that is too tight loses its power due to less mobility.

7. Ligaments, having no inherent contractile property, need full joint motions to maintain their integrity.

8. Random tightness diminishes the stretch reflex and the body therefore loses its efficient functioning.

9. Internal organs dependent upon vascular flow may not perform optimally as a result of structural misalignments.[5]

Contrary to popular belief, muscles do not stretch. Rather, they relax as a neurological reflex in reaction to the contraction of their opposing muscles. What we feel when we say we are stretching is the release of residual muscle contraction and the stretch of the fascia fibers surrounding the muscle tissue. Sometimes, the feeling of stretch is more the sensation of heat or even of a burn. Jane Fonda is well known for her instruction to go for the burn sensation during exercise. This burn is the experience of the connective tissue fiber that surrounds each muscle releasing its hold on the adjacent muscle's connective tissue fibers. It is a "good hurt," as it provides more freedom of joint motion.

---

[5] Jean Couch, "In Defense of Stretching," *Yoga Journal*, July/August, 1983, pp. 11–12.

Chapter 10

CLARIFYING INTENTIONS
AND SETTING GOALS

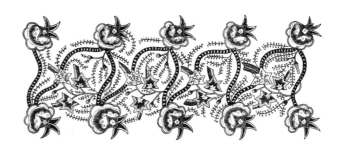

We all bring to our yoga practice a set of expectations and goals that we hope to attain. Perhaps you have a friend who tried yoga and felt better about themselves. Perhaps you thought that you could relieve your stress. Having an objective marker for where you are now and for the goal you aim to achieve will make it easier to determine whether or not progress is being made.

A yoga student, Louise, asked me about the strong emphasis on athleticism placed on yoga today. She asked for advice, since this goal did not match her desires. I suggested that she look at her own priorities. From knowing your own values, you can see where athleticism fits with your priorities.

One method I use for examining priorities is to imagine that you are in prison and the guards tell you that your freedoms are about to be taken away. You are assigned the task of writing all the qualities that freedom possesses for you. You must then choose 12 values that you can keep in this limited new social structure. You tear up that list into 12 sections and write your 12 values. After some time has passed, imagine the guards deciding that they were too liberal. They now tell you to make a decision to eliminate half your freedoms. The next week, they continue this process, again taking half your freedoms, leaving only the top three priorities in life. Finally, they say you must choose just one. I highly recommend you do this exercise to establish the goals you want to achieve with yoga practice.

Coming to know your ultimate values is a way to access your inner voice. According to yoga philosophy, sound is the first act of creation and, hence, the closest sense to the inner Self. Tension is a sign of the betrayal of the Self.

Many of the benefits of yoga are subjective and, therefore, difficult to measure. There are, however, objective benefits that can be verified as well. A thorough assessment of where you are as you begin yoga practice is, therefore, useful. You may very well find improvement in areas you considered unchangeable. Plan to be surprised!

Many yoga courses are designed around an eight-week format. This gives sufficient time to observe the effectiveness of yoga practice. Many studies and surveys have been conducted over a two- to three-month period. For a summary, see Table 2, page 73.

Setting Your Goal

To set a realistic goal, bear in mind what previous students and studies have shown to be plausible. Setting goals will allow for more accurate evaluation as you proceed, using a reference point by which to gauge yourself. An ideal is to have both objective goals that can be easily monitored and subjective goals that are best evaluated by psychological factors. Some examples follow.

IMPROVING POSTURE

If your goal is better posture, take photos of yourself from three sides before practice, then again after eight weeks. When you think of being depressed, imagine what your posture would look like. In the opposite manner, feeling good will tend to improve your posture. Improved posture is a subjective high. You may find friends telling you that you look better or seem more upright without being able to talk specifically about the changes they perceive. It is not uncommon for some yoga students to grow taller after several months of practice. Students have been known to regain as much as two inches in former height.

For more specific guidance, follow the procedures in chapter 11 to help you understand your specific misalignments, then proceed to chapter 19 to develop an individual therapy plan.

INCREASING STRENGTH

If your goal is increased muscular strength, begin with the test in chapter 18, "Muscle Strengthening Using the Joint-Freeing Series," to determine your individual muscle stamina. This baseline measure will help you evaluate the outcome of your yoga program.

Measure your ability to stress a muscle in an isolated muscular motion. If you wish to see if your back is stronger, first do Cobra Pose and time yourself to see how long this can be maintained without trembling. Compare this to the time you can maintain it after yoga practice. This can determine strength and endurance of the erector spinae, a deep layer of spinal muscles used during Cobra posture.

To test hip strength, in a modified Locust Pose, bend your legs at the knee and lift them one at a time. Time how long you can hold this lift before the leg begins to tremble or unstable breathing occurs. Use the opposite motion with the Upward Extended Leg Pose and test your stamina there as well. In this manner, you can evaluate opposing (antagonistic) muscle groups. A specially trained yoga therapist or physical therapist can do more specific evaluations. A subjective means of testing strength is to sense your endurance in routines that typically bring fatigue.

FLEXIBILITY/JOINT FREEDOM

If your goal is more flexibility, have a range-of-motion analysis done to determine the exact number of degrees lacking in the arc of a joint measured against what is normal. Follow the practice and evaluation of the Joint-Freeing Series (Pavanmuktasana) in chapter 15. A more accurate method is to have an accomplished "body reader" determine where and how much you are lacking in joint freedom. Practice the Joint-Freeing Series, using those specific motions for the joints you want to free, twice daily. Re-evaluate yourself in eight weeks. Allow at least this much time before you expect a noticeable change.

DIGESTIVE HEALTH

The organs of absorption (stomach and small intestine) and the organs of filtration and elimination (kidneys, liver, and large intestine) are all positively affected by yoga practices. The most effective practices include inversion poses, spinal twists, and purification exercises like Cleansing the Fire (Agnisar Dhouti Kriya). These organs will benefit from as little as two months of practice, although true change in their functioning takes 6 to 12 months. Be patient and persevere. You'll be delighted with the changes, internally as well as externally. While you may not lose much weight, you will normalize your weight and proportions.

MANAGING STRESS

If your goal is to manage stress, start by having your health-care provider administer a stress test to determine your resting and stressed heart rate, blood pressure, cholesterol level, etc. Be sure to monitor your blood pressure, because it is a standard measure of cardiovascular strength. The natural rhythm of your breath and breath-holding time are also excellent indicators of your body's tolerance for stress. A subjective means of monitoring your stress manageability is to sense your ease under normal pressure of family and work. Gauge your respiratory rate, heart rate, and subjective muscle tension on a scale of 1 to 10—1 being barely noticeable and 10 being when you're ready to run out of the room or scream. Eight weeks after beginning regular yoga practices, retest to determine the efficacy of yoga for you.

In general, a sense of increased comfort with your body may not necessarily be indicated by less pain, but by more tolerance of pain. Cancer and AIDS patients who are taught yoga principles may not have remissions and full recovery, but they may come to accept their lives as they are and defuse the emotional/mental stress of their physical pain.[1]

---

[1] Susan Jacobs with Jason Serinus, "Living with AIDS," *Yoga Journal*, July 1987, p. 30.

The Power of Intention

Doing yoga without a clearly stated goal is beneficial, yet it is like going for a drive without knowing where you want to go. The optimist will find beauty and adventure, regardless of where they go, while the pessimist may experience that their time is being wasted in foolishly rambling around an unknown terrain. Being optimistic *and* being directed is ideal.

By a willingness to observe your mind, you can uncover what it is you seek, as well as your natural optimism. When you find these, you have the two crucial elements that create the power of intention.

Whatever you look for you'll find.

Program yourself to look for subjective qualities such as love, joy, and beauty. Use your power of intention for developing physical, quantifiable qualities like improved postural alignment, strength, fullness of breath, and stamina. Through this power, you can develop nurturing friendships by looking for them. You can also use this power for the spiritual goal of being more connected to a loving Divine Presence.

If there is a will, there is a way.
If there is no will, there is no way.

What I have seen over and over in myself and in my clients is that a strong will is needed to make a lasting transformation. It is possible to make dramatic changes in our lives, in our physical, as well as in our emotional and mental, states. If you have the will to make a postural change, Structural Yoga Therapy™ can provide the means to that end. Remember, however, that the more important factor is your will, your desire for change. In the same way the inverse is also true.

If you lack the will for change
there is no one who can show you the way.

There is no barrier to change. Even pain is not a barrier to change. Indeed, it is more often than not an aid, an incentive, to change. As you dig down deep into yourself, you are likely to uncover pre-existing pain that you postponed experiencing at some previous point in life, because it was too intense, or because you lacked the support to fully understand the messages the pain was delivering. Now is the best time to make a change. By allowing yourself to receive the support of yoga, you assure your continued growth.

THE POWER OF TRANSFORMATION

Practicing yoga helps us to overcome obstacles within ourselves that may be preventing us from fully enjoying life and responding in beneficial ways to the variety of situations we encounter daily. Although substantial change in our detrimental reflexes, especially those below our level of consciousness (be they physiological or psychological), takes time and patience, practicing yoga with concentration and devotion can bring noticeable changes in our circumstances almost immediately.

Chapter 11

BODY-READING

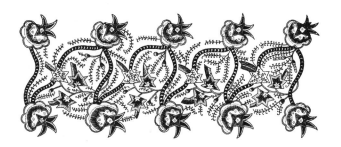

In 1973, a Hollander named Tinbergen won the Nobel Prize for studying how posture affects every system of the body, not only the neuro-muscular system, composed of joints, bones, ligaments, muscles, and nerves, but all the other physiological systems as well. This means that the endocrine system, immune system, and respiratory system reflect changes in posture as well. A simple example is found in the fact that when people are depressed, their chests tend to collapse. They tend to underbreathe, making their respiratory system less efficient. Depressed people also smile less often.

Another example is that an imbalance in leg length of even a quarter of an inch, which might come from ligamentous tension, muscle tightness in the hip flexors, or a spinal problem, can change the actions of the jaw muscles. This, in turn, can create an overbite. A tilt of the pelvis can be carried upward from the hips to increase the tension on one side of the jaw. If this postural change is not corrected, over time it can create temporomandibular joint (TMJ) problems, headaches, orthodontic problems, or even impaired speech.

Reading body language is instinctive, something we each do subconsciously, a way of "tuning in" to others and ourselves. Each of us does this in our own way, as a way to "get a sense of" another. Postural language contains a wealth of psychological information that we use daily to gauge the effectiveness of our communication and to express emotions. Elevated shoulders may tell us someone is "up tight." Rounded shoulders may tell us someone is "depressed or perhaps closed-minded." This type of body-reading has been discussed in depth in such books as *The Body Reveals* and *The Language of the Body*.[1]

---

[1] Ron Kurtz, *The Body Reveals* (San Francisco: HarperSanFrancisco, 1984) and Alexander Lowen, *The Language of the Body* (Old Tappan, NJ: Macmillan, 1971).

Another form of body-reading involves evaluating muscular tension. Freedom from tension allows us to more naturally express happiness and health. Subjectively, we know that improved posture indicates positive changes. We take advantage of our subjective nature in yoga by changing our posture, first with yoga asanas and then with other practices. We are not overly concerned about what happens in our outer lives when we do yoga. Our focus is on the joy of the practice.

Certain postural imbalances—knock-knees, a high shoulder, or minor scoliosis (a lateral spinal curvature)—are not correlated to changes in psychological states. One does not need to be professionally trained in body reading to notice these deviations from the norm. Such "abnormalities" are often due to heredity. In a few instances, recreational activities and work habits may stress the musculature in such a manner as to enhance such pre-existing conditions. In the case of knock-knees, for example, using specific motions and becoming adept at an activity causes other muscle groups to lose their tone. Soccer players, for instance, develop an increased tone in their hip flexors from kicking the ball and running. Bicyclists often show an increase in the size and strength of their quadriceps and gastrocnemius (calf) muscles due to the repetitive bending and straightening of the knee. Their hip flexors are often weak in comparison to soccer players or runners.

Postural changes may also occur simply as a response to stress. When someone says, "You look stressed out," he or she is reading your postural cues. A stress-related condition may have prevailed for so long that the individual doesn't realize that the associated muscular tensions have created postural changes that have gone unnoticed. Consequently, messages from those muscles tend to be ignored. Your mind may simply translate those muscular messages to mean that you're stressed and need to relax. Your yoga practice can help you become more sensitive to warning signs indicative of the approach of discomfort, which may bloom into disease if you fail to read them as encouragements to taking positive steps to maintain optimal wellness.

The prominent theory that migraine headaches are a genetic disorder involving an imbalance of brain chemicals has been disputed by one medical doctor who believes they are muscular in origin and related to posture.

"It runs in families," Dr. Bo Thomas Brofeldt, an assistant professor of surgery and emergency medicine at the University of California, Davis says. "When I lecture I say, if your mom or grandma were here in the audience, I could identify them. It's an anatomical predisposition."[2]

Brofeldt suggests a migraine sufferer is more likely to have a posture in which the head is held forward, never allowing certain jaw and neck muscles—"headache muscles"—to rest. Once the postural problems are identified, he gives patients specific exercises and advice about reorganizing their work environment.

The process of Structural Yoga Therapy™ is similar. Any pathological condition or stress creates a change in muscle tension and posture. By identifying these specific tensors, a structural yoga therapist can prescribe yoga postures as well as breathing exercises

---

[2] Bo Thomas Brofeldt, "Rebel with a Cause," in *Sacramento Magazine* (June, 1997), p. 31.

tailored to your present situation. By following the advice given and continuing to learn to adapt to your body's response to the relief of tensions, these stresses will continue to lessen and, in most cases, disappear entirely. With this relief of chronic tension often come insights into other aspects of your life that need change. The resulting transformation can leave you without the dis-ease that brought you to yoga in the first place. Truly successful students continue this process of self-examination in quest for insight and learn to transform many aspects of their lives into optimal learning situations. For many students, yoga practice becomes a long-term commitment, no longer tied to disease symptomology.

Many postural abnormalities, such as knock-knees, spinal curvature (structural scoliosis), or fallen arches, were either predisposed from birth or were shaped by our upbringing. One article points out that, "In a worldwide survey of postural habits, Gordon Hewes showed that we sit, kneel, stand, recline in ways that are socially determined. It's now clearly established that human posture, physique, motor habits, and body image, as well as emotions and thought patterns, are culturally shaped."[3]

Although "perfect posture" is somewhat subjective and illusive, postural imbalances do create musculo-skeletal tension to which we unconsciously adapt. Often, our adaptation involves a lack of awareness of the muscular tensions and the associated messages they reflect. We have learned to "live with" our "aches and pains," accepting them as normal, and teach our children to expect the same.

What gets lost in this context is the human capacity for transformation. To change our posture without a change in consciousness is not the goal of yoga. Classical Yoga is rooted in transformative experience. Please keep an open mind as you hear these words. You already know you can change, that postural change is inevitable. What you may have yet to consider is how you can transform the underlying patterns that created the "aches and pains" with which you've lived. The scope of the process is not necessarily to change what was given from birth. However, given a passionate desire for liberation from your present condition, it is possible to transform your body predisposed to stress.

A cardinal rule of Structural Yoga Therapy™ is
"If it ain't broke—don't fix it."

What I mean by this application of the great motto is that, if there is no pain or discomfort associated with the region of a postural change, don't try to change that aspect of your posture. Yes, bring attention to that area; make certain that your practice increases your strength and awareness of postural differences of which you weren't aware before body-reading. But don't worry about them. Many postural changes are due to the body's attempt to find balance following a trauma, accident, or injury. Emotional, or even psychic, traumas can create postural change.

If you know you were traumatized in your shoulder area, for instance, you may have developed a high shoulder and a rotation of your face away from that shoulder. This is a clear example of avoiding pain and of your body attempting to protect vital regions

---

[3] George Leonard and Michael Murphy, *The Life We Are Given* (New York: J. P. Tarcher/Putnam, 1995), p. 188.

from the trauma. If you approach yoga for the purpose of unwinding this trauma, you may find the pain level increases, until your multidimensional nature has integrated the new experience of being free of traumatic memory. For this type of yoga therapy to proceed, students must be comfortable with and trust their teachers enough to let them know their intention, so that they can help them pace the unwinding process. Be aware of your uniqueness. You are not only physically different from anyone else, you also have your own personal way of responding to real-life situations.

Because bodies are infinite in their variety of shape and size, everyone's experience varies when practicing yoga postures. Your unique postural alignment and how you have learned to react to tension will differ markedly from others. Yoga training will change more than what you feel. With accurate and compassionate instruction, it will teach you how to attend to the sensations of your body. Practicing yoga under skilled supervision will definitely improve both your physical and psychological posture.

As these changes take place, you will find that your goals may also change. You may want to pursue a different direction than the one that originally brought you to yoga. It's been my experience that you can uncover more of your potential through yoga than through any other discipline. The first step is to get to know your body and its posture as it is today.

Preparation for Body-Reading

Five factors are needed for a thorough body reading:

1. Perception—To be able to see not only what is obvious, but what needs to be unveiled at this point in time. Observe your high shoulder, tilted head, or your arms held differently, from a completely objective perspective. The objective is to see clearly and gather data without interpretation or moving quickly into recommendations to "fix it."

2. Concentrated Awareness—The ability to focus and, at the same time, to be free of distractions from the immediate environment. This requires the capacity to be present and nonjudgmental—to just perceive, free of goals.

3. Self-Study—The continuous process of knowing your own body/mind's signals and messages, of its progress toward balance, symmetry, and homeostasis. Learning the signs of tension that is developing strength, as opposed to tension that is developing stress. Knowing the difference between symmetry with ease, and manipulation toward balance.

4. Anatomical Understanding—An evolving knowledge of general anatomy and kinesiology, as well as familiarity with your own personal experience of your body's stresses, misalignments, and attempts toward balance. There is much to learn about anatomy and a distinction needs to be made between gaining objective knowledge and knowledge of knowing yourself.

5. Technique—A personal practice that assists you in getting to know yourself better. The ideal practice will not only bring improved health and vitality, but heightened sensitivity to those areas of yourself that have been less conscious.

A part of my training included studying Lomi Bodywork with Bob Marrone, Professor of Psychology at California State University, Sacramento. While involved in this training I practiced the art of looking and seeing. A master of this Lomi Bodywork process, Richard Heckler shared some of his ideas about perception. He describes the elements of perception as essentially the practice of selective conscious awareness. I have adapted his notes into a sequence that has been useful to me in reading my own body and those of my clients:

1. Look at yourself as a whole and see what comes to the foreground. Then look at that aspect in a general manner. Don't try to look for specifics just yet.

2. Look to see what is the most obvious, then contrast that with what is somehow subtly related.

3. See what parts seem to have less maturity, strength, or development, and contrast that with the parts that are more mature or stronger.

4. Notice the relationship of your body to gravity and your anatomical position.

5. Determine where the burden of tension is being carried.

6. Discover what part of your body contracts or avoids feeling when you are under stress.

7. See how you take up space, either filling it up or shrinking from your actual physical size.

8. Observe yourself in motion. Watch for the relationship of rhythm, power, flexibility, and balance/symmetry.

9. Question whether you work in or out of harmony with yourself.

10. Watch your respiratory pattern and look especially for overworked regions and the contrasting underdeveloped areas. Explore how your breath comes in and in what sequence it proceeds to flow through your torso. Is it regular or unstable?

Self-Examination

The information in Table 3 on page 103 summarizes the findings of this chapter. It shows the most common tendencies for muscular imbalances that may be present. The more you train your body toward balance and symmetry, the less these indicators will be present. General yogasana recommendations for postural imbalances can be found in Table 6 (in chapter 22, page 266). To the extent that you are unique, you may need a more personalized program created by comparing your body-reading findings with this Table. Then you can compose a list of muscles to strengthen and stretch. Use Chart 1 (page 106) to list them.

When doing your body reading, do your best to be objective. Consider that you are not looking at yourself, but at someone unfamiliar. Most of all, be easy on yourself. Criticism and judgment do not help in getting an accurate reading. It is important to evaluate in terms of change from the anatomical upright and open position, not in terms of good or bad. A perfect posture is actually a rare phenomenon subject to change. Those who possess it also go through changes as they adapt to life changes.

Remember that posture is not merely physical tone and structural symmetry. Posture also is an indicator of your psychological state. You can open your tendency to slouch and this will make a dramatic change in your mood and self-esteem. When you are depressed, you cannot help but slouch, rounding your shoulders and dropping your head forward. Your respiration becomes shallow and quite restrained. When you are proud, you will inevitably stand taller, your shoulders will thrust backward and your chest will elevate. Respiration becomes full and lifted. In doing your body reading, take into consideration your present mood and bring yourself to a more neutral tone before you begin. If you cannot change your mood immediately, wait to do the body reading on a more average day.

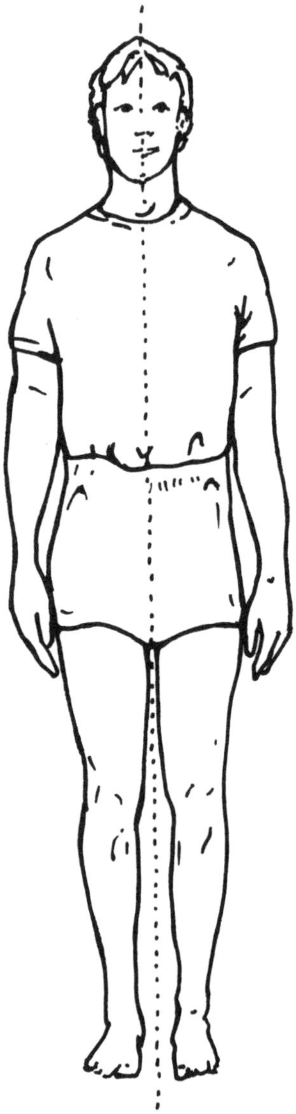

Let's begin by evaluating your standing posture as it is now. Have a good look at yourself wearing only underwear or without clothing in a full-length mirror. Look for evidence of postural changes from the anatomical position. At first, look to see what is most obvious. Pay special attention to those areas of repeated muscular tensions or where you have been injured. Reflect on what you would like to change about yourself to the vitality level you have or want to possess.

You are probably aware of some changes from this perfect posture. As you look carefully, you may find other changes that are more subtle. As you proceed, pay particular attention to those areas where you carry tension, where you love being massaged. Reflect on the differences in your clothing and how they wear. If you know that you have a leg-length difference or recall that your tailor hems one pant leg differently than the other, look to see if your knees line up and if the crests of your hips are even. If you are constantly adjusting sweaters or blouses to keep them from slipping to one side, it may be that one shoulder is higher. If your shoes wear unevenly, this may tell you about curvature in the legs. If your soles wear out on the outside, you may have bowed legs. If they wear out on the inside, check for knock-knees.

In the perfectly aligned standing posture, your body will be symmetrical when a plumb line is dropped down its center (see figure 7). The plumb line will pass evenly between your feet and knees, and through your navel and breastbone, and the center of your nose and head. Lines drawn parallel to the floor will reveal an evenness in shoulder and waist height. Your kneecaps will face directly forward, while your

Figure 7. The perfectly aligned standing posture.

feet will point straight ahead or with a mild turn-out. Your hands should be at the same level on your thighs, with palms facing inward.

Viewed from the back, the center plumb line will run evenly between your legs, through the center of your buttocks, sacrum, and spine to the middle of the back of your head. Viewed from the side, it will run from just in front of your anklebone and pass through the center of the side of your knee and your hip joint, then through the center of your upper arm to your ear canal.

Chapter 12

COMMON POSTURAL MISALIGNMENTS

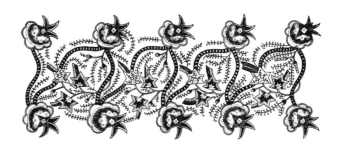

This chapter will explore common postural imbalances in detail. Refer to Table 3 on page 103 for an analysis of which muscles are likely to be involved in your postural imbalances. You will also find a diagram of the major surface muscles discussed in this book (see figures 17 and 18, pages 104 and 105). Record your postural self-examination findings on the final page of this chapter. This will serve as a reference point to measure the effect of yoga practice on your bodily tensions. For more detailed evaluation take a full body photograph to save and re-evaluate in six to eight weeks. Be sure to mark your calendar for the re-evaluation point when you take the photo, so you will have a reminder. Recommended yoga poses to correct these imbalances are cited in chapter 22, page 265.

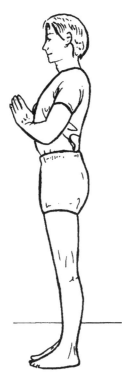

Figure 8. Naturally aligned centered posture.

Lateral Balance

Taking in the entire person with one view is the aim during this initial phase of body reading. Do not attempt to see details, just get a sense of whole-body balance to determine whether it moves forward or backward of the plumb line. After evaluating, begin to look for the possibility of segments that have shifted, such as the pelvic or shoulder region.

When viewed from the side, a naturally aligned centered posture looks as shown in figure 8. A vertical line goes through the center of the ear, shoulder, hip, and knee, ending slightly forward of the ankle.

A forward, or anterior, posture is the most common lateral deviation, usually with the pelvic and lower abdominal region moving ahead of the chest.

A backward, or posterior, posture is rarely seen. In this posture, the upper body seems to fall back from the waist.

Head and Shoulders

In the case of rounded shoulders, there may also be a hollow or sunken appearance in the space between the shoulders and the chest (see figure 9). The muscles between the scapula are weakened, while the chest muscles, the pectoralis major, are constricted. In addition, the head may hang forward. The arms tend to fall forward of the centerline as well, and are often internally rotated, with the palms facing backward. This posture and a high shoulder are often accompanied by chronic neck tension or headaches.

Another common deviation is high shoulder. In figure 10, the left shoulder is markedly higher than the right. Often, the shoulder is pulled, not only up, but also in, making the upper arm hug the side of the torso. With a high shoulder, the upper trapezius muscle is constricted chronically tight. When this is seen, one should also look for rotation in the head, neck, or upper back as these factors may reveal a lateral spinal curvature or mild scoliosis. In general, well-balanced shoulders present a smooth downward sloping line from the base of the neck.

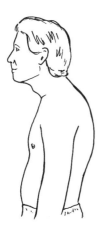

Figure 9. Round shoulders and forward head.

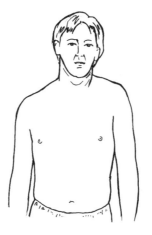

Figure 10. High shoulder.

Spine and Back

In winging of the shoulder blades (not shown), the scapulas do not lie smoothly against the posterior rib cage. In this instance, the medial border of the scapula is more posterior than the back of the arms. When standing with your back to the wall, the shoulders will be forward and only a small portion of the inner shoulder blades will touch the wall. The rhomboids and middle trapezius muscles will tend to be weakened. Rounded shoulders will often also be present. This condition often restricts full respiration in the chest and increases abdominal breathing, which tends to be sedative.

A flat back posture occurs when the spine lacks its natural posterior curvature in the upper two-thirds of the body (see figure 11). The spine may be seen as progressively straighter from the lower back and lumbar spine, to the neck. While normally this is an inherited trait, it is often developed during adolescent ballet training. The most common side effects of this posture are stiffness of the thoracic spine and tightness of the neck region.

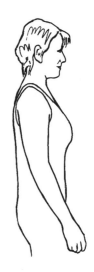

Figure 11. Flat back, no thoracic curve.

A lateral curvature, or scoliosis, is more common in women. It has several distinguishing features. The most marked is the double, or even triple, change in the direction of the spinal column. Other features can be high shoulder, a forward region of the rib cage and uneven hips. When you are not clear if a scoliosis exists, you can perform a more detailed analysis by having someone watch you in a gradual forward bend and observe how the spine rotates or remains even, one region at a time. In figure 12 left, the subject has a right thoracic scoliosis in which the right shoulder is high, the right arm is held more forward of the torso, the head turns to the right, and in a forward bend, the right middle thoracic region is higher than the left (see figure 12, right).

There are two types of scoliosis. Structural scoliosis is an inherited trait. Often the same sex parent has a similar curvature. This type of scoliosis may increase in severity with age. In a worst case scenario, which is quite rare, the spinal curves distort the shape of the rib cage to such a degree that the lungs become constricted. Surgery may be advised to implant metal rods to prevent further degeneration of curves above 40 degrees. In my experience, curvatures below this degree may be markedly improved by 30–50 percent with Structural Yoga Therapy™. The best results occur with motivated clients who are willing to progres-

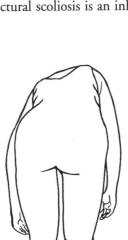 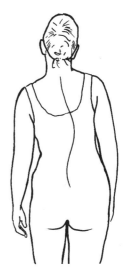

Figure 12. Lateral curvature or scoliosis.

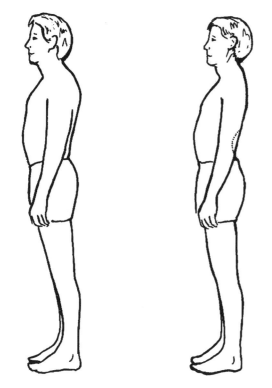

Figure 13. Khyphosis.

Figure 14. Lordosis.

sively develop the structural yoga asanas required to change the shape of their skeletal structure.

The other type is called functional scoliosis, which is developed by doing one-sided activities like waiting tables and carrying trays on the same side, bowling, golf, tennis, or baseball pitching. In these cases, persons who spend long hours developing their skills create a spinal curvature and rotation of the ribs that makes them more proficient at their activity. This type is easier to correct once the person has completed their athletic training. It is possible to diminish the residual tension following these twisting activities, yet maintain the stamina for athletic performance.

Khyphosis (see figure 13), commonly called hunchback, is revealed by a large posterior deviation, usually in the upper thoracic region. With this deviation, the shape of the ribs as well as the spine will be affected. The resulting posture may appear to be a sunken chest with depressed respiration and exaggerated rounding of the shoulders. This posture is possible to change in a motivated student, but becomes more difficult to change after the late 30s.

Lordosis (see figure 14), an excessive lower back, lumbar, curve, will be seen when the shape of the lower back is not visible from the side. The arm will hide the shape of the back. The depth of the curve is much greater than normal. Many different muscles will be involved, including thighs, hips, and abdominals. The major muscle involved is a constriction of the psoas, which runs from the groin, internally, through the pelvis, to the anterior lumbar spinal column (see figure 2, page 51). The degree of correction is dependent upon the individual case presented.

Knees

The knees are hyperextended when the lateral view reveals a posterior line at the knee joint (see figure 15, left). Knee position may be an inherited condition or one developed by being encouraged to press your knees back during the adolescent years. In this case, there has been an overstretching of the knee joints ligaments and not the musculature.

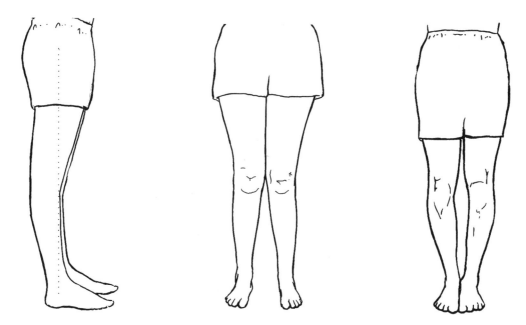

Figure 15. Hyperextended knees, knock-knees, and bowed legs.

This condition is often characterized by tight hamstrings and weakened lower quadriceps. It is often accompanied with an increased lumbar curve, and weak abdominals and/or hip flexors. Some people with this feature have excessive mobility in other joints, especially the elbows.

Knock-knees appear when the knees touch without the inner ankles touching (see figure 15, center). Often, the whole of the inner thighs will also be in contact. The adductors will tend to be tight and the hip abductors (gluteus medius and tensor fascia lata) weakened. In most cases, the shape of the bones is altered, though it is possible to correct with diligent practice, as in my own case.

Bowed legs occur when the inner knees do not touch, but the ankles do (see figure 15, right). This is the reverse of the previous condition, thus the inner thigh muscles, the adductors, will tend to be weak and the outer hips, abductors, tight. Changing the stamina of the weakened muscles will permit greater joint flexibility and, with persistence, the postural stance will improve markedly.

Tibial torsion (not shown) is indicated when the knees face inward when the feet face directly ahead. To gauge this, look carefully at the flat surface of the kneecap to see that it is parallel to the mid-line of the body. This condition is due to bone structure and will not respond to strengthening or stretching of the musculature.

Hip rotation (not shown) is revealed when the stance is more comfortable, with the legs pointing outward and the toes to the sides, while the knees are aligned directly ahead. This is different from tibial torsion, even though the knee and hip relationship appears to be the same. This posture may be altered by the Structural Yoga Therapy™ realignment process.

Legs inward (not shown) is noted when the natural comfortable stance is with the feet turned inward, commonly called a pigeon-toed posture. This condition comes from an increase in internal hip rotation and may be corrected by strengthening the external hip rotators located in the deep gluteal region and the psoas.

Ankles and Feet

Pronated ankles tend to collapse inward, causing weight-bearing to move from the sole of the foot to the inner anklebones (see figure 16, left). There is a weakness in the anterior tibialis muscle. This can be improved by lifting and spreading the toes, which will elevate the arch.

Sometimes flat feet accompany this posture. True flat feet do not respond to muscular toning. If they are associated with pronated ankles, however, the arch can be heightened. Fallen arches, or flat feet, place the longitudinal arch closer to the floor than normal. The opposite condition, high arch, raises the top of the foot as well as the arch.

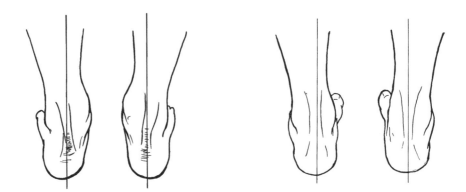

Figure 16. Pronated ankles and normal ankle line.

Table 3. Muscular Imbalances Revealed by Posture.

POSTURAL CHANGE	TIGHT MUSCLES	WEAK MUSCLES
Body leans forward	Tibialis anterior, psoas, rectus abdominis	Gluteus maximus, thoracic erector spinae
Body leans backward	Reverse of above	Reverse of above
Forward head	Sternocleidomastoid (SCM)	Upper trapezius
Round shoulders	Pectorals, serratus anterior	Middle and lower trapezius, latissimus dorsi
Tilted head	SCM and upper trapezius	Same on opposing side
High shoulder	Upper trapezius, levator scapula	Lower trapezius, latissimus, pectoralis sternal
Palm turned forward	Teres minor, infraspinatus	Pectorals, latissimus, teres major
Palm turned back	Reverse of above	Reverse of above
Winging scapula	Serratus anterior, pectorals, anterior deltoid	Middle trapezius, rhomboids
Flat back	Middle trapezius, rectus abdominis	Lumbar erectors, psoas, hip flexors
Lordosis (excessive lumbar curve)	Reverse of above	Reverse of above
Scoliosis (lateral curve of spine)	Psoas, erectors, latissimus dorsi, abdominus oblique	Same as opposing side
Khyphosis (hunchback)	Rectus abdominis, pectorals, upper trapezius	Thoracic erector spinae, middle and lower trapezius
Hip elevated	Quadratus lumborum, psoas	Same as opposing side
Hip twisted	Abdominus oblique, psoas, tensor fascia lata, sartorius	Same as opposing side
Hyperextended knee	Hamstrings, gastrocnemius	Lower quadriceps, popliteus
Knock-knees	Adductors	Tensor fascia lata, gluteus medius
Bowed legs	Reverse of above	Reverse of above
Tibial torsion	Tensor fascia lata, gluteus medius	Gluteus maximus, sartorius, tibialis anterior
Feet turned outward	Psoas, external hip rotators, sartorius, gluteus maximus	Fascia lata, gluteus minimus
Feet turned inward	Reverse of above	Reverse of above
Pronated ankles	Peroneals	Tibialis anterior, tibialis posterior
High arch	Reverse of above	Reverse of above
Flat foot	Tibialis anterior	Tibialis posterior

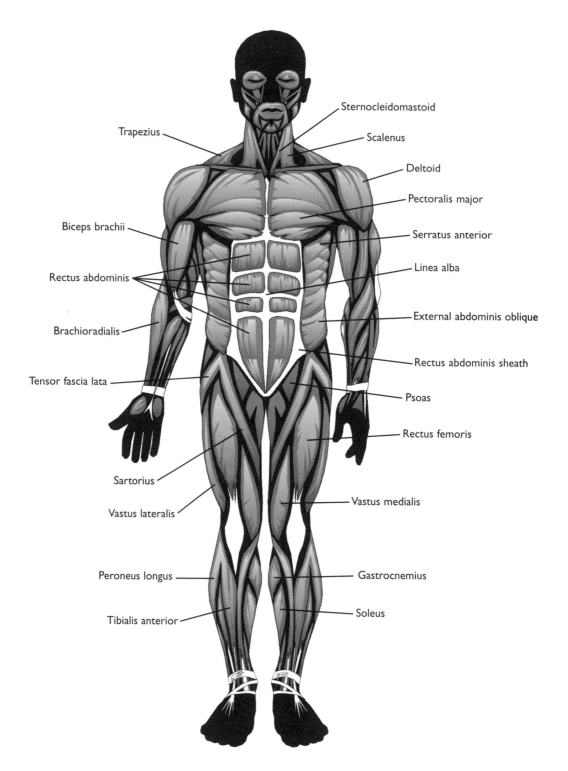

Figure 17. The muscular system—anterior view.
(Chart from Ananda Yoga Teacher Training program, used by permission.)

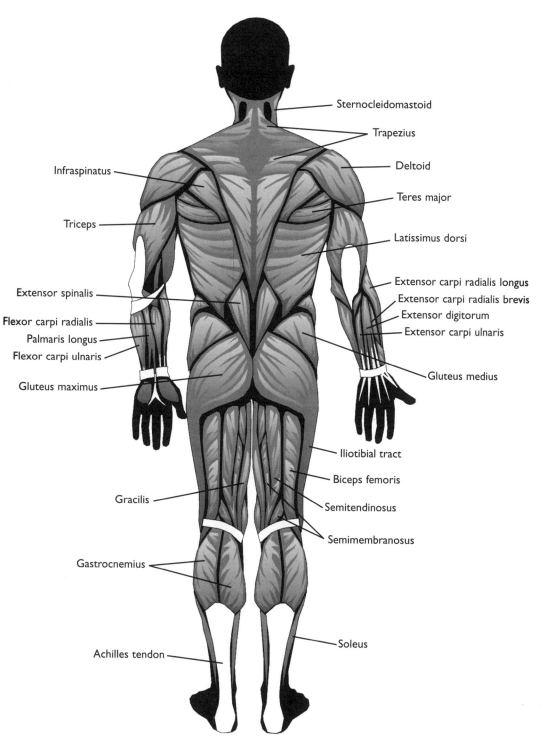

Figure 18. The muscular system—posterior view.
(Chart from Ananda Yoga Teacher Training program, used by permission.)

CHART 1
BODY-READING RECORD

DATE: _____

Where is your discomfort or pain and what is its intensity level? (Circle level on a 1–10 scale)

Side Balance: 1   2   3   4   5   6   7   8   9   10

Head: 1   2   3   4   5   6   7   8   9   10

Shoulders: 1   2   3   4   5   6   7   8   9   10

Shoulder blades: 1   2   3   4   5   6   7   8   9   10

Spine: 1   2   3   4   5   6   7   8   9   10

Knees: 1   2   3   4   5   6   7   8   9   10

Ankles and Feet: 1   2   3   4   5   6   7   8   9   10

Goal—What would you like to change about your posture? _____
_____
_____

SUMMARY OF FINDINGS [*Replicate these findings in Chart 4 on page 187 to create a program for improved posture.*]

Muscles to Stretch	Muscles to Strengthen

PART FOUR

Anatomy and Yoga

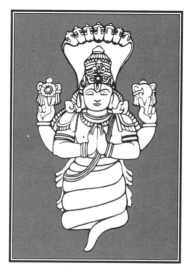

*This body is a world, a universe just like the one outside and
that is why Satpurushas (great beings) all say to look there,
inside. If you look outside of yourself, you
won't find anything. . . .
But what is it that has its eternal source in God? Certainly
not the body. The scriptures talk of the angustha purusha
(thumb-sized person) which dwells in the heart.
Within it are contained all the stored desires and
deeds of the individual soul.*

—SWAMI PRAKASHANANDA

INTRODUCTION

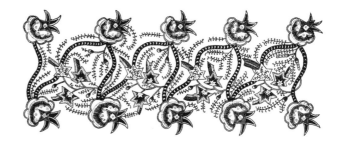

Everyone knows that exercise is an important factor in maintaining lifelong health. Without proper exercise, we not only lose muscle tone and joint flexibility, we may also discover that our aches and pains are seeping out of our body and into our personality. Motivation for exercise can come from its positive benefits or the negative consequences due to neglect. Since we cannot move to a better location, let's do what we can to learn about the house we live in, so we can practice optimal maintenance.

With this in mind, I have written the next section to acquaint the reader with the hidden terrain under your skin. By learning about the unknown—your body—it will be easier to deal with the experiences that it brings you. In many ways, facing the unknown about yourself requires courage, yet it produces such freedom from fear once you take the time to remove your misconceptions, that you'll wonder why you didn't do this before!

There are three major factors in getting a well-rounded exercise program. Everyone needs to cultivate strength, stamina, *and suppleness*. To accomplish these goals, it is important to know something about the boundaries and limitations of movement that define the arena of health. Not having enough of these three factors will negatively impact health. On the other end of the spectrum, developing too much strength or stamina is not likely to pose a problem unless you stop exercising. Developing too much flexibility can be a problem, unless it was given as your constitution at birth. In this next part I will present a series to help you more precisely evaluate yourself for these three factors so you can design a personalized yoga program.

Chapter 13

WHAT IS

JOINT FREEDOM?

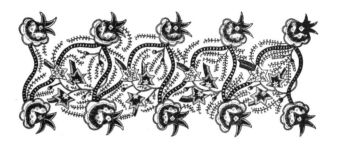

Joint freedom is the ability of each joint to move freely through its full range of motion without cracking, muscular stress, discomfort, or causing movement in the adjacent joints. It is not a common phenomenon, even in trained athletes or yogis, and is dependent upon several factors. Among them are a balance of muscle tone with elasticity, healthy connective tissue, which surrounds muscles to define their shape, keeps their muscular activity independent of adjacent muscles, and serves to bind muscles to bones and keep healthy bones free of extraneous material (bone spurs and/or arthritis). The resulting flexibility varies from person to person according to several criteria—the activities we engage in (and how coordinated and balanced we are while active); our age, sex, weight, genetic postural imbalances, injuries, pain, body conditioning; and our emotional mood state.

For example, running makes hamstrings stronger and tighter, which in turn lessens our standing forward-bending (hip flexion) mobility. Continually running can prevent the opposing muscles from working freely. Over time, this may change your posture. Our optimal age for joint freedom is ages 3 to 5, but for some people, it is maintained into the preteen years. Women are known to be more flexible than men.[1]

You may have been born with knock-knees, which will lessen the distance you can open your legs (hip abduction). If you have asthma, you'll tend to have less ability to reverse the curve of your upper back (thoracic extension). When people are depressed,

---

[1] R. D. Bell and T. B. Hoshizaki, "Relationship of Age and Sex with Range of Motion of Seventeen Joint Actions in Humans," *Canadian Journal of Applied Sports Science,* 6(4), pp. 202–206.

they tend to collapse forward, rounding the upper back and caving in the chest. This not only makes breathing shallow, it also tightens the chest muscles (pectorals), diminishing the capacity of the shoulders to be pulled backward (shoulder extension).

There are many benefits to yoga. Yoga exercises that maintain your suppleness may be a factor in extending lifespan. My favorite Hatha Yoga teacher is Indra Devi. She is known as the Mother of Yoga in the Americas, as she was the first woman teacher in the Western Hemisphere. She is a foremost student, in fact, the first woman student, of the master teacher Prof. Krishnamacharya. Indra Devi, born in Latvian Russia in 1899, is a great example of vitality and longevity. I was recently in Buenos Aires, Argentina, to celebrate her 100th birthday with 3000 of her closest students. While no longer teaching yoga, she still does a yoga practice and is a radiant example of her message to "send love and light to everyone you know—friends and enemies." Her teacher also lived past his 100th birthday. Many yoga practitioners are cited in Paramahansa Yogananda's classic *Autobiography of a Yogi* as having been blessed with long healthy lives.[2]

Anatomy of the Joint

In order to take full advantage of our body's capabilities, we need to learn more about our anatomy. Let's first consider our joints. Where bones meet at a joint, they are tipped with cartilage that serves to cushion the meeting of bones in their movements. A joint capsule, a membrane containing synovial fluid that lubricates the surfaces to provide smooth movement, surrounds the joint. When healthy, the synovial fluid and cartilage allow for complete ease and freedom of motion without aches or pains.

During normal motion, muscles contract on one side of the joint, while the antagonist muscle on the opposite side relaxes. Hence, half our muscular activity is created by tension. The other half is a simultaneous relaxation. Lacking either component will create lack of coordination. Muscular tension compresses the joint space. When a person's nervous system has not learned to relax during motion, the muscular tension can cause damage to the cartilage or joint capsule. The signal that we are experiencing change begins with subtle messages like the feeling of being stiff. If ignored, these become feelings of tiredness, awkwardness, lack of coordination, then progress to aches, pains, and disease.

In following Classical Yoga guidelines, we are encouraged to seek positions in which we continually experience our body to be "comfortable and steady." The loss of comfort begins a spectrum from discomfort, to pain, to pathology. When we fail to listen to this message and make a change in how we experience our bodies, we move away from yoga. Problems can arise from several factors:

- We don't know where the joint is, so in order to move, we exert misdirected tension that accumulates in the muscle belly;
- We don't know how to minimize the tension involved in muscular action;
- We don't know what is normal mobility;

2 Paramahansa Yogananda, *Autobiography of a Yogi* (Los Angeles: Self-Realization Fellowship, 1998).

- When we are not in alignment during motion, it causes detrimental stress;
- There is loss of the sensations of being comfortable and steady in our bodies.

The last is the most critical of all. For yoga to be effective we must be conscious and aware of the differences between comfort and discomfort. Yet consciousness is not enough. There must also be a discipline toward freedom from discomfort and disease. To practice yoga is to refine our awareness consistently over the span of a lifetime.

We need to learn all of these factors to be free of joint pain. By creating a healthy sense of joint space, working in alignment, and training ourselves to minimize the tensions of muscular activity, movement can become so natural that we again enjoy the glow of circulatory health.

Freedom of the joints can provide for independent movement at each joint. Without this, the body may move unnecessarily in other joints. For instance, when you raise your right arm above your head, your left shoulder may lift up, creating excessive stress around your neck. This creates a tremendous waste of energy and increases the wear and tear on joint tissues. Besides, it doesn't feel good to accumulate tension.

By learning to create relaxation, alignment, and space during motion, you bring about a transformation in your experience of living in the body home. In order to understand the mechanics of motion, you must be trained to feel your body in unfamiliar ways. Learning how to do yoga poses is not enough. *The student of yoga also needs to learn how to feel himself or herself.* Teachers will ask,"What do you feel when you do a yoga pose? Where do you feel the movement or the holding of a position?" They will also inform you as to the correctness of this feeling. If you are feeling tension in a part of your body that should be relaxing, they will assist you to shift your effort to more beneficial areas. If the tension is appropriate, they will assist you in learning what that signal means, as well. You will learn the difference between muscle and nerve sensation, strength and stretch sensations, good and bad pain.

This education of the feelings is a natural part of the yoga class curriculum. Learning to listen to your body's messages can be taught by a good yoga teacher who gives you pauses during the instructions so you can sense and feel your way back into proper relationship with your body's multitude of parts. The body's mass is composed of 60 percent muscle and skeletal tissues. This is a tremendous amount, and the major portion of our body's signals come from sensors located in these tissues. While visual stimuli make up the majority of our sensory input, the messages from muscles, joints, and skin are also significant.

Functional Anatomy—Kinesiology

To deepen your mind's interface with your body's anatomy, you can begin to apply the study of anatomy to understanding how muscles move joints and create function. This is the study of kinesiology. This is not the same as applied kinesiology (a chiropractic reflex treatment method). In kinesiology, we learn how specific muscles and joints react during movement. We can learn which muscles contract, which ones stretch, and whether they move too far or not far enough. It is ideal to be able to move each joint both independently and in combination with other motions.

Through this study, you can predict which yoga poses will be difficult. If you've had an injury or postural abnormality and know the structures involved and how they normally move, by the application of kinesiology, you can predetermine exercises that will need remedial work before you attempt more challenging and complex motions.

Scientists of physical medicine have studied normal range of motion since 1910. Acceptable standards for the direction of movement and mobility of each joint have been established in the professions of physical medicine, physical therapy, and orthopedics. They differ slightly as to what amount of flexibility is considered normal for each joint.[3] Joints move through a specific range of motion, as delineated by studies of physical medicine and orthopedics. Motions within this optimal range maintain the natural flow of synovial fluid for lubrication of the joints, as well as normal strength and flexibility of the antagonistic muscles on opposite sides of the joint. When this range is exceeded, by overstretching, poor posture, injury or skeletal deformity, the joint becomes hyperextended, less stable and potentially more vulnerable to injury. Conversely, when the range of a joint has been diminished, the resulting rigidity in the joint and postural muscles supporting it places more stress on neighboring joints and muscles.

While I have consulted all the physical medical association standards of joint mobility, the standards set here are, in general, an average. I have found that increasing the range of external rotation of the hips by 10 to 20 degrees (to 55 or 65 degrees) is more beneficial to the health of the spinal column and longevity of hip joints. The angles of mobility are presented using the Joint-Freeing Series to evaluate your joint freedom.

All movements are based upon the amount of shift in position from the basic anatomical position. In yoga, this posture is a modification of the Mountain Pose (Tadasana), with the palms facing forward and fingers extended. The measurements for each joint movement are in degrees of arc. The motions are described both in this manner, and by body-position relationships for the full normal range of motion.

For students seeking a more accurate measurement, you can purchase an instrument called a goniometer at a medical supply house or medical bookstore. These protractor-like instruments are available for $5 to $30. A more precise evaluation can be obtained by having a trained practitioner examine you using range-of-motion analysis and muscle testing to isolate the strength of specific muscles. An accurate analysis will often reveal lack of joint freedom in which adjacent joints move to compensate for lack of mobility of the neighbor joint. An accurate muscle-testing examination can show weakness due to compensation by accessory muscles doing the task of weakened prime-mover muscles. These skills are offered in Structural Yoga Therapy™ training courses.

---

[3] For a physical therapy persepctive see Lucille Daniels and Catherine Worthington, *Muscle Testing—Techniques of Manual Examination* (Philadelphia: W. B. Saunders, 1980). For an orthopedic perspective see Stanley Hoppenfeld, *Physical Examination of the Spine and Extremities* (New York: Appleton-Century-Crofts, 1976).

Chapter 14

HOW IS MOVEMENT CREATED?

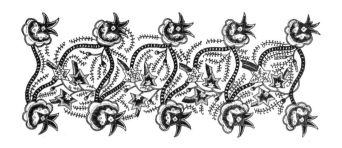

First, let us consider the anatomical structures that make motion possible. A fundamental type of tissue is called connective tissue. This is tissue that serves to connect, support, and bind body structures together. Examples include fat, fascia, cartilage, bone, ligaments, and tendons. In all connective tissues except cartilage, there are many blood and lymph vessels and nerves.

A joint is the meeting of the ends of two bones. There are approximately 206 bones that meet at 180 joints. I say approximately, as anomalies are not uncommon in the human body. Some people are blessed with additional bones, muscles, and/or joints. The ends of bones that meet at a joint are surrounded by a capsule. The termini of the bones are covered with hyaline cartilage, which lubricates and protects the smooth surfaces for fluid articulation. This area also contains various sensory elements. The sensors give proprioceptive awareness to our brain via fine nerve fibers, so that we are kept constantly informed about movements and the position of each joint.

The joint has its own stability, provided by another type of connective tissue called ligaments. Ligaments are fibrous bands that allow certain motions and prevent others. They will be lax in the direction of motions they create and reach the limit of their mobility to restrict motions that would otherwise injure the joint or surrounding muscle tissue. Ligaments can be tightened by injury or repeated muscular contractions, as in developing muscular stamina. They can also be stretched, though usually only with effort applied consistently. Some physical medicine specialists object to yoga students holding stretches too long, thus creating stretch, not in the muscles, but in ligaments. They fear this training may be a source of additional patients and potential surgery.

Ligaments can also be torn in the case of forced motions or accidents that go beyond normal joint mobility.

"The muscles are protected from injury by two kinds of nerve cells," Evjenth writes, "'muscle spindles and tendon spindles'. Muscle spindles prevent muscle cells from stretching too much when an unexpected movement occurs. They do this by making the muscle contract. This happens automatically and protects the muscle from over-stretching. Slow, intentional stretching is not prevented by the muscle spindles. Tendon spindles tell the brain, via nerve fibers, how tense the muscle is. If tension gets too high, tendon spindles send signals to stop the muscle contracting. These signals make the muscle relax."[1] In conversation with my colleague in Unity in Yoga Conferences, William Beer, M.D., he explained that "about 30 percent of our nervous system ener-vates these structures, which are responsible for our underlying learned messages regarding our posture. Because these neurons are operating at a subconscious level and therefore cannot be accessed by the mind, it is only through the breath that these struc-tures will release and 'reset' the muscle concerned at a more happy state."[2] Indeed, Dr. Beer makes an excellent point for the importance of breath awareness in learning to relax muscle tissue and both heightening awareness of the present moment and to maintain the ideal of where one wants to go in yoga practice.

It is important to distinguish between yoga and stretching. While stretching is a feel-ing sensation, Classical Yoga is not concerned with these sensations. The keywords in describing the physical sensations of yoga poses are steadiness, comfort, and relaxation of effort. Nowhere does it say that yoga consists of stretching exercises. Many writers engage in conscious stretching, done to purposely lengthen a muscle by holding a stretch-ing position with a high degree of tension for a sustained period of time. As a result, the muscles are in fact, injured. There is a resultant increase in muscle-resting length from the tearing of muscle fiber. *This is not Classical Yoga.* Many people are under the mistak-en impression that yoga is focused upon stretching muscle fiber.[3] While this may be true in some systems of yoga, let me repeat that this is not following the guidelines of Classical Yoga, nor my contemporary adaptation called Structural Yoga Therapy™.

There are three types of muscle tissue. The most common—comprising 99 percent of the body's muscle mass—makes up approximately 430 skeletal muscles that attach the skeleton together and maintain postural integrity. These are also called voluntary mus-cles, as they are responsible for all types of controlled conscious motion. They are also involved, however, in automatic reflex motions, such as running and walking. The next major group is smooth muscles, which make up many internal organs and blood vessels. The third group is the cardiac muscle, located only in the heart. Altogether, muscles make up about 60 percent of our body's mass.

Crossing over each joint are one or more skeletal muscles. Motor nerves coming from the spinal cord activate skeletal muscles. An electrical impulse from the nerve end-

---

[1] Olaf Evjenth and Jern Hamberg, *Auto Stretching* (Alfta, Sweden: Alfta Rehab Forlag, 1997), p. 243.
[2] William Beer, M.D., personal conversation.
[3] Thomas Griner, *What's Really Wrong with You—A Revolutionary Look at How Your Muscles Affect Your Health* (Garden City, NY: Avery, 1996), p. 25.

ings spans the gap to the muscle surface via a chemical secretion of acetylcholine. The muscle will stay in contraction until an enzyme that neutralizes acetylcholine is produced to create relaxation. Thus, muscles have only two properties—they contract, which strengthens them, or they relax. "Individual muscles can act only to shorten, and not to lengthen, the distance between two attachment points—they can pull but not push. For movement in the opposite direction, another muscle must be activated."[4]

Skeletal muscles are made up of two types of fibers—dark, or slow-twitch, fibers and white, or fast-twitch, fibers. Thomas Griner says that only slow-twitch muscle fibers can metabolize fatty acids, and that this is desirable for several reasons. First, fat metabolism is aerobic, it burns cleanly, and it doesn't make lactic acid. It can also draw directly on stored body fat and help reduce it. The fast-twitch muscle fiber can only metabolize glucose, so during heavy exercise, this process will be aerobic, but most of it will produce lactic acid and actually be anaerobic. The more vigorous your exercise program, the more you are going to engage fast-twitch fibers, while leaving the slow-twitch fibers behind. This means you burn less fat and produce more lactic acid. Slow movement is of more benefit in that it uses both the fast- and the slow-twitch fibers, thereby activating all your muscles.[5]

Slow steady-paced yoga practice based on the tradition of Patanjali is an efficient form of exercise for burning fat and reducing lactic acid. Patanjali states guidelines that, in effect, minimize the effort involved during the practice of asana.[6] Scientific research has also discovered that this type of stretching, characterized by low force yet long duration, produces a plastic or permanent deformation in the muscle tissue. The opposite type of stretching, with high force and short duration, was shown by the same researchers to produce elastic or recoverable deformation in muscle tissue.[7]

Skeletal muscles have at least two attachments. The attachment portion at either end of the muscle is called its tendon. One end is connected to a more freely mobile limb called the insertion, the other to a less-moveable attachment called the origin. When a muscle contracts, it exerts a pull on both ends toward the middle of the belly of the muscle, which usually moves the insertion toward the origin. In the case of the biceps brachii, its origin is on the shoulder and insertion on the upper forearm. When it contracts, it pulls the forearm toward the shoulder, as in the action of picking up an object. This is the more natural movement of the insertion moving toward the origin. It can also contract, by pulling the body toward the forearm, as in the pull-up or chin-up exercise motion. In this case, the origin is moving toward the insertion.

Muscles have two basic ways of working, Evjenth tells us:

1. *Concentrically,* when the muscle fibers *contract or shorten* so that the origin and insertion come closer to each other.

2. *Eccentrically,* when the muscle fibers *lengthen* so that origin and insertion

[4] Emmett Keeffe, *Know Your Body—The Atlas of Anatomy* (Berkeley, CA: Ulysses Press, 1999), p. 40.
[5] See Thomas Griner, *What's Really Wrong with You*, pp. 155–156.
[6] Stiles, *Yoga Sutras of Patanjali*, chap. II, sutra 47.
[7] C. G. Warren, et al., "Elongation of Rat Tails Tendons: Effect of Load and Temperature," *Archives of Physical Medicine and Rehabilitation*, 52(3), pp. 465–474.

move away from each other. When a muscle contracts without changing its length we call it *isometric contraction.*[8]

Many muscles work in pairs. The muscle that contracts in the most direct line of a specific motion is called the agonist or the primary mover. Other muscles helping in the motion are called secondary movers. A muscle that relaxes to allow the motion (this may be felt as a passive stretch) is called the antagonist. For instance, when the biceps brachii contracts, it bends/flexes the elbow. This can only happen if the antagonist muscle, the triceps brachii, relaxes/stretches. Conversely, to straighten/extend the elbow, the triceps brachii will contract, if the biceps brachii relaxes.

Sometimes the work of contraction is more than the muscle is accustomed to. Then there will be a residual contraction. In the example above, if the biceps brachii is overworked, once relaxed, the elbow will remain partially flexed. Afterward, you may find yourself complaining of stiffness in the biceps. This will commonly occur when a muscle has been used extensively. For instance, when you curl weight from a straight arm position, bringing it toward the shoulder, you contract the biceps strongly. After overexertion in building the muscle, the arm will hang at the side with a perpetual bend/flexion of the elbow joint. This is often the case of weight lifters who do not balance the full range of toning of the triceps brachii with toning of the biceps brachii. The residual contraction of the biceps has not been balanced relative to its antagonist muscle, the triceps.

In order for the complete range of motion to occur, the triceps brachii must fully relax so that the biceps brachii can fully contract. This is what we are seeking in yoga-based movements—a mobility that is within acceptable medical standards for joint health and is also smooth, steady, and comfortable, to produce a heightened sensitivity.

To understand the principle of antagonistic motion is to understand balance and symmetry. When any muscle is fully contracted, its antagonist muscle or muscles will necessarily be fully relaxed and stretched to their end points. This principle creates full range of motion. Whenever there is lack of mobility, there is necessarily an imbalance in antagonist muscles. The contracting muscle is weak and its antagonist is too tight. By getting to know the antagonist muscles, a student can learn to balance flexibility with strength.

A common problem we all face is in maintaining the health of our muscle tissue. Since muscles comprise so much of our body, nearly three-fifths of our mass, Griner points out, their health "has a direct effect on the nervous system and the circulatory system and impacts every function of the body—every organ and gland. When a muscle is in spasm, it adversely affects nerves and blood vessels and is a crucial though little understood factor in illness and disease. . . . when excess lactic acid becomes trapped in a muscle, the muscle will eventually develop an abnormal, sustained contraction known as hypertonic spasm. . . . It is extremely important to realize that we all have muscles in spasm. But, although spasm causes pain, most of us are not aware of it. This is because when muscles become spastic, the body releases its own painkillers called endorphins.

---

[8] Evjenth, *Auto Stretching*, p. 244.

Endorphins block the pain of muscle spasm from reaching your brain.[9] Griner goes on to say that spasms can be so bad they can cut off circulation and sensation in nearby nerves. The nerves become blocked and you don't feel any pain because the area is numb. Muscle spasm can create other physical problems, whether or not you feel the pain. You may develop bone, muscle, and joint problems, as well as other problems ranging from allergies to blocked arteries. You may experience cramps or tics, or more violent muscle spasms, but Griner was discussing the more serious spasm because it is permanent unless it is treated.

Some muscle structures are not involved in spasms. There are two types of skeletal muscles: flat and round. Griner tells us that flat skeletal muscles and their tendons are arranged in sheets that attach to the bone in a line. The tension is distributed evenly in a plane when a flat muscle contracts. Flat muscles are not subject to insidious spasm because they cannot trap lactic acid. Examples of flat muscles are the latissimus dorsi of the middle and lower back, and the gluteus maximus of the buttocks.

Round muscles and their tendons attach to bone between two points. So that tension can be evenly balanced around the line and between the two points, all muscle fibers must be arranged in concentric cylinders with that line at their center. When a round muscle contracts, it closes like a fist around the blood vessels, and traps lactic acid. For example, the biceps is a round muscle, and the pectoralis major (in the chest) and the deltoids (shoulder) are both made up of flat and round sections. All flat and round skeletal muscles, and their tendons, could become spastic at their attachments. Why? Because muscle attachments curve inward just before they attach to the bone, which in turns allows lactic acid to become trapped. The deeper muscle tissues are insensate; they lack pain sensing nerve fibers. Any pain felt from a spasm is the result of some kind of irritation transmitted to superficial muscles.[10]

"Lactic acid is our villain," Griner concludes. "It is the cause of hypertonic spasm. Lactic acid is produced when an animal cell metabolizes sugar anaerobically—without using oxygen. Whenever your muscles are at work—and that's all the time—they produce lactic acid. The harder and more sustained the muscle activity, the greater the output of lactic acid." [11]

By learning how to focus attention to the specific muscles that, when contracted, create joint mobility, the body moves efficiently and the mind is given a concentration point for direction, a dharana. In addition, when you train yourself to have an additional point of awareness upon the conscious relaxation of the antagonist, the stretching muscles, there is a deep relaxation reflex that occurs, promoting proper effort without stress.

As an example, in Cat Pose, when going into spine flexion and lifting the spine, if no attention is given to contracting the rectus abdominis muscle, the major muscle of trunk flexion, the movement of the back will not be full. Once you learn where the muscle is and how to focus your attention on a full contraction of the entire muscle, your lumbar and thoracic spinal regions will be given a full flexion motion. This movement

---

[9] Griner, *What's Really Wrong With You*, pp. 8, 43–44.
[10] Griner, *What's Really Wrong With You*, p. 47.
[11] Griner, *What's Really Wrong With You*, p. 53.

Table 4. Muscle Pairs and Their Corresponding Movements.

MUSCLE	MOVEMENT	ANTAGONIST	MOVEMENT
Sternocleidomastoid (SCM)	Lateral neck flexion, rotation	SCM on the opposite side	Opposite lateral flexion, rotation
Sternocleidomastoid	Neck flexion	Upper trapezius	Neck extension
Middle trapezius	Scapula adduction	Serratus anterior	Scapula abduction
Anterior deltoid	Shoulder flexion	Posterior deltoid	Shoulder extension
Biceps brachii	Elbow flexion	Triceps brachii	Elbow extension
Flexor carpi radialis/ulnaris	Wrist flexion	Extensor carpi radialis longus	Wrist extension
Rectus abdominis	Spinal flexion	Erector spinae, latissimus dorsi	Spinal extension
Gluteus maximus, hamstring	Hip extension	Psoas, rectus femoris	Hip flexion
Gluteus medius	Hip abduction	Adductors, gracilis	Hip adduction
Gluteus minimus, tensor fascia lata	Hip internal rotation	Psoas, external hip rotator group	Hip external rotation
Hamstrings	Knee flexion	Quadriceps	Knee extension
Gastrocnemius, soleus	Ankle plantar flexion	Tibialis anterior	Ankle dorsiflexion

can become even greater, though it is subtle, by an additional awareness that promotes conscious relaxation of the deep spinal muscles, the erector spinae. In this manner, by learning functional anatomy, you will definitely increase your joint freedom, muscular stamina, concentration, and capacity to relax.

Movement results from muscles contracting through a specific pattern of motion to pull the bones in various directions to open or close the joints (see Table 4). In any given movement, the forces involved include both the primary and secondary movers. The primary movers exert their contractile forces in a pattern corresponding to the line of their muscle fibers from beginning tendon, called the origin, to end point tendon, called the insertion. The secondary movers exert their forces at an angle to the motion and are hence less efficient. In learning anatomy, it is helpful to learn the primary movers of joint action. Knowledge of the secondary movers' effects upon motion is only necessary for advanced Structural Yoga Therapy™ training.

Chapter 15

THE JOINT-FREEING SERIES: PAVANMUKTASANA

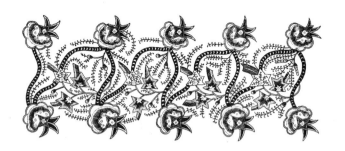

Ideally, before beginning your daily yoga asana practice, you will check in with the your body. This series accomplishes this goal and systematically loosens all joint movements. The Pavanmuktasana series moves each joint gently and systematically through its full and natural range of motion. The series starts with the feet and ankles, moves up to the knees, hips, torso, and spine, and finishes with the neck. The motions described in this series represent all the basic motions of the body.

Kinesiology, the science of the analysis of motion, defines 45 specific directions of possible body movements. To determine the average range of motion for each joint, experts in physical medicine analyzed each movement. These are the normal minimal ranges of mobility for each joint. If you follow these standards for joint mobility during yoga practices, you will be less likely to strain or injure muscles and joints. Students with injuries or chronic pain benefit immensely from adjusting their practices to these standards.

Your first performance of the series should be an evaluation of your joint suppleness. Keep a record of how your mobility compares to the standards of range of motion shown in the illustrations that accompany each movement in chapter 16.

This series can also be performed to serve several other purposes:

1. To heighten awareness and distinction between stretching and contracting muscles. Many people do not know the difference between the feeling sensations of stretching and those of strengthening a muscle. This training can, with the help of a trained teacher, be used to clarify the exchange between body sensations and mental understanding. It can "ground" your awareness into your physical body.

2. To move each joint through specific anatomical directional ranges of motion, which can enhance joint mobility and often relieve joint pain and stiffness. If a joint is stiff, it lacks full mobility. The feelings will tell you that the muscles involved in creating the motion are weak and/or that the contrasting antagonist muscles are tight. By practicing with an awareness of the specific imbalance you have, you can apply more force to develop muscle strength and joint mobility.

3. To observe and diagnose areas for comparative freedom. By maintaining mindfulness as you do the series you can discover, for instance, that when you flex your right wrist, the joint moves smoothly, while the left wrist creates a rotation with flexion. This comparison may reveal an underlying chronic tension in the rotator muscles, which may be a factor in the early phases of carpal tunnel syndrome due to excessive keyboarding.

4. To isolate muscles and test for comparative strength and stamina. This is dealt with more specifically in chapter 17 on isolating muscle strength, but a mild comparison is possible with this series.

5. To alleviate conditions associated with poor circulation. By focusing on making the complete motions of each joint systematically, the joint-freeing series moves synovial fluid within the joint capsule and enhances vascular circulation.

6. To allow you and your teacher to see what basic movements are at the root of difficulties that may arise in asana practice. As yogasanas are composed of combinations of individual joint motions, your instructor can more accurately predict which postures will need the most attention.

7. To be able to follow the guidelines of Patanjali's Classical Yoga, as stated in his *Yoga Sutras* (II, 46), that yoga poses should be "comfortable and steady." This series often removes the causes of "discomfort and instability." I have repeatedly had students tell me that this series alleviated their pain.

8. To provide a series that is especially beneficial for those with limited mobility due to injuries or arthritis. Students with arthritis often report that this series is all they need to be relieved of their worst symptoms. While not necessarily a cure for arthritis, it can be of major help when combined with Ayurvedic dietary counseling.

9. To uncover motions that are boring. Often, these motions indicate a movement in which the student "spaces out." This may reveal a site of unconscious chronic tension or weakness. The specific posture at the point of trauma or injury often holds a chronic trigger for the mind to go unconscious. By bringing to consciousness the feelings held in the body posture, the subconscious patterns can be released.

This last perspective comes from another translation for the term Pavanmuktasana—as "energy-freeing practices." This comes about through persistent conscientious practice of this series with coordinated breathing. This frees prana (the energy hidden within the breath) to flow into the region being exercised. The series enhances awareness of a subtle-body physiology that is the memory storehouse for all events. The subtle body is called the pranamaya kosha, literally the "sheath veiling prana." It is composed of energy flowing from a central wand of light, called the sushumna, in the subtle body superimposed on the physical spinal cord. From this wand of light emanate luminous vortices (chakras) that spread through subtle nerve-like channels called nadis. Awareness of the subtle body comes with a variety of experiences, ranging from heat, light, visions, recalling lost memories, feelings of a spiritual presence, or intuitive flashes of guidance. (For more about this, see chapter 6, "Remembering the Big Picture." For an overview of the Joint-Freeing Series, see figure 19, pages 132–133.)

• • •

When performing the Joint-Freeing Series, repeat each motion six times. Go at your own rate. Adjust your level of effort so that you can sustain the sequence rhythmically, in harmony with your natural breath rate.

The Ujjaye breath pattern (see page 55) used in all yoga asana practices is easily learned through regular practice of the joint-freeing series. The pattern is to inhale when extending or straightening the joint, and exhale when flexing or contracting. For motions of the torso, this means to exhale whenever the abdomen is contracted, and to inhale when the chest is expanded. The regular practice of harmonizing the breath with motion increases self-awareness. This in turn can be reflected in all activities of life.

The first four exercises that follow begin in Stick Pose (Dandasana). Sit on the floor with your legs extended together, toes toward the ceiling, arms straight with the palms flat and fingers turned back behind or beside your hips (whichever is more comfortable for your arm length). Keep your arms straight.

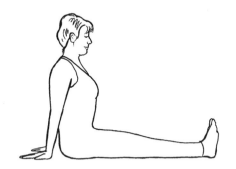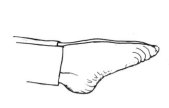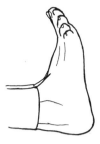

1. ANKLE PLANTAR FLEXION—DORSIFLEXION
(Stretch the top of the foot. Stretch the sole of the foot.)

Inhale as you point your toes (plantar flexion).

Exhale and flex the top of the foot back toward your body (dorsiflexion). As you continue, curl the toes on the Inhale and spread the toes on the Exhale.

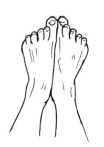
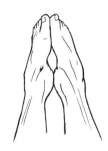

2. ANKLE EVERSION—INVERSION

(Side of foot turned out. Side of foot turned in.)

Inhale as you rotate the soles of the feet outward, drawing the little toes toward the head (the inner ankle bones may touch). This is called eversion.

Exhale, as you draw the soles of the feet toward each other so the big toes are pulled toward the head and the inner ankle bones are spread as wide as possible. This is called inversion. As you continue, move only your ankles and feet, with a minimum of rotation in your legs. Keep your feet upright, toes pointing to the ceiling.

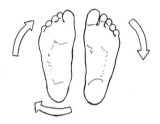

3. ANKLE ROTATION

(Rotate feet right. Rotate feet left.)

Inhale, with legs separated about 12 inches, as you rotate the ankles to the right and then point the toes forward.

Exhale as you rotate the ankles left and draw the toes up toward the head. As you continue, make a smooth circle with the toes. Restrict the movement to the ankles by keeping the thigh and knee from turning.

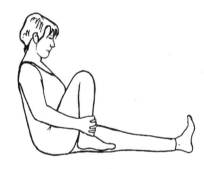
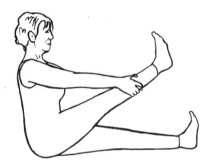

4. KNEE FLEXION—EXTENSION

(Bend knee. Straighten knee.)

Exhale as you grasp your lower right shin with both hands. Bend your knee, and draw your heel close to the center of your buttock. This is knee flexion.

Inhale and straighten your knee, lifting your right leg by holding lightly to the back of your mid calf. The action of straightening of your knee is extension.

5. HIP EXTERNAL AND INTERNAL ROTATION

(Thigh turned in. Thigh turned out.)

Begin in Stick Pose, then move your hands wider and farther back than in the standard position so your arms support your back.

Inhale as you turn your right leg out at the hip (forming external hip rotation) so your knee and foot are pointing to the right side. Swing your leg open to the side. Keep your foot about six inches from the floor.

Exhale as you turn your leg in (knee pointing to *left*) swinging your leg back to touch the left leg (internal hip rotation).

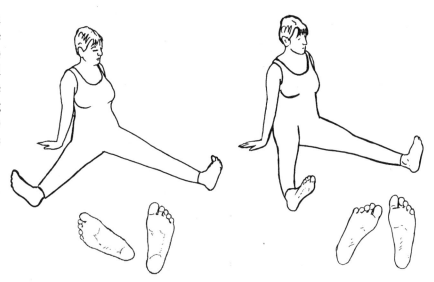

The next three poses begin on hands and knees in Cat Pose (Marjarasana), knees hip-width apart, hands wider than shoulder width.

6. SPINE EXTENSION—FLEXION

(Backward bend. Forward bend.)

Inhale and let your spine drop toward the floor. Relax your abdomen while raising your head. Contract the space between your shoulder blades, pulling your spine down toward the floor.

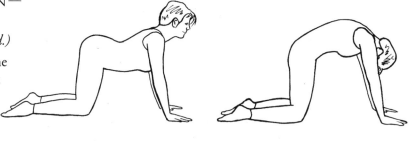

Exhale as you contract your abdomen and round your back upward. Let your head come down. Stretch your upper back to open the space between your shoulder blades.

7. HIP EXTENSION—FLEXION

(Thigh toward back. Thigh toward abdomen.)

Inhale, lifting your head as you extend your right leg straight out along

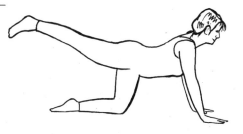
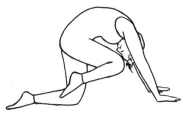

the floor. Then lift your leg, keeping your knee straight, until your foot is higher than your hips (hip extension). This is called the Sunbird Pose (Chakravakasana).

Exhale, pulling your chin toward your chest as you bend your knee. Pull your thigh close to your abdomen, causing your spine to round (hip flexion).

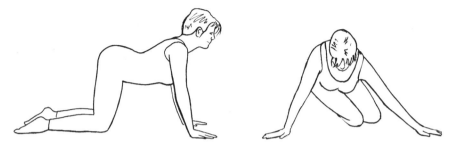

8. HIP ADDUCTION—ABDUCTION

(Thighs pull to center. Thighs pull away from center.)

Begin in the Cat Pose, with your knees together, hands wider than shoulder-width, then gently sway your hips from side to side.

Exhale, moving your hips straight to one side.

Inhale, coming back to center. Continue to alternate sides while you press your knees firmly into the floor.

The next six poses are done while sitting on the shins in Hero (Virasana) Pose. If this is uncomfortable for your knees or ankles, sit in a gentle cross-legged or Easy (Sukhasana) Pose.

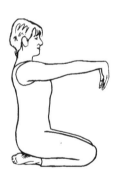 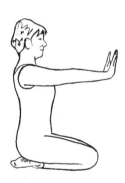

9. WRIST FLEXION—EXTENSION

(Palms of hands move toward forearms. Backs of hands toward forearms.)

Begin with your arms extended straight in front of you, parallel to the floor and to each other, palms down.

Exhale, pulling your hands down, palms toward your body.

Inhale, pulling your hands up, with the backs of your hands facing your head.

VARIATION:
- **Inhale** as you spread your fingers. **Exhale** as you close your fingers. As you continue, notice that not all your fingers can be opened fully.
- Isolate the opening of the spaces between each finger.

10. WRIST RADIAL DEVIATION—ULNAR DEVIATION

(Hands move away from the midline. Hands move toward the midline.)

Keep your hands flat and palms up, with your fingers together.

Inhale while pointing your wrists and fingers out.

Exhale while pointing your wrists and fingers in.

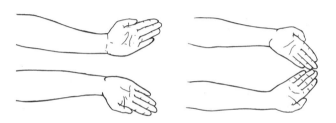

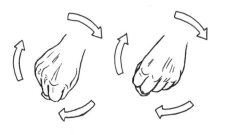

11. WRIST ROTATION

(Rotate upward. Rotate downward.)

Inhale as your fist is brought up.

Exhale as your wrist goes down. Rotate the fists in slow circles. Do both arms simultaneously, in rhythm, without movement in your upper arms. Repeat three times clockwise, then three times counterclockwise.

12. ELBOW EXTENSION—FLEXION

(Straighten. Bend.)

Begin with your arms straight in front, palms up.

Inhale, stretching out your arms, extending your elbows and fingers.

Exhale, closing your hand into a fist. Bend your arms, placing your knuckles on your shoulders.

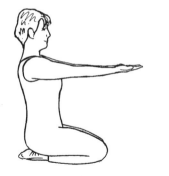

13. SHOULDER ABDUCTION—ADDUCTION

(Arms open to sides. Elbows close together.)

Begin with your knuckles resting on your shoulders, elbows straight ahead at shoulder height.

Inhale, opening your elbows and pulling them behind your shoulders.

Exhale, pulling your elbows inward, touching them in front of you.

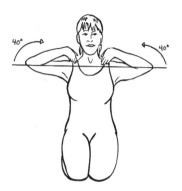

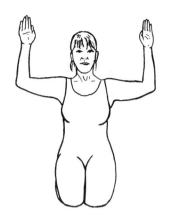
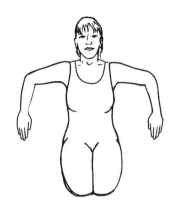

14. SHOULDER EXTERNAL AND INTERNAL ROTATION

(Rotate upward. Rotate downward.)

Begin with your arms out to the side of your shoulders, parallel with the floor.

Inhale as you bend your elbows to a right angle, palms forward beside your head (external shoulder rotation).

Exhale, swinging your forearms down beside your waist by rotating your upper arms in the shoulder socket. Your palms will face backward (internal shoulder rotation).

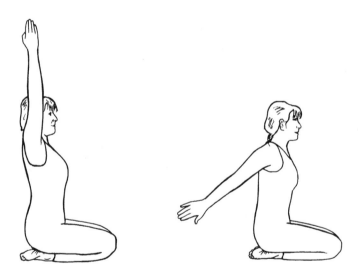

15. SHOULDER FLEXION—EXTENSION

(Arms raised forward. Arms raised backward.)

Begin with your arms straight down at your sides, wrists and fingers straight.

Inhale, lifting your arms overhead until they are beside your ears (shoulder flexion).

Exhale, lowering your arms and reaching back and up behind you (shoulder extension). As you continue, be aware of your spine staying immobile, so the benefit can go specifically to your shoulders.

The next three positions are done in any comfortable cross-legged position, hands upon knees.

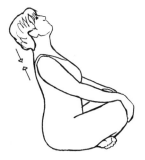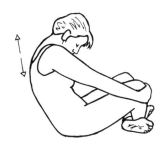

16. SPINE EXTENSION—FLEXION
SCAPULA ADDUCTION—ABDUCTION

(Back arched. Shoulder blades together. Back rounded. Shoulder blades spread.)

Inhale, and arch your back forward, so that your chest is lifted, squeezing your shoulder blades together.

Exhale, and reverse the movement, rounding your spine, spreading your shoulder blades wide apart.

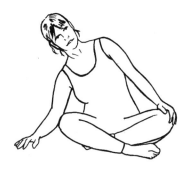

17. SPINE—LATERAL FLEXION

(Side bend.)

Inhale, and extend upward as you elongate, from your tailbone to the top of your head.

Exhale, and bend directly to the right side, allowing your elbow to come toward the floor. Continue to inhale to center, then exhale and bend left.

18. SPINAL ROTATION

(Rotate to each side.)

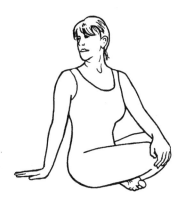

Inhale, and bring your left hand to your upper right shin, putting your right hand flat on the floor 12 inches behind your right hip. Lift your chest with an arch to your midback.

Exhale, and pull with your arms, turning your head and shoulders to the right.

Inhale, and face to center. Reverse your arms and lift your chest.

Exhale, and repeat the twisting motion to the left side.

For the last three exercises, reverse your legs, placing the opposite leg in front.

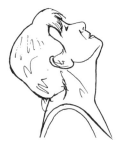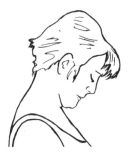

19. NECK EXTENSION—FLEXION

(Facing up. Facing down.)

Inhale, sitting with your head and spine erect (neutral position).
Exhale, letting your head bow slowly forward (neck flexion).
Inhale, bringing your head back to the starting position.
Exhale, then let your head gently extend backward (neck extension).

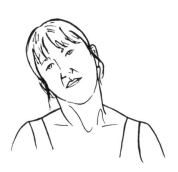

20. NECK LATERAL FLEXION

(Facing forward, ear toward shoulder.)

Inhale, with your back and head erect.
Exhale, letting your head tilt straight toward your right side, your ear falling toward your shoulder.
Inhale, moving your head to a neutral pose.
Exhale, relaxing your head to the left.

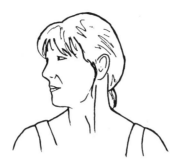

21. NECK LATERAL ROTATION

(Head level, turning to either side.)

Inhale, with your head erect.
Exhale, twisting your head to the right.
Inhale, with your head to the center.
Exhale, twisting your head to left.

RELAXATION AND ABSORPTION POSE

At the end of the Joint-Freeing Series (Pavanmuktasana), lie down on your back, opening your arms and legs a comfortable distance, for three to seven minutes to allow the benefits to be absorbed fully throughout your body and mind. This practice of deep conscious relaxation is more fully described as the Corpse Pose (Savasana) in Part Five (see page 240).

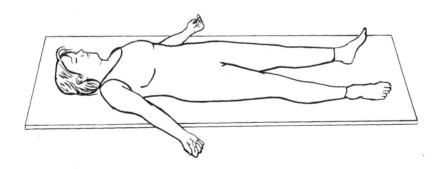

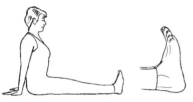 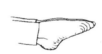 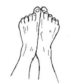

1. Stick Pose–*Dandasana*
Exhale, feet toward
head, toes spread
Dorsiflexion 20°

Inhale, point foot,
curling the toes
Plantar Flexion 50°

2. **Inhale,** soles face out,
keep feet upright
*Dorsiflexion with
Ankle Eversion 20°*

Exhale, soles face in
*Dorsiflexion with
Ankle Inversion 45°*

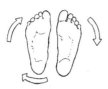 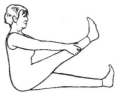 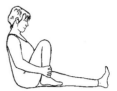

3. **Inhale,** circling out
Exhale, circling in
Ankle Rotation

4. **Inhale,** with mild arm
effort, straighten knee
Knee Extension 0°

Exhale, hold lower shin,
pull heel to thigh
Knee Flexion 150°

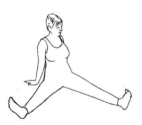 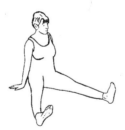 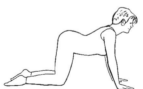 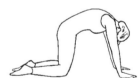

5. **Inhale,** turn leg out
and swing it wide open
Hip External Rotation 45°

Exhale, turn leg in and
swing it back
Hip Internal Rotation 35°

6. **Inhale,** head up,
spine down
Spine Extension

Exhale, back up,
abdomen in
Spine Flexion

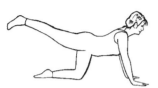 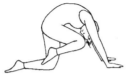 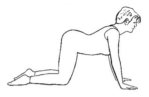 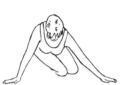

7. **Inhale,** stretch leg
back and up, spine level
Hip Extension 30°

Exhale, bring knee
toward chest, spine lifted
Hip Flexion 135°

8. **Inhale,** center pose,
squeeze thighs

Exhale, hips to side, feet
opposite, toes forward
Hip Adduction (right) 30°
Hip Abduction (left) 45°

Figure 19. Overview of the Joint-Freeing Series.

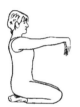 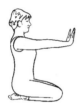 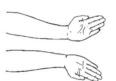 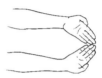 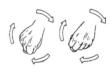

9. **Exhale** hands in
a fist, curled
toward forearms
Wrist Flexion 90°

Inhale, hands up,
fingers toward head
and spread
Wrist Extension 80°

10. **Inhale,** palms flat
and out
Radial Deviation 20°

Exhale, palms flat
and in
Ulnar Deviation 30°

11. **Inhale,** fists out
Exhale, in 3 times,
then reverse circles
Wrist Rotation

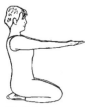 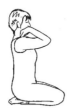 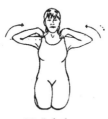 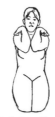 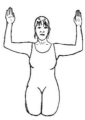 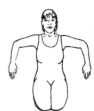

12. **Inhale,** arms
straight, palms up
Elbow Extension 0°

Exhale, knuckles
to shoulders
*Elbow
Flexion 145°*

13. **Inhale,**
elbows wide apart
*Shoulder
Abduction 40°*

Exhale, elbows
together
*Shoulder
Adduction 130°*

14. **Inhale,** arms up,
palms facing forward
*Shoulder External
Rotation 90°*

Exhale, arms
down, palms back
*Shoulder Internal
Rotation 80°*

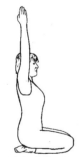 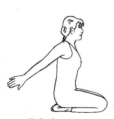 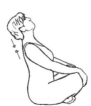 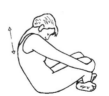 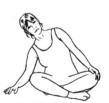

15. **Inhale,** arms
up, palms facing in
Shoulder Flexion 180°

Exhale, arms
behind back
Shoulder Extension 50°

16. **Inhale,** arch
back, squeeze blades
*Scapula Adduction
Spine Extension*

Exhale, round back,
open shoulder blades
*Scapula Abduction
Spine Flexion*

17. **Inhale,** erect
Exhale, side bend
Spine Lateral Flexion

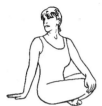   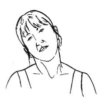

18. **Inhale,** sit erect
Exhale, spinal twist
Spinal Rotation

19. **Inhale,** head up
Neck Extension 55°

Exhale, head down
Neck Flexion 45°

20. **Inhale,** sit erect
Exhale, head to side
Neck Lateral Flexion 45°

21. **Inhale,** center head
Exhale, rotate head
Neck Rotation 70°

Figure 19. Overview of the Joint-Freeing Series (continued).

133

Chapter 16

ANATOMY AND MOBILITY ASSESSMENT

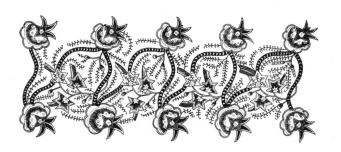

The following series will provide you with details of the Joint-Freeing Series and describes the muscles contracting to create the motion and the normal range of suppleness. The drawings of the Joint Freeing Series are repeated with angles and degrees of arc to indicate the direction of motion from the baseline of the standing posture Mountain Pose. On the last page of this chapter you will find a place to summarize your findings as you evaluate yourself for increased or diminished range of motion (see Chart 2, page 154). From this information you can determine which muscles are short and which might be weak. You can use a form that will reference the affected muscles to specific yogasanas (see chapter 21, pages 250–251). This information will enable you to personalize your practice.

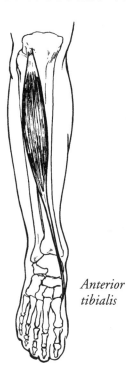

Anterior tibialis

1. ANKLE DORSIFLEXION

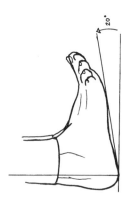

Normal range of motion is 20 degrees. One way to analyze this is to sit in Stick Pose and place the sole of your foot against the wall. Then pull the ball of your foot away from the wall, while keeping your heel against the wall. These muscles are assisted by the peroneus (fibularis) longus and peroneus (fibularis) brevis detailed on the next page. Normal flexibility would create a one-inch space (less than two finger-widths) between the wall and the ball of your foot. Attention should be maintained to keeping the rest of your leg motionless, especially your knee. The **tibialis anterior** muscle originates from the upper, lateral portion of the shin (tibia) and attaches at the base of the ankle, well above the great toe. When it contracts, it pulls the foot toward the shin and inverts the big toe. It is especially involved in running or walking uphill, and is aggravated in the creation of shin splints.

Ordinary activities of this motion are walking uphill and lowering your heels as you step down from a ladder.

PLANTAR FLEXION

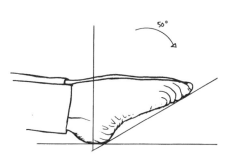

Normal range of motion is 50 degrees. This creates a straight line from the top of the foot, even with the shin (tibia) bone. Two muscles are involved in creating plantar flexion, a surface calf muscle called the **gastrocnemius** (shown in the drawing to the left) and a deeper muscle, the **soleus** (right drawing). Both muscles attach to the Achilles tendon at the heel. The gastrocnemius begins above the knee on the posterior side of the thigh (femur). Hence its contraction will also flex the knee. The origin of the soleus is upon the posterior head of the outer shinbone (fibula) and the middle third of the posterior tibia. Because of the leverage exerted at the ankle, these two muscles are tremendously strong for their size.

Ordinary activities include walking, as you momentarily lift your heel to balance on the ball of your foot and toes.

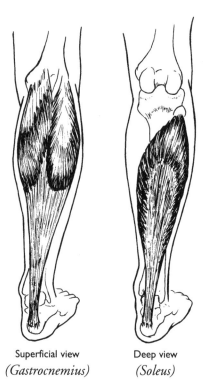

Superficial view
(Gastrocnemius)

Deep view
(Soleus)

2. ANKLE EVERSION

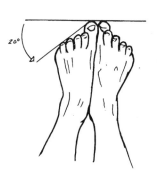

Normal range of motion is 20 degrees. In this motion, the outer foot is pulled toward the head about an inch. The movement is usually accompanied by adduction, giving the ankle more flexibility. The foot everters consist of the **peroneus longus** and the deeper **peroneus brevis**. These two muscles originate on the upper and middle lateral surface of the fibula and attach beneath the lateral side of the foot. They assist in ankle plantar flexion.

Ordinary activities of this motion include kicking a ball sideways, or the action of the upper ankle when walking across a sloped hill.

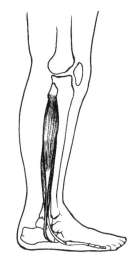

Peroneus longus and Peroneus brevis

ANKLE INVERSION

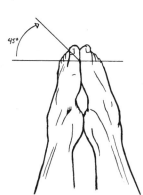

Normal range of motion is 45 degrees. In this motion, the inner surface of the foot near the great toe is lifted about one inch toward the head. This motion is done with abduction, giving the ankle greater mobility. The ankle is the most commonly sprained joint in the body. The muscles involved in ankle inversion are on the opposite sides of the lower leg. On the right is a drawing of the **tibialis posterior**. This is an accessory muscle to the previously seen **tibialis anterior**, located on the front of the shin. The tibialis posterior originates on the upper half of the adjacent surfaces of the posterior tibia and the fibula. It inserts at the bottom of the foot, forming the long arch of the foot.

A *common motion* in soccer would be a sideways kick with the inner foot.

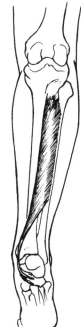

Posterior Tibialis. The deep right calf.

3. ANKLE ROTATION

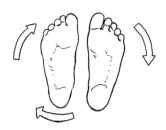

This movement combines the muscles and ranges of all the previous motions. Provided those motions are normal, this circling of the ankles will allow your feet to reach the floor on both sides with a smooth motion. Go slowly to incorporate all the muscle groups involved, including your toes.

4. KNEE EXTENSION

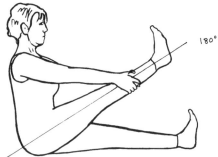

Normal range of motion is 0 or 180 degrees, a straight line. In the Stick Pose, the ability to lift the heel more than one inch while the back of the knee stays stationary on the ground indicates a hyperextended knee, one that is too flexible. The muscles that straighten the knee are the **quadriceps**, meaning "four heads"; that is they are four muscles that all insert into the patellar tendon, in which the kneecap rests. They are assisted by the tensor fascia lata (see hip abductors).

1. **Rectus femoris** "king of the thigh," is the major muscle originating above the hip joint on the lower border of the pelvic rim (ilium). It also serves, with the psoas, as a hip flexor.

2. **Vastus intermedius** (shown with a dotted line) lies beneath the rectus femoris, beginning on the upper two-thirds of the anterior femur.

3. **Vastus medialis** occupies the inner (medial) and lower portion of the thigh.

4. **Vastus lateralis** lies on the lateral femur.

A *common use of this motion* is getting up from sitting in a chair or the act of straightening your knee during walking.

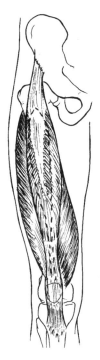

Front of right thigh—quadriceps

KNEE FLEXION

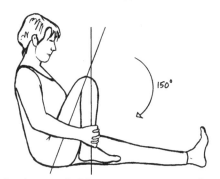

Normal range of motion is 150 degrees. At this range, the heel will come within the width of your hand to touching the back of your buttock. The major muscles involved in knee flexion are the **hamstrings**, which are composed of three separate muscles. They share a common origin on the base of the sitz bone (ischial tuberosity). The **gastrocnemius**, the surface of the calf detailed in exercise one, plantar flexion, also flexes the knee. In addition, the gracilis (see adductors) and sartorius (not shown) assist in this motion. Looking from right to left at their insertions on the back of the lower leg, the hamstrings are:

1. **Biceps femoris**, with two origins on the ischial tuberosity (sitz bone) and the central portion of the posterior femur. It is the only hamstring attaching to the lateral surface of the lower leg at both the fibula and the tibia.

2. **Semitendinosus**, inserted on the front inner surface of the tibia.

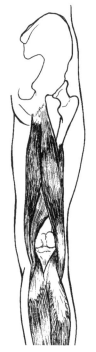

Back of the right leg—hamstrings

3. **Semimembranosus**, ending just above the previous section on the posterior medial section of the tibia, it is medial from the semitendinosus.

Common motions include bending of the back knee during walking or lowering yourself to sit in a chair. Sitting on your heels requires full knee flexion and is normal mobility.

5. HIP EXTERNAL ROTATION

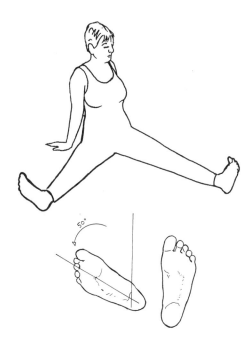

Normal range of motion is 45-60 degrees. In full mobility, the kneecap can rotate halfway to the lateral side. This motion is the outward rotation of the thighbone (femur) within the hip socket. The **hip external rotators** are a group of six deep muscles located beneath the **gluteus maximus,** which is also an external rotator. They all insert on the posterior of the femur and originate at various points on the posterior or internal pelvis. Viewed from top to bottom the muscles are:

1. **Piriformis** (below it lies the sciatic nerve)

2. **Gemellus superior**

3. **Obturator internus**

4. **Gemellus inferior**

5. **Quadratus femoris**

6. **Obturator externus** (not shown, it lies deep to the quadratus femoris muscle)

The **gluteus maximus** (shown cut on both sides of the deeper rotators) is a potentially powerful external rotator. Simply taking a greater stride as you walk can increase its strength. Its fibers originate on the posterior iliac crest, sacrum, and coccyx and insert on the upper posterior femur, as well as the iliotibial band of the tensor fascia lata muscle. The posterior portion of the **gluteus medius** (see hip internal rotation) assists in the motion.

Common activities of this motion are ballet's turnout and crossing your ankle over the opposite knee while in a seated position.

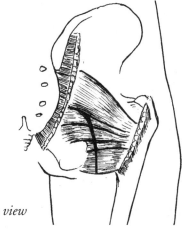

Right hip, deep view

139

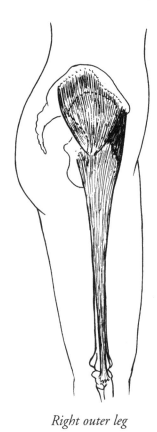

Right outer leg

HIP INTERNAL ROTATORS

Normal range of motion is 35 degrees. With full motion, the kneecap can turn nearly halfway inward, while the hip remains stationary. The three major muscles involved in internal rotation are the **gluteus minimus**, the **tensor fascia lata**, and the anterior portion of the gluteus medius. The **gluteus minimus** (deep in the center of the lateral hip, below the gluteus medius) originates on the middle lateral surface of the ilium and inserts at the anterior surface of the head of the thighbone. The **tensor fascia lata** muscle (shown darker) is short, usually about 6 inches long, and begins just forward and above the gluteus minimus. However, because it inserts into the longest tendon in the body, the iliotibial band, its full length is greater than that of the thighbone. This tendon, in turn, inserts at the lateral head of the tibia.

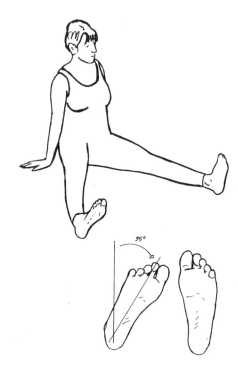

Common activities include the motions of the outer hip in turning a corner.

6. SPINE EXTENSION

There are no standards set in physical medicine for this motion. From a yogic point of view, we look for symmetry and fullness in back-bending and for a lengthening of the spinal column. In this sense, all segments of the thoracic region can be reversed, and the lumbar region can elongate, thus narrowing your waist. The principal muscles involved in extending the spine are collectively called the **erector spinae**. They are composed of six primary segments:

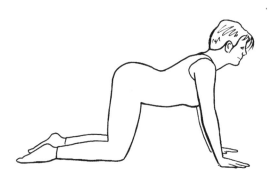

1. **Semispinalis capitis**

2. **Splenius capitis**

3. **Splenius cervicis**

4. **Iliocostalis**

5. **Longissimus**

6. **Spinalis**

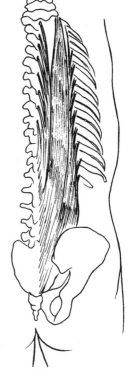

Deep musculature of the back

These muscles are assisted by the **latissimus dorsi** when the arms are actively assisting, while being held posterior to the shoulders (as in the Cobra Pose using the arms).

Common motions include sitting up straight, arching your back to look at the ceiling, or raising your chest and upper back from a prone position.

SPINE FLEXION

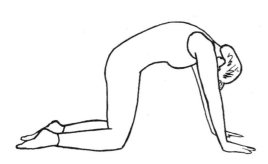

There are no standards of the range for spine/trunk flexion. A yogic view is that, if the tone of the spine flexors is balanced to the opposing muscles, the erector spinae, the spine arcs evenly, creating a symmetrical semicircle. The major muscle involved is the **rectus abdominis** ("king of the abdomen"). It originates on the cartilage sections of the fifth, sixth, and seventh ribs. Shaped like a "V," its attachment is located on the crest of the pubic bone. The paired muscles are connected by a central line of fascia called the linea alba ("white line"). This muscle is divided into four segments by connective tissue. Each of the segments can act independently, thus abdominal tone can vary from upper to lower regions. When good tone is maintained, it supports the position of the digestive organs and maintains healthy spinal posture, thus minimizing pressure on the spinal discs. Among the *most common activities* are sitting up, forcibly rounding your back to stretch it, and curling into "spoon pose" for snuggling your teddy bear or sleeping on your side.

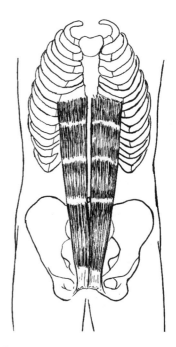

Abdomen—superficial view of rectus abdominis

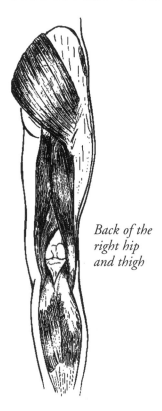

Back of the right hip and thigh

7. HIP EXTENSION

Normal range of motion is 30 degrees. In this motion, the knee rises above the level of the buttock. Analysis of this motion is deceptive, since lumbar flexion accompanies hip ex-

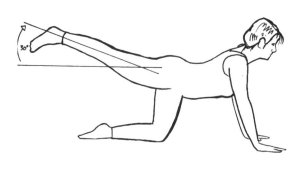

tension and accounts for half the motion (15 degrees). The major muscles performing hip extension are the **hamstrings**, previously shown under knee flexion and the **gluteus maximus**. The gluteus maximus is a potentially powerful hip muscle that also externally rotates the hip. It attaches along the outer portion of the femur and connects through fascia to the iliotibial band of the tensor fascia lata, which also assists in knee extension.

Common motions are the crawl stroke in swimming, and the action of the backward leg during walking and running.

HIP FLEXION

Normal range of motion is 135 degrees. With this free-dom, the thigh can come within two inches of touch-ing the lower ribs. The major muscles are the psoas (tech-nically the combination of the illiacus, which lines the inside of the iliac pelvic bones and psoas attaching to the spine are functionally

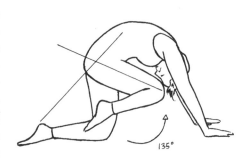

called the iliopsoas) and the rectus femoris (knee extensor) and seven other muscles (five adductors, sartorius, and the tensor fascia lata). The psoas runs from the front to back of the body, from the front groin to the anterior lateral sec-tions of the lumbar spine. The psoas originates from the lateral bodies of the last thoracic (T12) and the first four lumbar (L1–4) vertebrae. The iliacus (adjacent to the psoas) terminates on the internal crest of the pelvis and the lateral bor-der of the sacrum. It also assists in external hip rotation. Just lateral to the psoas is the quadratus lumborum, connecting the iliac crest to the lowest ribs. It serves to elevate the pelvis and laterally flex the spine.

Common motions include squatting, sitting, and lifting your thigh to walk up stairs.

Front of the body, with internal muscles

8. HIP ADDUCTION

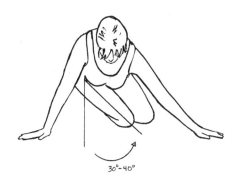

30°-40°

Normal range of motion is 30-40 degrees. In the drawing at left, the left thigh is in abduction, while the right thigh is in adduction. This position creates a contraction of the outer left hip abductors, while the right adductor is contracted. In the full motion, the thigh crosses the centerline to the opposite side. Adduction contracts the groin muscles. The **hip adductors** located in the groin have the most mass of the thigh muscle groups. They all originate from the lower border of the pelvis at the ischium and pubic bones, making them hip flexors. With the exception of the gracilis, which terminates on the tibia, they insert along the femur. The muscles making up this group (viewed from the front uppermost to inferior) include:

1. **Pectineus**

2. **Adductor longus**

3. **Adductor brevis** (behind the pectineus and adductor longus, shown with a dashed line)

4. **Adductor magnus** (the largest, extending from above and behind the pectineus to just above the patella)

5. **Gracilis** (the longest, it is also a knee flexor)

Among the most *common motions* are crossing your thighs when seated, squeezing your thighs while riding horseback, and standing in a long line waiting for the restroom. The yoga posture Face of Light/Cow (Gomukhasana) is normal full range of motion for hip adduction and external rotation.

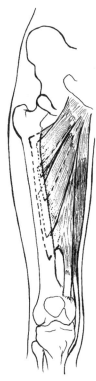

Front of the right thigh

HIP ABDUCTION

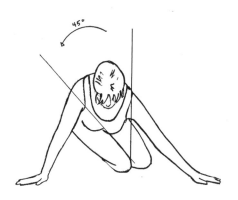

45°

Normal range of motion is 45 degrees. In the drawing at left, the left thigh is in abduction, while the right thigh is in adduction. This position is created by a contraction of the outer left hip abductors, with a mild stretch of the right adductors. The major abductor muscle is the **gluteus medius**. Located anterior and below the gluteus maximus and shaped like an open fan, the gluteus medius originates along the upper outer surface of

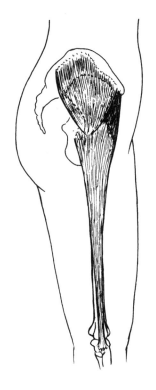

the ilium and attaches on the upper lateral surface of the head of the femur. This muscle's anterior fibers also perform internal hip rotation, while the posterior fibers do external hip rotation. Assistance in this motion comes from the **psoas, sartorius, gluteus minimus, gluteus medius,** and the **tensor fascia lata.**. This latter muscle is shown as the darkest shade attaching to the longest tendon in the body, ending at the lateral tibia.

Common motions include swinging a leg out of a car or spreading your thighs to make a wide sideways step.

Lateral view of right hip

9. WRIST FLEXION

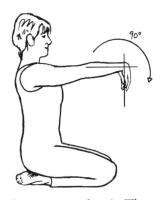

Normal range of motion is 90 degrees. The wrist flexors move the hand though an arc, taking the palm of the hand toward the elbow. Full motion will make a right angle between the forearm and the hand. The major muscles contracting to create this motion attach on the hand. Viewed from their insertions left to right (thumb to little finger), they are the **flexor carpi radialis, palmaris longus** and the **flexor carpi ulnaris**. These are located on the palmar surface of the forearm, originating from the inner bone of the upper arm (humerus).

Common motions are combing your hair and curling weights to your chest with your palms upward.

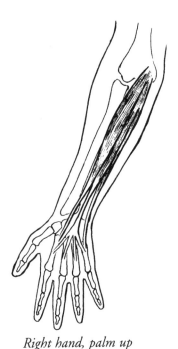

Right hand, palm up

WRIST EXTENSION

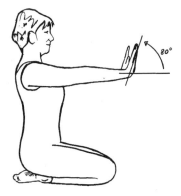

Normal range of motion is 80 degrees. This is stressed by the hyperextension required in certain yoga poses such as Stick, Front Body Stretch (Purvottanasana), and Camel. The usual placement in these poses can aggravate carpal tunnel conditions. To avoid overstretching this motion, I recommend reversing your fingers to point them away from your body during these poses. The major muscles involved are, shown from left to right on page 145, the **extensor carpi ulnaris**, the **extensor carpi radialis brevis**, and the **extensor carpi radialis longus**. All originate on the lateral elbow at the humerus. The ulnaris ends at the wrist base of the little finger. The brevis ends at the wrist base of the middle finger. The longus ends at the base of the 2nd metacarpal bone.

This *motion* is used to indicate "stop." These muscles are constantly contracting during keyboarding activities.

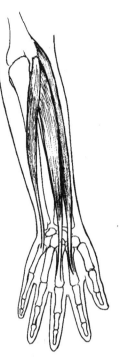

Back of the right hand

10. RADIAL DEVIATION

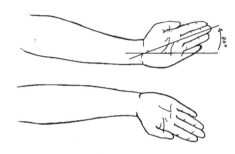

Normal range of motion is 20 degrees. The movement is an arc from a neutral position. The thumb moves toward the radial bone. The muscles strengthened by the movement are the flexor and extensor carpi radialis; both were cited previously in wrist flexion and wrist extension.

A *common motion* is cleaning the outermost sections of a table-top or window.

ULNAR DEVIATION

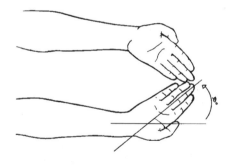

Normal range of motion is 30 degrees. The little finger moves toward the ulnar bone. The muscles strengthened are the **flexor** and **extensor carpi ulnaris**, shown previously under wrist extension.

A *common motion* is turning a dial clockwise with the right hand.

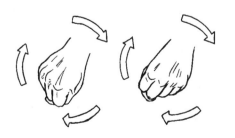

11. WRIST ROTATION

Wrist rotation is a combination of the four preceding motions utilizing all the muscles previously cited. To create a fluid motion, the full range of carpal joints must be free.

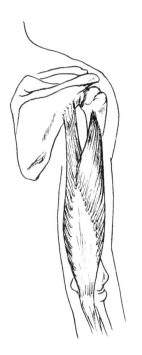

Back of the right shoulder and arm

12. ELBOW EXTENSION

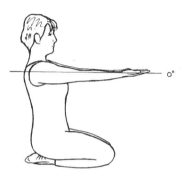

Normal range of motion is 0 degrees—a straight line, with the upper arm level to the forearm. It is fairly common to see women who have a hyperextended elbow, in which the elbow goes above the adjacent segments, often unaccompanied by pain or discomfort. The major muscle contracting to form elbow extension is the **triceps brachii**. Triceps means "three heads," referring to three origins of the muscle. The superior head of the triceps is the lower lateral border of the scapula; the other "heads" are on the upper sections of the humerus. The insertion point is the point of the elbow (ulna's olecranon process). The triceps brachii also performs shoulder extension.

Among the *common movements* are putting down a weight carried in your arms, the end of a golf or baseball swing, and throwing a ball.

ELBOW FLEXION

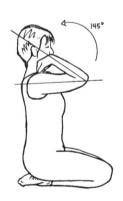

Normal range of motion is 145 degrees, a point at which the biceps will make contact with the forearm. It is common for women to have a carrying angle in which the forearm deviates from making a straight line with the upper arm. Usually, there is no discomfort associated with this, though it may give a leverage disadvantage in attempts to strengthen the elbow flexors, the biceps and shoulder flexors, and the deltoids. The **biceps brachii** of the upper arm has two heads or origins, both located on the front surface of the scapula. The terminus of the muscle is on the upper medial section of the radius. Due to this attachment point, the muscle also contracts to supinate the forearm, turning the palm up.

Another muscle in elbow flexion is the **brachioradialis** extending the length of the forearm. Due to its leverage advantage over the biceps, it is a comparatively stronger muscle.

Common activities involving this motion are picking up a bag of groceries or a child, hugging a friend, and embracing.

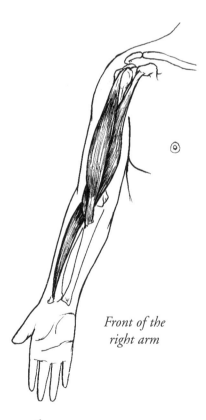

Front of the right arm

13. SHOULDER ABDUCTION
(Horizontal Extension)

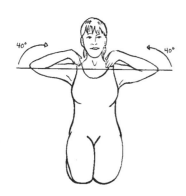

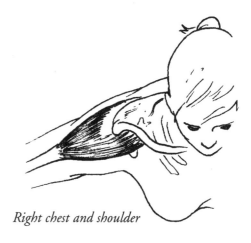

Right chest and shoulder

Normal range of motion is 40 degrees in a posterior direction. In a full motion, the upper arm will move backward, completely out of sight, when facing directly forward. The muscle contracting is the posterior **deltoid**. It originates from the front outer third of the collarbone and connects to the back along the spine (ridge line) of the shoulder blade. Its fibers are involved in all lifting and rotating of the arm. This is a commonly weak muscle, often associated with chronic neck tension. To test it, hold your arms straight out for one minute without lifting your shoulders.

This is often the *first motion* of the day, the morning yawn and stretch. When you reach up overhead to get something from a high shelf, you are contracting your deltoids.

SHOULDER ADDUCTION

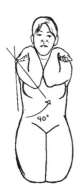

(Horizontal Flexion)

Normal range of motion is 130 degrees, allowing the elbows to touch, and also cross each other in front of the chest. This is the motion required to complete the Eagle Pose (Garudasana). In this pose (not shown in this book), the arms are crossed above the elbow then intertwined in front of the chest.

The muscles contracting to form the motion are the **pectoralis major** and the **anterior deltoid,** assisted by the biceps brachii and coracobrachialis. The pectoralis major covers the entire chest, originating from the central third of the collarbone, the breastbone, and the cartilage of the first six ribs. It lies beneath the breast tissue and helps to support their shape. It also contracts during shoulder internal rotation and shoulder depression. The **anterior deltoid** creates the rounded contour of the front of the shoulders.

Common activities using this motion are when you reach across the chest to your opposite side. It is unfortunately used as a means to protect our emotional and physical hearts.

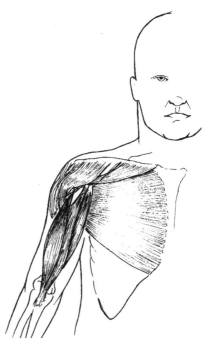

Right chest and shoulder

147

14. SHOULDER EXTERNAL ROTATION

Normal range of motion is 90 degrees. If this motion is done against a wall, the entire shoulder, arm, and hand lie flat to the wall. The prime movers are, from top to bottom, the **posterior deltoid, infraspinatus** and the **teres minor.**

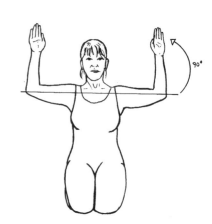

1. **Posterior deltoid** lies in an oblique line from the spine of the scapula to the lateral arm (humerus).

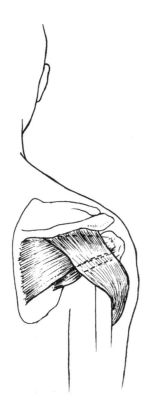

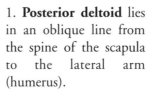

Back of the right shoulder

2. **Infraspinatus** covers the basin of the shoulder blade. It starts on the inner two-thirds of the basin and inserts on the lateral head of the arm.

3. **Teres minor** begins on the armpit border of the shoulder blade and attaches just below the infraspinatus to the posterior humerus.

This is the windup *motion* of throwing a ball, or the action of your arms as they reach back to remove a coat.

SHOULDER INTERNAL ROTATION

Normal range of motion is 80 degrees. When performed sitting with the back and head against a wall, the shoulder and elbow would remain on the wall, but the wrist does not touch. The primary muscles contracting to form the motion are the **clavicular** portion of the **pectoralis major, latissimus dorsi, anterior deltoid** and the **teres major.** The pectoralis major and anterior deltoid were covered in shoulder adduction. The latissimus dorsi and the teres major were covered with shoulder extension.

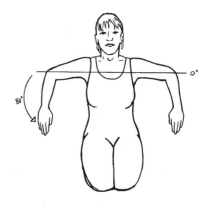

Movements include putting on your coat, putting your hands on your heart, or attaching your bra behind your back.

15. SHOULDER FLEXION

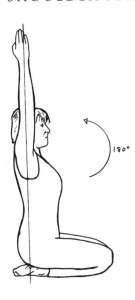

Normal range of motion is 180 degrees. Full range is achieved when the arm is in a straight line with the torso and directly adjacent to the ear. The prime movers to this position are the **anterior deltoid, biceps brachii, coracobrachialis,** and the **upper** or **clavicular** section of the **pectoralis major.** With the exception of the coracobrachialis, located below and medial to the biceps brachii, these muscles were shown previously in shoulder adduction and elbow flexion.

This *movement* is used to reach overhead and is often seen on winter Sundays signaling a touchdown.

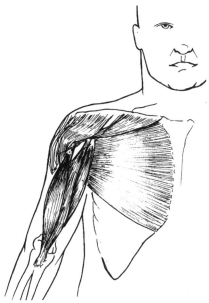

Right chest and shoulder

SHOULDER EXTENSION

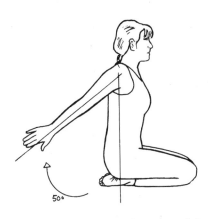

Normal range of motion is 50 degrees. In this vertical motion, the arm is brought back and upward, halfway toward the horizontal. The primary movers are the **latissimus dorsi, triceps brachii,** and the **teres major.** The latissimus also internally rotate the shoulder. These muscles are assisted by the posterior deltoid and infraspinatus (both shown under external rotation).

1. Latissimus dorsi covers two-thirds of the middle and lower back. It originates from the central points of the lower six thoracic (beneath the trapezius), lumbar, and sacral vertebras, and the medial half of the pelvic crest (iliac). It ends in a groove located just below the medial head of the upper arm (humerus).

2. Teres major originates from the lower section of the shoulder blade (above the latissimus) and terminates just behind the latissimus on the upper arm.

This *motion* is the backswing windup of bowling, the backstroke of sawing, or pulling a ski pole behind you for more speed.

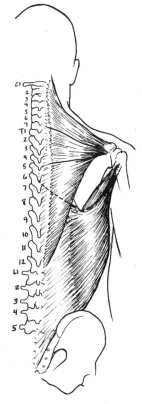

Back of the right side

149

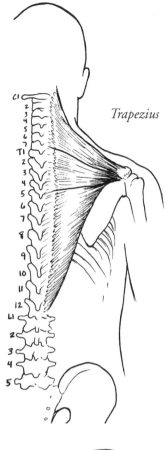

Trapezius

16. SCAPULA ADDUCTION

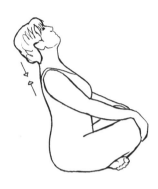

Normal range of motion is not established. A full movement squeezes both shoulder blades close enough that the spine is not visible between them. The model in the drawing to the right is also doing spinal extension. The major mover for this motion is the **middle trapezius**, between T1–T5. The **upper trapezius**, between C1–C7, pulls the scapula in and upward, while the **lower trapezius**, between T6–T12, pulls the scapula in and downward. The trapezius originates from the points of the seventh cervical and all the thoracic vertebrae, and from the occipital ridge at the base of the skull. It inserts on the full-length upper border of the scapula's spine to the acromion. An assist in the motion comes from the **rhomboids** (not shown), located below the middle trapezius. This muscle elevates the scapula as it adducts them.

This *motion* is used in bringing the body down during a pushup and in pulling the shoulders together to stretch the chest, a good idea following a long drive.

SCAPULA ABDUCTION

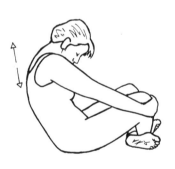

Normal range of motion is not established. The movement, in this case, is accentuated by adding spinal flexion. The primary mover of scapula abduction is the **serratus anterior**. The muscle literally wraps around the rib cage, with its insertion on the underside medial border of the scapula. Its origins are the upper borders of the first eight or nine ribs. Due to individual differences, some people have a larger muscle that extends further. When the shoulders are fixed, it can become an accessory muscle, aiding deep respiration.

This *motion* is utilized in the lifting phase of a push-up or Cat Lift Pose, and the embrace of a big teddy bear. To develop its full strength, you must exaggerate the rounding (flexion) of the thoracic spine. In so doing, this often releases chronic shoulder, upper back, and neck pain.

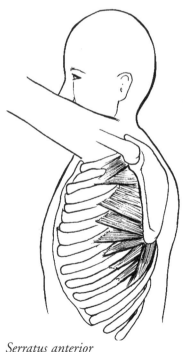

Serratus anterior

17. SPINE LATERAL FLEXION

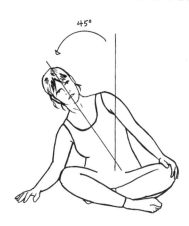

Normal range of motion is not established (though it appears to be 45 degrees). With this mobility, the breastbone comes nearly halfway to the floor, while the shoulders stay vertically aligned and the pelvis stationary. There are four principal muscles involved, to create flexion to the right. All the muscles on the right side contract.

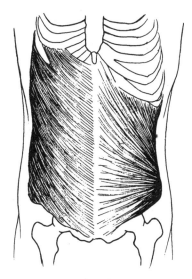

External and internal abdominis obliques

1. **External abdominis oblique** (shown on the left of the anatomy drawing), which originates from the lower edge of the eight lower ribs and inserts into the front half of the pelvic (iliac) crest, the pubic bone, and the abdominal central tendon.

2. **Internal abdominis oblique** (shown on the right), which begins on the lower border of the cartilage of the lower three ribs and inserts just beneath the external oblique on the iliac, the central tendon, and the lumbar fascia.

3. **Quadratus lumborum** (shown under hip flexion, lateral to the psoas) begins on the posterior iliac crest and inserts into the middle half of the lowest rib and the transverse processes of the first four lumbar vertebrae.

4. **Erector spinae** (shown under spine extension).

5. **Latissimus dorsi** (shown under shoulder extension) will assist when the shoulders are actively extended.

We use this *motion* to pick up something from the floor beside our chair, or during the "wave" at ball games.

18. SPINE ROTATION

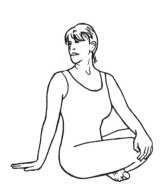

Normal range of rotation is not established. It is greater, however, in the upper segments of the spinal column than in the lumbar. From a yogic perspective, the shoulder girdle will rotate 45 degrees so that the center of the chest will face halfway to the hip joint. The muscles contracting to turn right are the **right latissimus dorsi**, **left external abdominus oblique**, and the **right internal abdominus oblique** (shown above, right).

This *motion* is used when reaching behind your car seat to get something in the back seat, loosening or cracking your back, and in twisting dance motions.

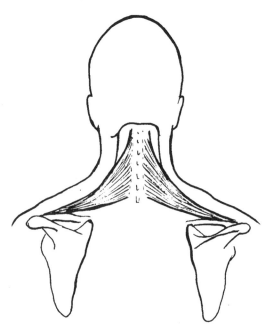

Upper trapezius muscles

19. NECK EXTENSION

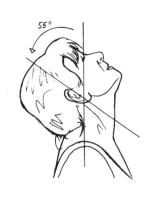

Normal range of motion is 55 degrees, enabling the forehead to come nearly parallel with the floor without moving the midback. At full extension, you can look at a point directly above you. The primary muscle contracting in cervical extension is the **upper trapezius**. It also elevates the scapulae. Accessory muscles in the movement are located deep to the trapezius.

What a rare *motion* to look up at the stars and wonder!

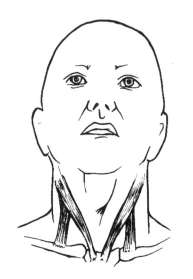

Sternocleidomastoid

NECK FLEXION

Normal range of motion is 45 degrees, which enables your field of vision to see your entire upper chest. The primary muscle contracting is the **sternocleidomastoid**, so named for the three bones to which it attaches. The muscle originates from the upper breastbone (sternum) and the upper middle collarbone (clavicle), to insert behind the ear on the skull (mastoid).

A most *common motion* is looking down at what's beneath us. Yet, with humility, looking down brings us to the sanctum sanctorum, that is our own Heart.

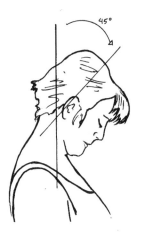

20. NECK LATERAL FLEXION

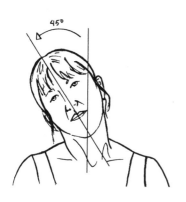

Normal range of motion is 45 degrees, or halfway to the shoulder. When the muscles and joints are free, this is done without rotating the face downward. The muscles contracting to tilt the head to the right are the right upper trapezius, the right **sternocleido-mastoid**.

While uncommon here in the West, except out of discomfort from tensions in one side of the neck, in India this motion, done quickly, means, "acha" (Hindu for "I understand," or "I agree").

21. NECK LATERAL ROTATION

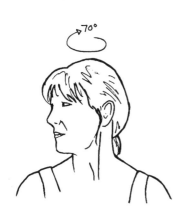

Normal range of motion is 70 degrees, which will enable you to look over your shoulder and see your upper shoulder blade. When the cervical motion is free, the head will remain level as it rotates. To rotate the head to the right, the primary contracting muscles are the **left sternocleidomastoid** and the **right upper trapezius**. Both muscles were detailed previously in neck flexion and neck extension, respectively.

The *motion*, often strained, of looking over your shoulder while your back is fixed as in a car seatbelt, or shaking your head to indicate "no."

CHART 2
SUMMARY OF
JOINT MOBILITY

DATE: _____

Movements that are limited _____

_____

_____

_____

_____

Muscles to be stretched _____

_____

_____

_____

_____

Movements that are excessive _____

_____

_____

_____

Muscles to be strengthened _____

_____

_____

_____

_____

Chapter 17

OPTIMIZING MOBILITY
AND STRENGTH

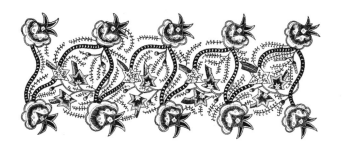

While a main purpose of the Pavanmuktasana series is to normalize the range of motion of each individual joint, some joints function most efficiently when used in combination with others. I have found that the following mobilizing exercises are quite helpful in learning to isolate individual muscles and functional groups. These exercises will enable you to isolate muscular strength within yoga poses, maximize your joint mobility, and heighten concentration. For instance, you will learn how to mobilize the lower back or pelvic girdle while the rest of your body is stationary. This permits a full range of motion of the back within every phase of entering, retaining, and coming out of the most common yoga poses.

An ideal for advanced students is to hold a yoga posture at any phase of the range of motion. Therefore, adept Hatha Yoga teachers are able to present their bodies at the level of flexibility and stamina of the students they are teaching. These exercises help them to adapt the movements to the level of their students, rather than just doing the yogasanas in a way suitable to their own personal practice. By learning how to adjust your own flexibility, you will find that you can challenge different muscle groups and combinations of muscles, thus building optimal strength. With practice, these exercises will enable you to focus strength to specific muscles, thereby enhancing the overall benefits of yogasanas. People who have mastered this principle often find that it makes them more adaptable in life.

As stated previously, muscles function by antagonistic motions—that is, when one muscle contracts, its antagonist must completely relax in order to activate the full potential for strength. When you become conscious of this symbiotic relationship between the two sides of movement, your muscles can be made stronger and will relax more effectively. From training in this manner, a yogi's body becomes sleek and slender, with well-defined muscle tone.

This short series is composed of movements that are not traditional yoga postures. These movements, however, can isolate the intricate motions of the spine, making the more challenging components of "advanced" yogasanas more easily attainable. I have found that, without these exercises, it often takes months for students to gain competency in the fundamental yogasana series.

The following sequence will reveal a way to do the Joint-Freeing Series with variations to isolate the challenge to strengthen commonly weak muscles. This series is particularly beneficial for students who have chronic tensions and pain. Without understanding what motions are restrained and what underlying muscles are weak, you will continue to avoid toning your weakened muscles. Often, weakness is due to the body compensating by over-utilizing adjacent muscles. Postural misalignments will continue, despite more attempts at physical fitness, because your body uses postural muscles in habitual patterns. This often occurs at the expense of efficiency, resulting in specific, chronically weak muscles. When weakened or tight muscles are balanced and made functional, all adjacent regions improve their functions. Our body was designed by the Master Creator for optimal efficiency. When we learn how it functions, we can regain harmony with the underlying creative force.

WALL HANG

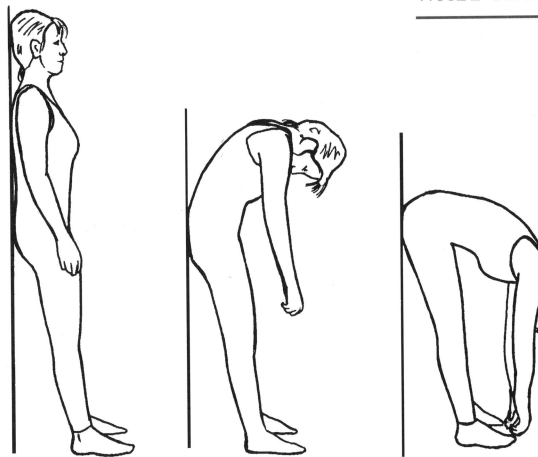

PRECAUTIONS

This movement is a powerful practice in releasing stress and lowering blood pressure. For some people the change in posture, coupled with changes in blood pressure, may be extreme. I have measured up to a 30-point drop in systolic blood pressure in students after doing the Wall Hang. It is very important that you breathe deeply and fully throughout the exercise. Changes in blood pressure may cause dizziness during forward bending. If you feel dizzy at any point in this process, squat or sit down. If dizziness persists, lie down and rest until it passes. If you have low blood pressure, hold your head up so that you are looking forward as you forward bend. With time, your baroreceptors, located in the sides of the neck in the carotid arteries, will begin to function better and regulate blood pressure changes due to body positioning.

If you have sciatic pain (i.e., shooting pain down your hip or the back of your thighs), do only the first two phases. Test yourself to see where the stretch feelings become uncomfortable. While it is important to learn to receive the benefits of this profound exercise, it is more important that you not overtax yourself. If this motion does not release tension, avoid the pose until it becomes effective.

BREATHING

Allow your breath to be deeper than normal, with a continuous flow throughout the exercise. It is very important that your breath be full throughout the exercise. Breathe through your nose, except when you feel increased tension. Then, breathe through your mouth, loudly and fully, making an audible sighing sound to help you focus on releasing stress and tension from the specific regions being affected at each phase of the forward motion.

INSTRUCTIONS

Stand with your buttocks, shoulders, and head resting against the wall. Place your feet 12 inches from the wall, keeping them parallel and slightly wider than hip-width apart. Until you are used to this exercise, keep your eyes open. Move slowly. The Wall Hang should take at least one minute to reach the limit of your forward bend and slightly less time to come back up. The spine is brought down slowly in four phases:

Phase One—The Head

Relax your face and jaw, releasing the lower jaw by opening the mouth for several breaths. Begin to move your head slowly off the wall without moving your shoulder blades. Let your head hang loosely forward as you take several deep breaths.

Phase Two—The Shoulders

Slowly round your shoulders, moving them forward off the wall. Stop when you feel the vertebrae of the upper and mid spine against the wall. Rest here for a while to release the holding patterns of your neck and upper back muscles. Let your arms hang freely in front of your thighs.

Phase Three—The Lower Spine

Tilt the top of your pelvis back, so that your lower back is pressed into the wall. Continue folding forward until only your lower spine is in contact with the wall. Your arms hang free and loose, with your hands below the knees. Breathe deeply and feel the pressure of the lower back into the wall. If your hamstrings feel tight, focus on rooting your feet into the floor, allowing gravity to increase its sucking effect from the bottom of your body toward the Earth. If the effect is experienced as a strain in your lower back, bend your knees. This will transfer the stretch to your hamstrings. It is important to keep the effect in your legs, as this minimizes potential strain in the back. The desired effect is to release the spine passively (not through actively stretching downward).

Phase Four—The Hips

Increase your pelvic tilt by contracting your abdominal muscles and pressing your lower back into the wall. This will allow your hips to slide up the wall, freeing your hamstrings to stretch and your lower pelvis to rotate foward and upward. Pause in the full forward-bending position until you feel rested. Let your breathing become regular and deep. For a few moments, bend your knees to allow your hands to touch the floor.

RELEASING THE POSTURE

Before you start to come back erect, bend your knees more to take the pull off your lower back and hamstrings. This causes your quadriceps and abdominal muscles to work harder. Your legs may even tremble at the effort. In coming back up, use your pelvic tilt to press, first your sacral area, and then your lumbar spine to the wall, one vertebra at a time. This must be accomplished by a strong contraction in your abdominal muscles, from lower abdomen, to navel, to upper abdomen.

Pause for a moment to stabilize your breathing at phase three, then gradually bring the rest of your spine back to the wall to rest at phase two, with your shoulders remaining open and your arms and head hanging freely. Then slowly roll the rest of your body to the wall until you are erect.

Once you are comfortable in the standing position, stretch your arms up the wall. Open your fingers to stretch the full length of your arms, shoulders, and spine. Inhale deeply and extend your arms out to the side, then down to a natural, relaxed position.

Common Errors:	*Correction:*
Going into the pose too quickly	Take a minimum of 30 seconds to go to full Wall Hang
Staying in the forward bend too long	*Adapt* the stay to your comfort level
Coming out of the posture too quickly	Take as long to come up as you do to go down
Strain in the lower back	Make sure you bend your knees more to work your quadriceps
Tension of the shoulders	Don't move too quickly in phases one and two, and make sure you drop your shoulders

BENEFITS

The Wall Hang is one of the most profound stress-relieving exercises. The inverted position of the neck and upper back reverses the gravitational accumulation of stress and tension along the spine and shoulders caused by gravity. The Wall Hang relieves tension even more rapidly than yoga's best-known relaxation posture—Savasana, the Corpse Pose. It is, therefore, ideal as a brief "stress break" during work hours. The benefits are well worth the brief time it takes to perform. The Wall Hang also trains you to become sensitive to the specific regions of stress along your back and shoulders. It can promote a release of deep-seated tensions of the erector spinae muscles located deepest to the spinal column. These muscles are active every time we sit or stand erect.

PREPARATION FOR

Extended Triangle (Utthita Trikonasana), Downward Facing Dog (Adho Mukha Svanasana), and in general for all forward-bending poses, whether done in standing or sitting positions. It is a good preparation for Intensive Stretch (Uttanasana).

HALF-FORWARD BEND

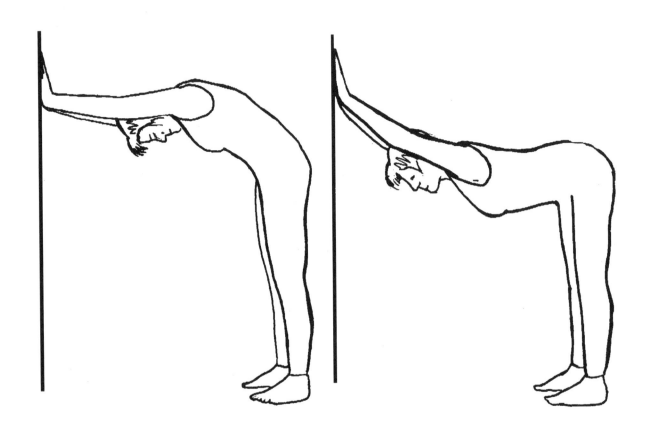

PRECAUTIONS

If you have sciatic pain (i.e. shooting pain down your hip or in back of your thighs), do only the first two phases. If this is not comfortable, avoid the pose until it is. (Focus instead on Cobra and Locust Poses.) If it is comfortable, go to phase three and hold this with steady breathing.

INSTRUCTIONS

Face the wall, standing about three feet from it. Place your palms on the wall at lower-chest height, with your hands about six inches wider than shoulder width. Exhale as you bend forward so that your legs are parallel to the wall and perpendicular to the floor. Your back and arms will be nearly parallel to the floor. Push the wall, while stretching your hips back. Stay for 6 breaths. Inhale as you lift your arms. Your hands will pull you up while your mid back resists the motion. Repeat three times.

VARIATIONS

1. Lift your upper back to relieve tension there and in your shoulders. Press down as you inhale and release as you exhale. Repeat the motion 6–10 times, in a manner similar to the flexing motions of Cat Pose, to develop strength in your upper back and flexibility in your shoulder joints.

2. Raise your head and look at the wall. Your upper back is to remain stationary, with only your lower back moving. As you exhale, contract your abdomen and thrust your pubic region forward, rounding your lower spine. As you inhale, tilt your lumbar spine forward to flatten and extend your lower back. Repeat 6–10 times. This isolates your lumbar spine and develops strength in the erector spinae and psoas muscles.

3. To stretch exceptionally tight hamstrings more gradually, start with your hands below standing shoulder height and bend your knees. Hold your upper back still, while creating movement in the lumbar spine as in variation number 2. Repeat 6–10 times.

Common Errors:	Correction:
Stressing your shoulders and neck	Place your hands wider and/or higher
Holding your head up	Look at the space between your feet
Straining your lower back	Bend your knees

BENEFITS

The full seated forward bends—Westside Back Stretch (Paschimottanasana) and Head-to-Knee Pose (Janu Sirsasana)—take time and persistence to master. Half-forward bend allows you to explore the intricacies of your spine. Over time, your spine will gain greater freedom of motion, allowing each individual vertebra independent motion.

PREPARATION FOR

Stick (Dandasana), Downward Facing Dog (Adho Mukha Svanasana), and all standing forward bends. The motion itself is essentially Half-Intensive Stretch Pose (Ardha Uttanasana). It develops the lower back strength necessary for sitting comfortably for sustained pranayama and meditation practices. It also opens your chest and shoulders in preparation for the Downward Facing Dog Pose (Adho Mukha Svanasana) and Warrior I (Virabhadrasana).

RUNNER'S STRETCH

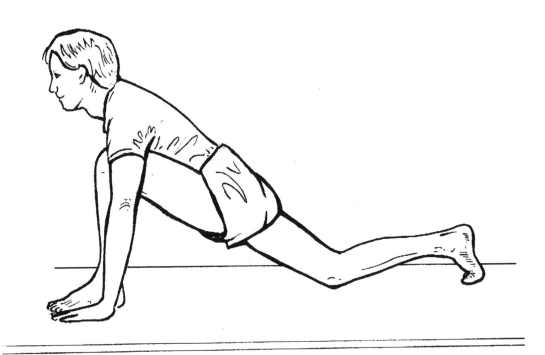

This is the fifth movement of the Sun Salutation (Surya Namaskar).

PRECAUTIONS

If you have low back pain, sciatica, or are in the last trimester of pregnancy, adapt this exercise by keeping your torso lifted. It will be safer if you lift your abdomen off your legs; i.e., do not lean forward over your legs. If necessary, you can place your hands on your thighs, to bring your pelvis lower than your knee joint.

INSTRUCTIONS

Begin on your hands and knees in the Cat Pose (Marjarasana), and then bring your left leg forward between your hands. Adjust the distance until your shin is at a right (90 degree) angle and your right leg is extended back as far as is comfortable. Your abdomen will be resting adjacent to your left thigh. Keep the toes of your right foot tucked forward. Use your hands to help support you as you slowly allow your weight to move forward and down. This may create a stretch in the front (quadricep muscles) of your right thigh and/or in the back of your left thigh (hip extensors—hamstrings and gluteus maximus). If your muscles release, your hip will lower and your left knee will extend beyond your ankle. In this event, move your foot and hands forward to maintain the 90-degree angle of your shin to the floor. Keep your chest and head lifted to create a mild arch in your middle back. Hold for 3–6 breaths.

VARIATIONS

This pose can also be done with the back knee extended, lifted fully from the floor. This variation will lift the pelvic region, which may also help to prevent stress around the inguinal ligament where the pelvis meets your thigh. Keeping your back leg lifted changes the effect on the quadriceps and hip flexors from a stretch to a strengthening action for the quadriceps.

Another variation of this pose is to move your hips and hands back, gently straightening your knee (not shown). Hold this position for 2–3 breaths, with your chest and head extended forward and down, to stretch the back (hamstrings) of your left leg. Repeat three times on each side. Make certain that the distance between your legs is the same when you repeat the movements on the other side.

Common Errors:	Correction:
Straining the groin of your front leg	Lift your torso off your thigh (use a support)
Compression strain of lumbar spine	Narrow the distance between your knees
Stress to the inner knee tendons	Align your knee above your ankle and check to keep your back heel above the ball of your foot

BENEFITS

Focusing the stretch to your hamstrings relieves the muscles of your lower back. In this way, your hip flexor muscles, their antagonists, can more easily develop tone. In turn, this permits your lower back and hip joints to move more freely. The motion also provides a stretch to the adductors, which are often neglected in stretching programs. Adductors are also hip flexors and external rotators; stretching them promotes hip mobility as well. A focus on the quadriceps stretch can deepen to a stretch of the upper groin, where your hip flexors, including the psoas muscles, are located. This can relieve chronic pressure on your lumbar spine. Together, these two stretches bring freedom of movement and length to the spine and are excellent before and after running or walking.

PREPARATION FOR

Closed-hip standing poses that tone the inner thighs and stretch the outer thighs, such as Intensive Side Stretch (Parsvottanasana) and Warrior I (Virabhadrasana).

GROIN STRETCH

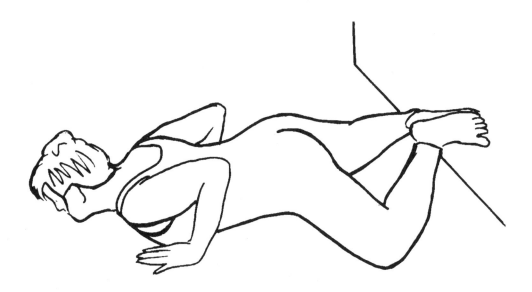

PRECAUTIONS

Move into and out of this stretch slowly.

INSTRUCTIONS

Begin in Cat Pose, then place your knees wide (up to three feet apart) and turn the soles of your feet flat together 6–12 inches up from the floor, pressing them against the wall. Slowly bring your pelvis forward and down. Raise your feet to a level that can accommodate the mobility of your groin. For most students, the pelvic region will not touch the floor when the feet are on the floor. Keep your soles together as you press your lower pelvis toward the floor. Adjust yourself so you feel a stretch, but not a strain. Relax into the pose by letting gravity and your weight stretch your groin. Stay in the pose for thirty seconds to one minute in the beginning. Turn your head to one side for half the holding time, then to the other side for the second half.

End the exercise by slowly raising your feet apart and sliding your thighs together. Reach back to grasp your ankles, then press your heels down near your buttocks. This creates a complimentary stretch to the front of the thighs (quadriceps) and releases the muscles of the groin (adductors). Hold this counter-stretch for fifteen to thirty seconds, with deep breathing. If you cannot reach your ankles, repeat the Runner's Stretch as a counter pose.

VARIATION

Support yourself on your forearms and rock your pelvic girdle back and forth about twelve inches. Repeat 6–12 times, holding any phase that reveals specific regional tension. This maneuver will tone the deltoids of the shoulders and provide a range of stretch across the five adductor muscles of your groin region.

Common Errors:	Correction:
Stress at the inner knees	Pad beneath your knee, check symmetry in the alignment of thighs to shins, with your toes turned out
Pain in hip or groin	Lessen the width of your knees, progress slower to full phase

BENEFITS

This motion provides a deep stretch for the groin adductor muscles and increases mobility of the hip joints. Freeing the hips often provides stress relief to the spinal column and major postural muscles. It is frequently beneficial for sciatica by relieving the compensatory tightness of the groin, which is directly opposite to the sciatic nerve. This practice often makes sitting erect in chairs or on the floor more comfortable. This exercise is especially recommended throughout pregnancy to facilitate natural childbirth, and minimize the need for an episiotomy.

PREPARATION FOR

Open-hip poses such as Extended Triangle (Utthita Trikonasana) and Warrior II (Virabhadrasana) as well as sitting and meditation poses.

PELVIC TILT AND THRUST

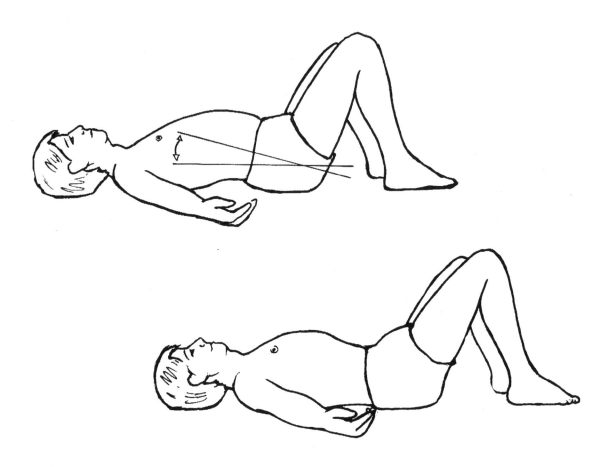

PRECAUTIONS

To keep the lumbar spine comfortable and not strain the sacroiliac joints, avoid over-arching your lower back when doing the upper movement (pelvic tilt).

INSTRUCTIONS

Lie on your back, knees bent, and feet on the floor, hip-width apart and close to your buttocks. As you inhale, let your lower back arch away from the floor (top figure) moving your tailbone downward. Your upper pelvis (iliac) and abdomen will roll forward, your tailbone (coccyx) backward. This phase is called pelvic tilt. As you exhale, contract your lower abdominal muscles and press your lumbar spine toward the floor (bottom figure), lifting your tailbone. This phase is called pelvic thrust.

Isolate the motion to your lower back, keeping the rest of your body relatively still. Focus on separating the five vertebrae of your lumbar spine so that a snake-like undulation is felt throughout your lower back into your pelvis. Repeat a minimum of 10 times.

Common Errors:	*Correction:*
Lifting the pelvis from the floor	Keep your buttocks on the floor
Overarching lumbar spine	If your lumbar spine is hypermobile, limit the range of your pelvic tilt
Shoulders and head moving excessively	Relax your upper body to confine motions to spinal column, yet allow a slight up/down motion of your chin

BENEFITS

The pelvic tilt and thrust stretches the lower back and strengthens muscles of the abdomen, the deep muscles of the lower back, and the pelvic floor. It develops the tone and freedom of the psoas muscle, which can lead to separate movement of the five lumbar vertebrae. The pelvic tilt and thrust in a standing position also strengthens the outer thighs and the muscles of the buttocks. By its capacity to tone your abdominal muscles, it can aid in regulation of breath. Regular practice of this motion can be highly beneficial for pregnant women, as it relieves lower back fatigue and can also be directed to tone the pelvic floor, thus promoting stamina and increased enjoyment of sexual intercourse.

Studies have shown that sexual pleasure increases with an increase in strength of the pelvic floor muscles, the pubococcygeal group, or the PC muscles (see figure 2, page 51). For childbirth and sexual enhancement, practice the root lock (Mula Bandha), which develops the tone of the rings of muscles surrounding the urogential and rectal region. This is done by contracting the PC muscles and buttocks as you exhale, relaxing them as you inhale. Begin slowly and build to 50 repetitions. Your Classical Yoga teacher can present many variations for individual needs. The combination of pelvic tilt and thrust motions are beneficial for many lower abdominal, pelvic, and hip disorders, such as constipation, dysmennorhea, sciatica, arthritis of the hip, and hemorrhoids.

PREPARATION FOR

Bridge (Setubandhasana), Supported Shoulderstand (Salamba Sarvangasana), and yoga breathing practices such as Head Shining (Kapalabhati), and Bellows (Bastrika).

ROLLING BRIDGE POSE

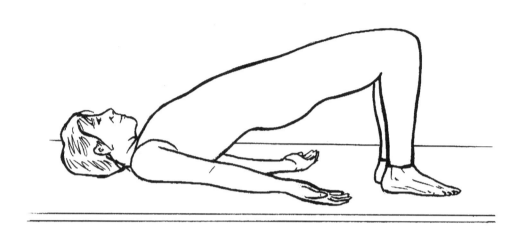

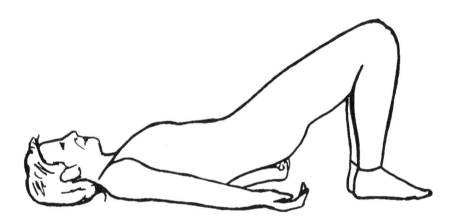

PRECAUTIONS

Avoid overarching your lower back. The effects should be felt in your buttocks or thighs, not in your lower back.

INSTRUCTIONS

Lie on your back, knees bent and feet hip-width apart. Keep your arms straight, palms up beside your hips. Perform the pelvic thrust and, while keeping your buttocks firm, lift your lower pelvis from the floor by leading from the pubic area (pelvic thrust). Come to a height such that the line of your thighs becomes straight and even with the front of your body. Hold the position for three breaths.

Come down by lowering your back from the top of your spine, vertebrae by vertebrae. About halfway down, strengthen the pelvic thrust (lifting your tailbone), lowering your lumbar region to the floor first, then your sacrum (the bone between your buttocks).

Repeat by rolling your spine up from the lower region, until your weight is carried in your shoulders, then roll back down, controlling your spine's flexibility through the strength of your thighs and buttocks. Ideally, coming up and going down will be accomplished by rolling your spine one vertebrae at a time, up and down. Repeat 10 times.

Common Errors:	*Correction:*
Feet misaligned to knees	Hold your knees over your ankles, shins perpendicular to the floor
Strain to inner or outer knee ligaments	Turn your toes outward, while maintaining the distance between your knees

BENEFITS

Practicing the sequence from pelvic tilt, to pelvic thrust, to Bridge Pose, to Rolling Bridge Pose gives flexibility and strength to your spine, hips, and thighs. First, the joints are freed, eliminating stress. Later, the spine and pelvic muscles develop the strength necessary to maintain good posture during prolonged periods of sitting or standing. The inversion also changes the position of the abdominal and pelvic organs, thus flushing them by changing vascular circulation. The Bridge Pose has been used in this variation to aid in prolapse of the uterus and colon, and for keeping the fetus happy during the early stages of pregnancy. It also aids in releasing those cases of lower back pain that may be due to loss of tone in the lumbar and gluteal muscles.

PREPARATION FOR

Bridge Pose (Setubandhasana), Supported Shoulderstand (Salamba Sarvangasana), and other inverted poses. It also tones the abdominal muscles and repositions the organs of digestion, increasing peristalsis and improving their functions. It prepares the body for more demanding practices of pranayamas, like Head Shining (Kapalabhati), Bellows (Bastrika), isolation of the rectus abdominis (Nauli), and cleansing the digestive fire purifications practices (Agnisar Dhouti Kriyas).

Chapter 18

MUSCLE STRENGTHENING USING THE JOINT-FREEING SERIES

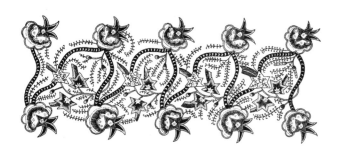

Physical therapists grade the level of muscle strength according to five degrees.[1]

Grade 5 (Normal)—This value is accompanied by the ability to complete a full range of motion and maintain the end-point range against maximum resistance.

Grade 4 (Good)—This value is used to designate a muscle group that is able to complete a full range of motion against gravity and can tolerate strong resistance without breaking the test position. The muscles will "give" out, losing their stamina at the end of its range with maximum resistance.

Grade 3 (Fair)—This level of strength can move through full range of motion against gravity, but mild additional resistance causes the motion to break.

Grade 2 (Poor)—The muscle at this level can complete the full range of motion in a posture that minimizes the force of gravity.

Grade 1 (Trace)—The examiner can detect visually or by means of palpation some contractile activity in one or more muscles that participate in the movement being tested. However, there is no movement as a result of this minimal contractile activity.

A physiologist named Sharrard counted alpha motor neurons in the spinal cords of poliomyelitis victims at the time of autopsy. "He correlated the manual muscle test

---

[1] Lucille Daniels and Catherine Worthingham, *Therapeutic Exercise for Body Ailment and Function* (Philadelphia: W. B. Saunders, 1977), pp. 4–6.

grades in the patient's chart with the number of motor neurons remaining in the anterior horns (of the spinal cord). His data revealed that more than 50 percent of the pool of motor neurons to a muscle group were gone when the muscle test result had been recorded as Grade 4 (Good). Thus, when the muscle can withstand considerable, but less than 'normal' resistance, it has already been deprived of at least half of its innervation."[2]

Based on the previously cited scale, I have composed a student self-evaluation scale for the Joint-Freeing Series.

> Grade 5. Full strength—an ability to hold the pose steadily and comfortably without trembling at any position along its arc of range of motion for 12 full breaths.

> Grade 4. Average Strength— an ability to hold the position steadily and comfortably at only the end point of full range of motion for 12 breaths.

> Grade 3. Fair Strength—the posture can be done for 6 to 12 breaths with the requisite muscles functioning fully, and is accompanied with mild discomfort and trembling.

> Grade 2. Poor Strength—the posture cannot be achieved with the designated muscles contracting. The body compensates and does a rudimentary resemblance of the pose using adjacent or accessory muscle groups to achieve the position.

> Grade 1. Trace Strength—the posture is done relying on the joints to hold the position. Minimal muscle strength is utilized. "Locked" or hyperextended joints especially characterize this posture, with soft muscle tissue opposing taut, overstretched muscle tissue. Often seen in hypermobile practitioners doing "advanced" yogasanas.

This scale can also be used to evaluate your progress in all the Classical Yoga postures. By keeping an accurate record of your practice, you can more readily determine your progress in making changes to your health and stamina. It may be ideal to have your instructor evaluate you according to these standards, especially if you are uncertain of your performance in the yoga poses, or to find out whether you are using the proper muscles meant to be utilized in the yogasanas.

Many of the joint-freeing motions can also be used as an evaluation of muscle strength for some of the major muscles of the body. By holding the following poses you can isolate the appropriate muscles and test their strength.

If, upon testing yourself with these motions, you determine the muscles are weak, repeat the test position as a way to develop stamina. For this type of regular practice, go in and out of the motion, while taking steady full breaths. Once a week, repeat the test, holding the poses, to determine how long you can hold the position steadily and comfortably.

---

2 W. J. W. Sharrard, "Muscle Recovery in Poliomyelitis," *Journal of Bone Joint Surgery* (1955): 37B, pp. 63–69.

If the region you find weak has been a source of pain, either acute or chronic, give yourself at least six weeks of regular practice, regardless of how quickly you reach the goal of holding the motion for twelve steady breaths.

Joint-Freeing Series Variations

The details for these motions can be found in chapter 15. The numbers assigned to the movements here correspond to those shown in figure 19 (pages 132–133). Test your progress against the above standards, then practice the movements regularly as necessary. Modify them as described to optimize the strength of the muscles cited. As a final step, summarize your findings on the Muscular Strength Evaluation form at the end of the chapter (see pages 182–183).

❖ LATISSIMUS DORSI MUSCLE

1. Stick Pose, lifting your chest with your hands turned backward behind your hips. Do this motion with your hands placed farther back and wider than the basic position to optimize the tone of shoulder and thoracic extension.

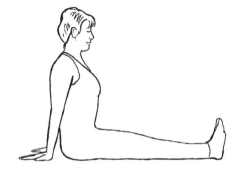

PREPARATION FOR

Extended Triangle (Utthita Trikonasana), Downward Facing Dog (Adho Mukha Svanasana), Bridge (Setubandhasana), Half-Supported Shoulderstand (Ardha Salamba Sarvangasana), and Camel (Ustrasana).

❖ HIP FLEXORS AND KNEE EXTENSOR MUSCLES (QUADRICEPS)

4. This is a straight leg lift without aid of the arms. In doing this motion to tone these muscles, avoid using your abdominals and keep your back still. Watch for a tendency to round your lower back. Only lift your leg to a height where your back begins to react. To work the hip flexor muscles, especially psoas and rectus femoris, bend your knee and continue to pull your thigh toward the torso.

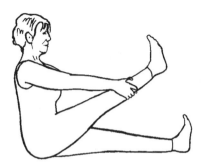

PREPARATION FOR

Upward Stretched-Leg Pose (Urdhva Prasarita Padasana), Supported Shoulderstand (Ardha Salamba Sarvangasana), and Complete Boat (Paripurna Navasana).

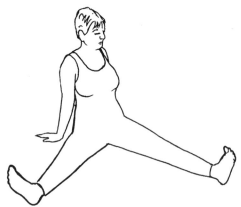

❖ HIP EXTERNAL ROTATORS, INCLUDING PSOAS

5a. From the Stick Pose, turn your thigh outward from your hip. Keep your foot 3–6 inches from the floor and your feet at least 36 inches apart. As you rotate your lower leg outward, you will be strengthening the major muscle of external hip rotation in the front of the body, the psoas. The external hip rotator group is located deep to the gluteus maximus and is more effective with the hip in extension than in flexion, as when you do this motion from the Sunbird Pose (#7 of the Joint-Freeing Series—Chakravakasana).

PREPARATION FOR

Extended Triangle (Utthita Trikonasana), Warrior II (Virabhadrasana), and Bound Angle (Baddha Konasana).

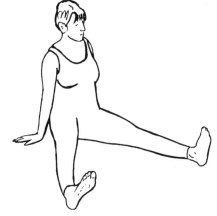

❖ HIP INTERNAL ROTATOR MUSCLES (TENSOR FASCIA LATA AND GLUTEUS MEDIUS)

5b. From the Stick Pose, turn your thigh inward from your hip. With this motion, your hip will tend to lift, to the point that your buttock may be lifted from the floor. To have an accurate test, keep your buttocks on the floor. The optimal position is as shown with your foot 3–6 inches off the floor.

PREPARATION FOR

Warrior I (Virabhadrasana), Side of Hip Stretch (Parsvottanasana), Abdominal Twist (Jathara Parivartanasana), and Spinal Twist (Marichyasana).

❖ SPINE EXTENSION (ERECTOR SPINAE)

6a. From the Cat Pose, let your spine sink to form a groove from base of your neck to your waist. While doing the Cobra Pose done without the aid of your arms is a better test of these muscles, this is nonetheless accurate for a basic assessment. Check to feel if your spine is evenly pulled downward, forming a symmetrical groove down the full length of

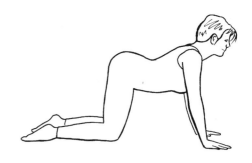

your back. Have a friend tell you if there are any visible differences from the base of your spine to your neck region. Often, a section only two to three vertebrae long may be weak. By focusing your attention on flexing this region, its stamina and mobility will be increased.

PREPARATION FOR

Extended Triangle (Utthita Trikonasana), Bridge (Setubandhasana), Supported Shoulderstand (Salamba Sarvangasana), Stick (Dandasana), Cobra (Bhujangasana), and Locust (Salambhasana).

❖ SCAPULA ADDUCTION (MIDDLE TRAPEZIUS)

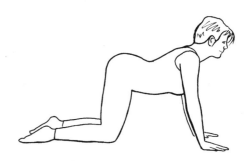

6b. This same motion (the Cat Pose) can be accentuated to assess scapula adduction. By squeezing your scapula together as you press your spine down, the middle trapezius is toned. The motion should be done with your neck lengthening, rather than pulling the back of your head toward your scapula to look up.

PREPARATION FOR

Bridge (Setubandhasana), Supported Shoulderstand (Salamba Sarvangasana), and Camel (Ustrasana).

❖ SCAPULA ABDUCTION (SERRATUS ANTERIOR) AND THORACIC FLEXION (ABDOMINUS RECTUS)

6c. Cat Pose with your spine pressed upward. In this variation, you keep your head between your arms, and your scapula spread. The arching upward of your spine indicates its flexion capacity. The ideal pose will create a smooth upward C, with the lower pelvis tucked forward, like a dog pulling its tail between its legs. There are two distinct regions active in this motion. Strength of the serratus anterior and a release of the trapezius create the upper back lift. Strength of the rectus abdominis rounds the lumbar spine.

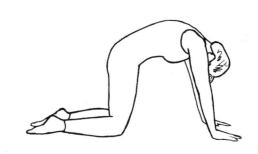

PREPARATION FOR

Fetal Pose (Garbhasana).

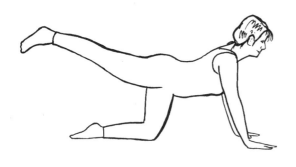

❖ HIP EXTENSORS (GLUTEUS MAXIMUS AND HAMSTRINGS)

7a. In the Sunbird Pose, lift your leg backward, with your foot held above your buttock. This motion tests the strength of your hip extensors one side at a time. As you do the motion, watch to be certain you do not compensate and use adjacent muscles. The back of your pelvis should remain level with the floor and the supporting thigh should remain still. Keep your knee straight and your foot only 6 to 12 inches above the top of your buttocks.

PREPARATION FOR

Warrior I (Virabhadrasana), Bridge (Setubandhasana), and Camel (Ustrasana).

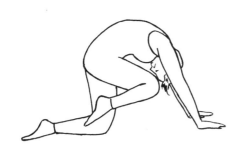

❖ HIP FLEXOR (PSOAS AND RECTUS FEMORIS)

7b. For the Sunbird counter pose, keep your thigh pulled forward, nearly touching your lower ribs, with your thigh pulled up into hip flexion. This exercise uses your abdominals as well, so, for a more accurate test, keep the tension focused to the top of your lifting thigh.

PREPARATION FOR

Side of Hip Stretch (Parsvottanasana), Extended Triangle (Utthita Trikonasana), Downward Facing Dog (Adho Mukha Svanasana), Upward Stretched Legs (Urdhva Prasarita Padasana), Head-to-Knee (Janu Sirsasana), Westside Back Stretch (Paschimottanasana), and Complete Boat (Paripurna Navasana).

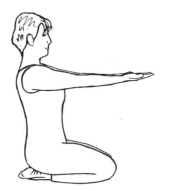

❖ SHOULDER FLEXORS (ANTERIOR DELTOID AND PECTORALIS MAJOR CLAVICULAR)

12. In the Hero Pose, hold your arms parallel to floor. The most accurate test is to keep your arms extended at the elbow rather than flexed. The tendency is to let your shoulders lift toward your ears during this motion, using the commonly over worked upper trapezius, resulting in neck and upper-shoulder tension. Oddly, this is often accompanied by a weakness in the adjacent

muscles, the deltoids. If this pattern is felt, pull your shoulders down and back, then lift your arms to a line parallel with the floor. Repeat the motion to develop stamina and take the effort from the sides of your neck to the tops of your shoulders.

PREPARATION FOR

Extended Triangle (Utthita Trikonasana) and Warrior II (Virabhadrasana).

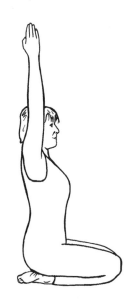

❖ SHOULDER FLEXORS (MIDDLE DELTOID)

15a. From the Hero Pose, move your arms straight up beside your ears. In this motion, the same tendency exists to overwork the upper trapezius and must be watched for. Keep your arms up at the elbows, but your shoulders pulled down and back from your ears.

PREPARATION FOR

Warrior I (Virabhadrasana), Balancing Tree (Vrksasana), Downward Facing Dog (Adho Mukha Svanasana), and Upward Stretched Legs (Urdhva Prasarita Padasana).

❖ SHOULDER EXTENSORS (TRICEPS BRACHII, LATISSIMUS DORSI, AND POSTERIOR DELTOID)

15b. In the Hero Pose, pull your arms straight backward and upward from your hips. Focus your attention on tensing and strengthening the back of your shoulders. If your chest is expanded fully and lifted, these muscles will be drawn into full tone.

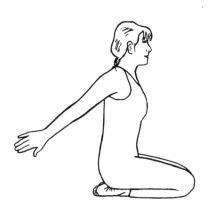

PREPARATION FOR

Bridge (Setubandhasana), Supported Shoulderstand (Salamba Sarvanghasana), and Camel (Ustrasana).

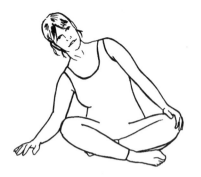

❖ THORACIC LATERAL FLEXION (ABDOMINIS OBLIQUE AND QUADRATUS LUMBORUM)

17. From Easy Pose, seated side bending on the lower side. This is a mild test of the muscles at your waist on both the front and the back. In an accurate test, your body will remain free of rotation. A stronger test of the muscles is to do the movement from a standing position.

PREPARATION FOR

Extended Triangle (Utthita Trikonasana).

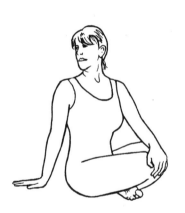

❖ THORACIC LATERAL ROTATION (ABDOMINIS OBLIQUE AND LATISSIMUS DORSI)

18. From Easy Pose, do a seated lateral twist of the upper body. For testing the muscles involved, use your arms only mildly. This will isolate the tone to the sides of your abdomen and back. Maintain the position, with your chest lifted and both scapulas pulled backward.

PREPARATION FOR

Abdominal Twist (Jathara Parivartanasana) and Spinal Twist (Marichyasana).

Additional Muscle Strengthening Poses

Following are some exercises that can help you to tone and strengthen commonly weakened muscles.

❖ SHOULDER STRENGTH
CAT BOW—MARJARASANA

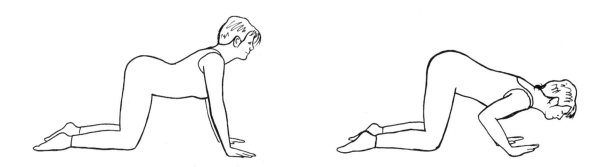

Kali Rae, of Tri Yoga International, to whom I am grateful, showed this movement to me. It has been of tremendous benefit to many students. It is a graded practice toward the sixth movement of the Sun Salutation, called the Eight-Limb Salutation or Ashtanganamaskar.

Begin on your hands and knees, hands shoulder-width apart, fingers pointing straight ahead. Inhale, arching your spine downward into a Cat Lift Pose. Exhale, bending your elbows and lowering your chest in a forward motion. Keep your head up, with your neck long, and your shoulders pulled back and down. Keep your elbows close to your sides. To muscle test, hold this phase of the motion and retain all its features.

After the test, inhale and return to the straight-arm pose. To develop strength, do the motions in rhythm with your breath, exhaling down and inhaling up. Over time, increase your repetitions to twelve to maintain full strength.

VARIATION

Begin as above, but with your hands turned inward, middle fingers aimed directly at each other, elbows going to the side. Repeat six bows, with your elbows aligned straight out from your shoulders. This tones the posterior deltoid and internal shoulder rotators.

BENEFITS

Developing strength in the back of the shoulders (triceps, middle trapezius, latissimus dorsi, and posterior deltoid), and lessening the tendency for rounded shoulders and poor posture. When developed sufficiently, it alleviates the major sources of discomfort during the shoulderstand and headstand, lessening the need for props.

PREPARATION FOR

Bridge (Setubandhasana) and Supported Shoulderstand (Salamba Sarvangasana), as it enhances the natural curve of the cervical region and strengthens the supportive muscles of the neck and head.

❖ NECK STRENGTHENING*

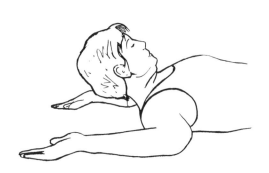

Lie on your back with knees bent and feet close to hips. Place your arms in external shoulder rotation, elbows directly out from shoulders and at right angles. Draw your shoulder blades together and down toward your pelvis to contract your middle and lower trapezius muscle.

1. Exhale and lift your head up, tucking your chin down toward your collarbone. Inhale as you lower your head. Relax all facial and neck muscles completely before you repeat. Repeat the motion gently, stopping when you feel fatigue or shaking. Optimal strength is twelve repetitions.

2. Turn your head to the left. Keeping your arms on the floor, exhale as you lift your head and watch your left elbow. Inhale as you lower your head. Optimal strength is six repetitions. Repeat the motions for your right side.

3. When the optimal level is reached, you may perform the more complex series. Combine the motions, exhaling while lifting your head to center. Keeping your head lifted, rotate to the right, then again to center. Repeat the movement to the left, back to center, and lower slowly while gazing down at your breastbone. Optimum is six slow repetitions.

BENEFITS

This exercise isolates the sternocleidomastoid muscles (see neck flexion, page 152). These muscles rotate the head and flex the neck. They are commonly weak, due to the stress that accumulates in their neighboring muscle, the trapezius. This exercise is of great benefit for chiropractic patients, often eliminating the necessity for frequent neck adjustments.

PREPARATION FOR

Extended Triangle (Utthita Trikonasana), Abdominal Twist (Jathara Parivartanasana),

---

*Precaution: In the event of neck injuries or extreme weakness wherein the head cannot be lifted, the muscles should be isometrically tensed. That is, tense the muscle, visualize the motion but do not actually perform the movement. With patience and persistence, tone will be created and the movement will come gradually to full range.

and Spinal Twist (Marichyasana). This exercise develops the muscle stamina and coordination necessary to maintain alignment of the neck and shoulders during these poses.

VARIATION FOR STABILIZING MISALIGNED VERTEBRAE

Often, people experience their neck going out of alignment. What is occurring is a strong pull on one side of the vertebral column, accompanied by a relaxation of the antagonist muscles on the opposite side. This can result in a slipping, or subluxation, of the vertebrae from adjacent bones. The motion can be lateral, or elevated and lateral combined. In the former case, the individual may experience their head leaning off to the side. When they lie prone, it may be more comfortable to turn the head to one side. In the latter case, the head will be tilted, in addition to being off center.

TEST FOR WEAKENED MUSCLES

Test the lateral rotators by lying supine and lifting your head not more than six inches, then rotating it to test the comparative strength of each side of the neck. The weaker side may tremble when you attempt to hold it still, and/or your chin may lift in an exaggerated fashion. These are signs of a weakness in the sternocleidomastoid on the elevated side of the neck.

REALIGNMENT AND STAMINA BUILDING

Once the position is achieved, hold your head up while it is turned to the side. Keep your shoulder blades back and down, with your arms at your sides. Hold the position as motionless as possible, while taking full deep breaths extending from your chest to your lower abdomen. After a few moments, muscle stamina will be exhausted and you will need to exert sheer willpower to hold your head up. Once this point is reached, you will likely experience trembling. Begin to take deeper breaths for three rounds, then slowly lower your head to center position, and relax, with full breathing, for several moments. Gently roll your head from side to side 3 times. Retest both neck rotators. The goal is to bring muscle tone into a greater balance on both sides. This is often accompanied by a spontaneous realignment of the vertebral column—without the normal cracking sounds associated with a chiropractic neck adjustment. The improved muscle tone gently slides the vertebrae back into alignment.

VARIATION

Sometimes, the vertebrae may have fallen posterior as well as lateral. In this case, the technique needs to be done with your head hanging off a massage or coffee table.

PRECAUTION

Holding the stamina-building position for an excessive length of time can create trembling, or even muscle spasm. Only hold as long as this doesn't occur, and until there is also full deep breathing. When either quality is compromised, relax and lower your head.

CHART 3
MUSCLE STRENGTH EVALUATION SUMMARY

REGION—MUSCLE   FINDINGS/DATES

ANKLE

Dorsi flexion (*anterior tibialis*) _____

Plantar flexion (*gastrocnemius, soleus*) _____

KNEE

Extensors (*quadriceps*) _____

Flexors (*hamstrings*) _____

ABDOMEN—SPINAL COLUMN

Spine flexion (*rectus abdominis*)_____

Spine extension (*erector spinae*) _____

Spine lateral flexion (*erector spinae* and *abdominis oblique*) _____

_____

Spine rotation (*abdominis oblique*) _____

HIPS

Internal rotators (*gluteus medius, tensor fascia lata*) _____

_____

External rotators (*gluteus maximus* and *deep external rotator group*) _____

_____

Extensors (*hamstrings, gluteus maximus*) _____

_____

Flexors (*psoas, rectus femoris*) _____

Adduction *(adductor group)* _____

Abduction *(gluteus medius)* _____

BACK, SHOULDERS, AND CHEST

Elbow extension *(triceps brachii)* _____

_____

Elbow flexion *(biceps brachii)* _____

_____

Shoulder abduction *(middle and posterior deltoid)* _____

_____

Shoulder adduction *(pectoralis major)* _____

_____

Shoulder flexion *(anterior and middle deltoid)* _____

_____

Shoulder extension *(latissimus dorsi)* _____

Shoulder external rotation *(infraspinatus and teres minor)* _____

_____

Shoulder internal rotation *(pectoralis, latissimus dorsi, teres major)* _____

_____

Scapula adduction *(middle trapezius)* _____

_____

Scapula abduction *(anterior serratus)* _____

_____

NECK

Extension *(upper trapezius)* _____

_____

Flexion, Rotation *(sternocleidomastoid)* _____

_____

Chapter 19

PERSONALIZING STRUCTURAL YOGA

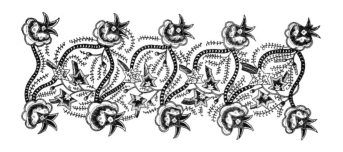

O nce you have examined and tested yourself through the optimizing strength practices, you may begin to see a pattern in these findings and in those from the body reading and joint-freeing analysis. You now have three sources of information that can help you evaluate your muscular balance and joint freedom—one static, through the postural analysis method, and two dynamic, through range-of-motion analysis and muscle-testing of the Joint-Freeing Series. The static method of self-analysis reveals tendencies toward muscular tightness, limited range of motion, and a pre-disposition for muscular weakness. The dynamic method reveals more specifically your limitations of mobility. From this you have created a list of muscles that need to be stretched or toned regularly, until their freedom creates more comfort in your natural daily activities.

There will be some overlap in these findings: some muscles may have been identified as being shortened from the static body reading and also from your practice of the Joint-Freeing Series. These double findings reinforce the need for additional attention to these muscles in determining your personalized program. You may find, on the other hand, that some of the findings seem to contradict each other. For instance, the postural body reading may reveal that your latissimus dorsi muscle is weak, but the Joint-Freeing Series tells you that this muscle is tight. Both are true. Indeed, a tight muscle is often weakened, in that it cannot pull your body through its full range of motion. In this case, you need to do exercises that both stretch and strengthen the muscle. Priority should be given to relieving any area of pain or chronic discomfort.

To put the work into a healthy prospective, focus your attention on creating a program that strengthens the major area you want to realign and also stretches the major area of stress. If you begin to work with this program unsupervised by a yoga therapist, I recommend a focus on no more than three muscles at a time. For many people, I find just working with three muscles makes a major difference in a surprisingly short period.

Summarizing Your Findings

The next step is to review the summary of your postural body reading and place the findings in Chart 4 on page 187. Then review the summary of your practice of the Joint-Freeing Series and add those findings. By joining the two groups together into a composite summary, you build an evaluation of your passive and active body readings. From this, you can more accurately determine what yogasanas to practice to improve your muscular-skeletal balance of strength and flexibility.

It is natural to find weak muscles accompanied by antagonist muscles that are tight. Compare your findings with the information given in Table 4 (page 120). Some common findings I have seen are shown below. Please note that these lists can be reversed and also be true. In this case, the muscles cited in the first column can be identified as weak, and weak muscles can be identified as tight.

Tight Muscles	*Accompanying Weak Muscles*
Hamstrings	Quadriceps
Psoas	Gluteus maximus and hamstrings
Adductors	Abductors and internal hip rotators
Pectorals	Middle and lower trapezius
Latissimus dorsi and/or Erector spinae	Rectus abdominis

It is perhaps surprising, but not uncommon, to find that weak muscles may also be found to be tight. In such cases, they will need to be given exercises for both functions.

ADDRESSING SPECIFIC POSTURAL IMBALANCE

As an example of how to create a regimen for a specific postural problem, let us consider working with knock-knees. In Table 3 (page 103), you will see a list of the specific muscles shortened and lengthened from knock-knees. The muscles needing stretch are the adductors and gluteus medius. The muscles needing to be strengthened are the gluteus medius and the tensor fascia lata.

Table 5 (pages 250–251) shows you various yoga poses for stretching and strengthening each major muscle. For clarification purposes, let us take just the first level of efficiency for each muscle cited. The respective stretches will thus be the Extended Triangle and the Side-of-Hip Stretch. The strengthening poses will be the Balancing Tree and Energy-Freeing Pose. Figure 20 shows the poses sequenced in the most beneficial order. Even when doing just a few poses, they should be sequenced in this manner. Placing the

CHART 4
COMPREHENSIVE OVERVIEW

Postural Body Reading Form (Chart 1, Chapter 12), from page 106.

Muscles to Be Stretched

_____

_____

_____

_____

Muscles to Be Strengthened

_____

_____

_____

_____

Joint-Freeing Series Evaluation (Chart 2, Chapter 16), from page 154.

Muscles to Be Stretched

_____

_____

_____

_____

Muscles to Be Strengthened

_____

_____

_____

_____

Muscle Testing Evaluation (Chart 3, Chapter 18), from page 182.

Antagonist Muscles to Be Stretched

_____

_____

_____

_____

Muscles to Be Strengthened

_____

_____

_____

_____

Summary

Muscles to Be Stretched

_____

_____

_____

Muscles to Be Strengthened

_____

_____

_____

practices for knock-knees in the proper practice sequence results in the following thera-peutic series—Side-of-Hip Stretch, Balancing Tree, Extended Triangle Pose, and Energy-Freeing Pose.

Figure 20 also cites the principal effects of the yoga poses when the body is aligned. Thus, people who have knock-knees may not feel the effects cited on this chart when doing the poses. They should focus instead on doing the poses that will strengthen their weakened muscles and stretch those motions that are less than normal. By moving the body toward postural alignment, students will feel the effects cited in Table 5. This is likely if they have made significant progress in the realignment process.

This principle can be applied to any postural change. Table 6 (page 266) summa-rizes the major postural imbalances. However I caution you to stay focused on your own body's sensations and learn to read its messages. As each body is unique, so also similar postural imbalances are individual. The specific muscular imbalances for each joint may be different from person to person, due to the same variety of factors that created the imbalances in the first place. In addition, the adjacent joints to your imbalances will tend to be personal. Therefore, while working to correct knock-knees using Extended Triangle Pose, some students may need to apply external hip rotation and others may not. By get-ting to know your own body, you can refine your sensitivity and personalize the prac-tice. I encourage you to determine your priority yourself and persevere to manifest your own goal.

BODY SCULPTING—A NEW YOU IS A REALITY YOU CAN ATTAIN

In Structural Yoga Therapy™, a realistic starting point is not to correct the postural devi-ation, but rather to lessen the tension it causes you. This first phase of restructuring will lessen your total physical stress level. At first, you may not experience that knock-knees is a "problem." There may not be pain, or even discomfort, directly from this condition. The only sign you may have is that you are dissatisfied with the shape of your legs and would like "prettier," shapelier legs. This is certainly a worthwhile goal to strive to achieve.

There may not be a functional handicap from the problem, unless you are a com-petitive athlete. In this case, the postural change of knock-knees will predispose the adductors to sufficient tightness that the muscular efficiency of the thighs and hips is compromised. Greater performance comes from a smoothly operating, aligned muscu-lo-skeletal body.

Upon working with the muscles involved with this medically "asymptomatic," knock-knee condition, many students report that the minor tensions they held in other parts of their anatomy are no longer present. Thus, unrelated lower-back pain may dis-appear or lessen from the shifting of the muscular structures of the hips and thighs. Thus structural yoga often relieves subjective symptoms that may not have been reported to either yoga teacher or physician. This is often the case with yoga practices when they are done diligently. The fact is that yoga is therapeutic for many subclinical stressors—psy-chological, physical, and spiritual.

HYPEREXTENDED JOINTS

A hyperextended joint is, by definition, one in which the ligaments have been over-stretched. The joint has become hypermobile, which gives the appearance of flexibility. In some cases, this is true. In other cases, the muscles surrounding the joint are actually short. This can only be determined by holding the joint in a neutral position and stretching the surrounding tissue. In some cases, the muscles surrounding the joint are weak. In my case, my hyperextended knees were accompanied by weakened lower quadriceps, in spite of the fact that I had been a competitive runner for over five years.

In general, too much flexibility can be a sign of diminished muscle strength and stamina. Maintaining proper alignment and holding the postures longer within the limits of your flexibility will help to overcome a lack of stamina.

It is my experience that, by correcting the muscle imbalances, hyperextended joints can be trained to maintain a neutral position. This will prevent further increases in hypermobility and potential ligament or cartilage damage. To achieve this takes an investment of determined effort, constant practice over a minimum of six months, and a willingness to change.

PART FIVE

The Practice of Yoga Asanas

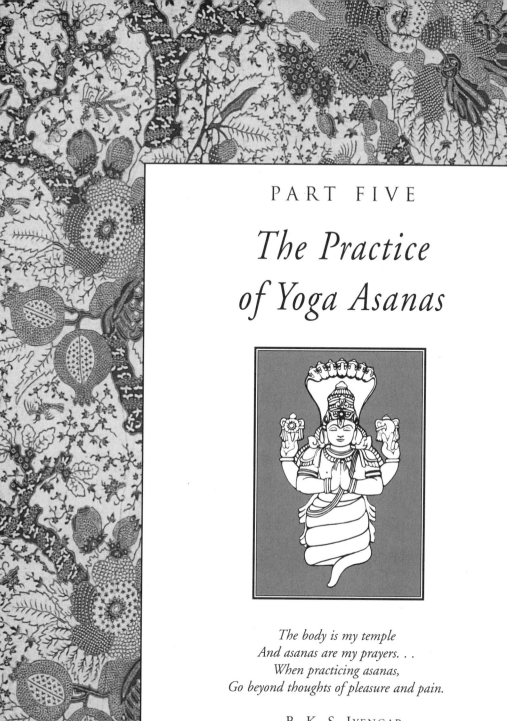

*The body is my temple
And asanas are my prayers. . .
When practicing asanas,
Go beyond thoughts of pleasure and pain.*

—B. K. S. IYENGAR

INTRODUCTION

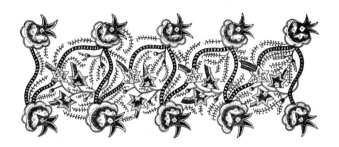

The main purpose of Structural Yoga™ is to be consistently reminded of the state of yoga through a variety of musculo-skeletal cues. Continue to reflect upon the story of Matsyendra, the first teacher of yoga and how he learned yoga. Read the *Yoga Sutras* and see how to integrate the insights gained from this into your practice. The key element from the *Yoga Sutras* is that yoga poses should be done comfortably and steadily. Several principles need to be kept firmly in mind during all yoga practice. Begin your practice with a relaxed body; start either with a relaxation pose or sitting quietly while feeling your heart of compassion. The following principles will help you establish a comfortable routine.

1. Adjust your body for comfort first, regardless of "looking good like a yogi should."

2. Always make an effort to extend your spine.

3. Relax the physical and psychic effort required to hold the posture.

4. Make a conscious scan of your body to relax all those areas of unnecessary tension. Become proficient in using only those parts required to attain and sustain the posture.

5. Breathe in a natural manner through your nose. With expanded practice, this can be deepened by ujjaye pranayama and personalized by your instructor to include Bandhas and Mudras adapted to your individual needs.

6. Hold the pose only as long as your body is opening. Once the limit of openness has been attained, several changes take place. Your spine will begin to shorten, your breath will lose its fullness, and your mind will no longer be held on one focal point of aware-

ness. By being alert to any one of these signs, you can optimize the benefits of yogasana practice.

7. It is ideal to hold the pose the same number of breaths on both sides. In general, hold two-sided poses half as long as single-sided poses.

8. In the stage of an asana where it can be held for more than ten breaths, or one minute, concentrate your mind on your breath or your given mantra. You can concentrate on any one of these pranayama techniques: the counting of your breath, on its location, on its rhythmic ratio, or on the sensation of the breath as it enters or exits your nostrils.

During your Structural Yoga training, there are several major points that you will need to learn to have a successful practice. Yoga books may assist you in learning these points, yet they cannot provide the benefit of a living instructor. Your instructor's objectivity, combined with your natural subjectivity, will help you get the most from practice. Some important things to remember while practicing Structural Yoga are listed below:

1. Evaluate your posture using body reading and the Joint-Freeing Series to determine probable muscular imbalances;

2. Realign your posture using specific poses that direct stretching and strengthening to the specific muscles needing extra attention;

3. Make adjustments for changes in your body's alignment as your strength and flexibility improve;

4. Work with the concept of counterpose and antagonist muscles when necessary, so that strong stretches are balanced with muscular contractions through the full range of joint motion;

5. Distinguish the feelings of contraction from those of stretch to refine your awareness during asana practice;

6. Isolate the movements of major muscle groups, so that your postures can be done with a minimum of effort;

7. Coordinate your movements into and out of the postures in a relaxed, yet alert manner harmonized with your breath;

8. Maintain steady, rhythmic wave breathing (ujjaye pranayama) and an awareness of the changes in your breath's movement patterns;

9. Move with an awareness of the position of your body without visual cues (a subcortical function called proprioception) and develop the process of focusing and withdrawing your senses from external objects (Pratyahara).

Chapter 20

STRUCTURAL YOGA ASANAS

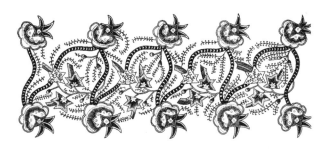

The twenty-four postures that make up the Structural Yoga asana sequence are a complete series. They form the foundation from which all other asanas are derived. They incorporate all the directions of motions your body can make and will sensitize you to reveal potential or current muscular and skeletal stressors. No additional postures are required. This series is based primarily upon a study of Iyengar Yoga poses to determine a series that can provide normal range of joint motion and develop tone and stamina in all the major muscles.

If you take the time to learn these poses thoroughly, your body will gradually realign itself into a better posture, most muscular stressors will subside, and many recurring health concerns will fall away.

MOUNTAIN POSE

Tadasana

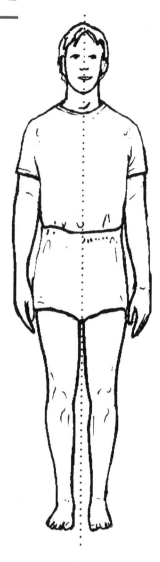

The Sanskrit root of tad is tat, *referring to "That," referring to the Eternal, which is unnamable and unmovable.*[1] *The pose is also called Samasthiti meaning "standing steady."*

INSTRUCTIONS

Stand erect, with your feet together, equal weight on each foot, no pressure on your toes. Your posture is erect and poised. Relax your arms, with your palms facing your sides.

---

[1] Swami Nikhilananda, ed. and trans., "Chhandogya Upanishad," *The Upanishads* (New York: Ramakrishna-Vivekananda Center, 1978), vol. 4, part 6, chap. 14, sutra 3, p. 321. One of the four Great Utterances (Mahavakyas) summarizing the teachings of the Vedas comes from the Sama Veda. It is *Tat Tvam Asi* (Thou art That. You are That which is unchangeable, eternal).

Your chest will be fully lifted, with a slight pelvic thrust, strong enough to produce a mild tone to your lower abdominal muscles. Allow your eyes to gaze steadily, yet softly (a practice called tratak), at a fixed spot, the focal point being either internal or external.

VARIATION

The pose is more stable when practiced with the feet 12 inches apart, directly under your hip joints.

FOCAL MOVEMENTS

A sense of poise for creating contemplation on being centered and grounded.

PRECAUTIONS AND COMMON ERRORS

The most common error is overworking in order to strive for "perfect posture." Remember, the classical guideline is to become steady, yet comfortable, make a relaxed, consistent effort, and remain open and receptive to your inner guide.

BODY READING

This and Corpse Pose (Savasana) are the most accurate postures for body reading, as it is the foundation pose from which all other postures derive. Take some time to review the body-reading concepts in chapter 11. A front view can reveal leg distortions, such as knock-knees, which prevent your feet from touching, bowed legs, in which the ankles touch but the knees are separated, or fallen arches. Signs of spinal curvature (scoliosis) may appear as a high shoulder, head turn, or one arm in front of the other. From the side view, one may find hyperextended (backward) knees, flat back, overarched lower back (lordosis), sunken chest with rounded shoulders, hunchback (khyphosis), or forward head.

BENEFITS

Good posture is not simply a matter of "standing tall." It is the result of genetically inherited traits and proper training in the efficient use of your body at all times. Yoga training can lessen the effects of inherited postural stressors and create internal room for organs to function normally, as well as for your vascular system to become more efficient. As a result of excellent training, your body is freed to move in all directions, effortlessly. This often results in a natural, spontaneous swaying motion during Mountain Pose, revealing energy freeing itself from habitual postural patterns. Should this occur, relax and permit the motions to run their course.

WARRIOR I

Virabhadrasana

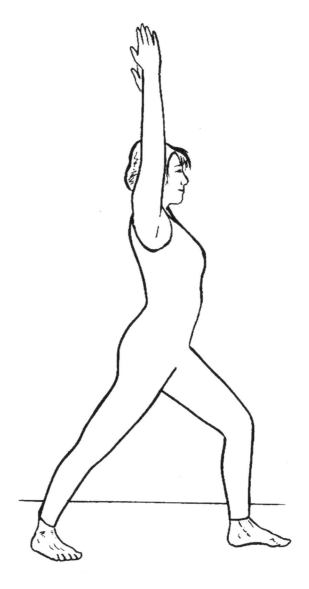

This pose is named after the vengeful hero created by Siva from his hair. The story is well told in Iyengar's Light on Yoga.[2]

INSTRUCTIONS

From Mountain Pose, step forward three feet with your right foot. Adjust your feet so that your right foot faces directly forward (12 o'clock) and your left foot points outward toward 10 o'clock.

---

[2] B. K. S. Iyengar, *Light on Yoga* (New York: Schocken Books, 1979).

Inhale, as you raise your arms adjacent to your head, your palms facing each other. Extend your fingers, keeping them together except for your thumbs, which are open.

Exhale, bending your right knee until your shin forms a line perpendicular to the floor (knee directly above ankle).

Inhale, adjusting your torso so that your pelvis and shoulders are squarely facing forward. Remain steady in the pose for a minimum of 6 slow, deliberate breaths.

Exhale, as you straighten your knee, returning to center position. Repeat on the opposite side.

VARIATION

A more challenging variation is to gradually move your forward thigh parallel to the floor. As you open the range of your external hip rotators, this becomes more possible. Remember, as always, to keep your shin perpendicular to the floor as you challenge your hip mobility.

FOCAL MOVEMENTS

Hip adduction and shoulder flexion. Feel the strength of your inner thighs (adductor muscles) and the top of your shoulders (deltoids). Feel the stretch of your calf (gastrocnemius muscle) in your back leg. This pose is called a closed-hip pose, as it tones the inner thighs, closing the inner line of the hips.

PRECAUTIONS AND COMMON ERRORS

Aligning your feet in standing position is for slender, posturally balanced bodies only. Most other people may need to position their feet with an increased side-to-side width for stability. This is because the center of gravity will be displaced from the normal pelvic center. Your back leg should be fully extended, without hyperextending your knee (which is felt as a stretch behind your knee joint). Your front leg should be aligned so your knee remains directly over your ankle. If your knee goes inward, losing its perpendicular alignment, a potentially harmful stretch of your inner knee can occur, stretching the knee joint's inelastic ligaments. Keep your hands active, so that attention can flow continuously through your arms to your fingertips.

BODY READING

Inflexibility of your outer ankle and weakness of your arch will prevent even weight distribution on your back foot. Weakness of your adductors will twist your pelvis so that it isn't at a right angle with your front thigh. A tightness of the hip flexors in the upper thigh and groin region can exaggerate the lumbar curve or reveal lordosis. The ankle of the back foot may pronate inward, indicating a weakness in the tibialis anterior muscle.

BENEFITS

This variation of the Warrior Pose encourages stimulation of the lungs and heart. The toning of the hip extensors (hamstrings and gluteus maximus) of the back leg may relieve discomfort of sciatica or lower back pain.

199

SIDE-OF-HIP STRETCH I

Parsvottanasana

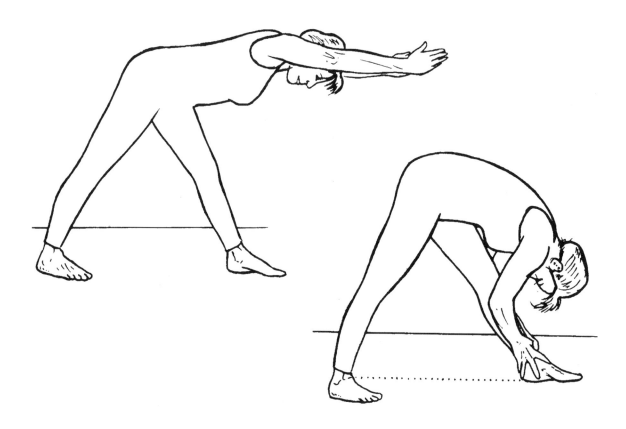

Parsva *means "side of the hip" or "flank."* Uttana *means "to stretch" or "lengthen intensively."*

INSTRUCTIONS

Begin in Mountain Pose. Step three feet forward with your right foot. Keep your hips and torso facing front, and your right foot at the 12 o'clock position. Turn your left foot out to 10 o'clock.

Inhale, as you raise your arms overhead, palms facing each other.

Exhale, bending forward from your hips, keeping your legs and back straight (figure on left). Reach out with your arms, then place your hands on your upper shin.

Inhale, as you extend your back, looking forward.

Exhale, reaching your chest forward and over your leg. Repeat the last two movements, gradually extending your hands down your leg toward the floor. End the pose with your head dropped between your arms, close to your shin (figure on right). Stay in the pose for a minimum of 6 breaths.

Inhale, as you lift up to center position.

Exhale, twisting to the opposite side. Place your left foot at 12 o'clock, and turn your right foot outward toward 2 o'clock. Repeat all the motions on this side.

FOCAL MOVEMENTS

Hip flexion and adduction. Feel the strength of your deep groin (psoas) and your inner thighs (adductors). Feel the stretch of the back of your legs (hamstrings) and hips (gluteus medius). This, like the preceding pose, is also a closed-hip pose.

PRECAUTIONS AND COMMON ERRORS

Aligning your feet in standing is for slender, posturally aligned bodies only. Most other people may need to position their feet with an increased side-to-side width for stability. This pose should be avoided when sciatica and other lower-back problems are present. In these cases, do this pose only under the supervision of an experienced yoga therapist. The pose creates an extreme stretch of the hamstrings and should be approached progressively, without a prolonged stay in the endpoint of the pose. To avoid strain at the immediate back of your knee joint or inner knees, allow your knees to bend.

BODY READING

This uneven forward-bending pose reveals any lack of symmetry in the waist, hip, and spine. The pose exaggerates lateral postural imbalances that may not be obvious in Mountain Pose. A small lumbar curvature will be revealed in the uneven height of the sides of the pelvis. Differences in hamstring flexibility can be readily disclosed. Proper adjustments will help to create better posture and improved muscle tone.

BENEFITS

With persistence of practicing this pose over months, restricted hip freedom due to short hamstrings is released. This tightness often prevents freedom of the spine. The deep stretch of the adductors and hamstrings releases stored-up energy, enabling an enhanced sense of vitality. Persons with bowed legs should aim to feel the pose stretching their abductors (outer thigh and pelvis). Those with knock-knees need to feel the stretch in the adductors (groin and inner thigh). For persons whose legs are aligned, the effect will tend to be in the hamstrings, at the back of the thighs. The pose can be individually adapted for a therapeutic program to lessen the curvatures of scoliosis. Over time, this pose can prove to be a key element in correcting uneven spinal curvatures.

BALANCING TREE

Vrksasana

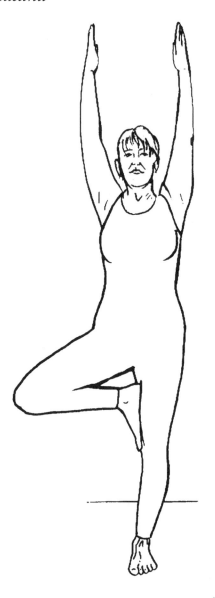

Vrks is Sanskrit and means "a tree." A tree's stability comes for a solid base, reaching into the earth yet having flexibility to adapt to change. Balancing Tree develops this stability and flexibility on all dimensions.

INSTRUCTIONS

Begin in Mountain Pose, with your hands placed, palms together, in front of your heart. This is called the Palm Salute, or Anjali Mudra. Gaze directly ahead at a fixed point throughout the pose. Maintain a squeeze of your inner thigh muscles, contracting your adductors.

Inhale, as you lift your chest, extending yourself to full height.

Exhale, bending your right knee forward, lifting your thigh as far as possible without the assistance of your arms.

Inhale, turning your right thigh outward, so that the sole of your foot rests against your inner leg.

Exhale, steadying your balance.

Inhale, extending your arms overhead, parallel to each other, while lifting your chest fully. Stay steadily for 6 rhythmic breaths.

Exhale, lowering your leg and hands to Mountain Pose. Repeat the motions for the opposite side.

FOCAL MOVEMENTS

Hip abduction, with external rotation and shoulder flexion. Feel the strength of your supporting leg's inner thigh (adductors), the upper buttocks (gluteus medius), and deep hip (external rotators) of your balanced leg. This pose is an open-hip pose, as it tones the outer thighs and stretches the inner thighs. Feel the stretch extending to lengthen your spine, while relaxing the space between your shoulders and neck.

PRECAUTIONS AND COMMON ERRORS

Balance is retained by maintaining a steady gaze. When bringing your foot upward, your pelvis should remain steady. As the normal range of hip abduction is 45 degrees, your knee should point outward only halfway to either side when in the completed pose. If you turn your bent knee further backward, your pelvis will twist, resulting in instability. By avoiding the tendency to pull your the leg farther up your thigh with your free hand, there will be more stability. Your foot should rest softly against your inner thigh to lessen the tendency to shift weight, thus also causing instability. Resist pushing your supporting leg with the weight of your bent leg.

BODY READING

Instability in balancing poses often comes from a combination of weakness in the foot arch, inner thighs, and buttock muscles, or from loss of concentration. To assist in toning the adductors of your inner thigh, place your foot on the gracilis muscle (an adductor, see page 143) and remain firm beneath your foot. Tightness of the chest (pectorals) and weakness of the shoulders (either in the trapezius or the deltoids) may result in the arms not being fully extended, or an inability to bring them beside the ears. Bent elbows indicate tightness of the biceps and weakness of the triceps.

BENEFITS

Balancing Tree Pose tones the postural stabilizing muscles: gluteus medius/maximus, hip flexors, and tibialis anterior. It fully expands the chest, enhancing deep breathing. The tailor muscle (sartorius) is toned by bringing your leg up and slowly down.

As mental poses, balancing asanas are helpful in regaining stability and flexibility. They can become postures of repose.

EXTENDED TRIANGLE

Utthita Trikonasana

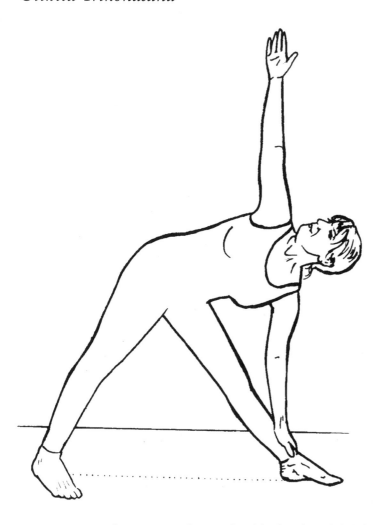

Utthita *means "extended" or "stretched out." Tri means "three" and* kona *means "angle." Trikona, therefore, refers to a triangle shape. This pose forms a perfect equilateral triangle, in which the length of the legs and the space between the feet become equal.*

INSTRUCTIONS

Begin in Mountain Pose. Step to the side, placing your feet three-and-a-half feet apart. Turn your right foot out 90 degrees, to 3 o'clock position, and your left foot inward halfway, to 45 degrees, to 2 o'clock. Keep the lift of your arch. Maintain a pelvic thrust throughout the pose.

Inhale, as you raise your arms out to the sides, bringing them even with your shoulder height, while lifting your rib cage out of your waist.

Exhale, moving your hips to the left, as you simultaneously extend to your right side, bringing your right hand to rest lightly upon your right shin.

Inhale, turning your head to face your upward hand, palm facing forward. Open your hand so that your fingers are extended together, with your thumb pulled open to a right angle with your forefinger. Keep your legs straight and firm. Stay steady and breathe deeply for a minimum of six breaths.

Inhale, returning to center, with your feet facing front. Reverse the pose to complete the other side.

FOCAL MOVEMENTS

Hip flexion and lateral flexion of the spine with external hip rotation. Feel the strength of the front of your thighs (quadriceps, especially the uppermost muscle, the rectus femoris), the sides of your abdomen (abdominis oblique), and the sides of your neck (sternocleidomastoid). Focus awareness on the stretch of your inner (adductors) and posterior thigh (hamstrings) muscles. This pose is an open-hip pose, as it tones the outer thighs as it stretches the inner thighs. Your arms are opened and lengthened, yet pulled down from their origin at the shoulders, toning your lower trapezius.

PRECAUTIONS AND COMMON ERRORS

Aligning the feet in standing is given for slender, posturally aligned bodies only. Most other people may need to position their feet with an increased side-to-side width for stability. If sciatica has been present recently, it is best to do this pose with a bent knee and not try to "polish" your alignment. The pose is intended to be a lateral, not a forward, bend of the spine. Thus, a common adjustment by teachers is to have students do the pose with their lower hip, shoulders, and head against a wall. While the lower hip will easily rest on the wall, the upper hip is pulled away from the wall. This variation will convey clearly any lack of vertical alignment.

Some teachers use the instruction to reach out to the side as you go into this pose. In this manner, students lose the symmetry of the arms being at a right angle with the spine. One side becomes unnaturally elongated and the head tends to resist the movement and moves away from the elongated lower side, with the head staying upright, due to the righting neurological reflex. This reflex keeps the head upright regardless of body posture, as a protective defense from an anticipated fall. By moving into the pose in this way, students will feel the stretch of the underside waist, then will experience the stress of a misaligned neck. Instead, go into the pose by first exaggerating the lift of the torso out of the waist on both sides, then tipping the pelvis, allowing for a slight rotation of the top hip forward to compensate for the lowering of the torso to one side. Aligning your arms with your torso throughout the pose can alleviate stress.

BODY READING

Tightness of the hip flexors (psoas and rectus femoris) results in the loss of pelvic thrust and an increased swayback that will cause the abdomen to expand. Weakness in the side of the neck (sternocleidomastoid muscle) will prevent the head from being aligned to the thoracic spine. In this case, the head may drop or rise in an exaggerated fashion, depending upon which side of the neck is weak.

BENEFITS

Extended Triangle tones the inner thigh muscles and promotes strength to the deep external rotation of the hips, improving sitting postures. This pose prepares you for inverted poses. It should be practiced frequently before training for the Shoulderstand or Headstand.

WARRIOR II

Virabhadrasana II

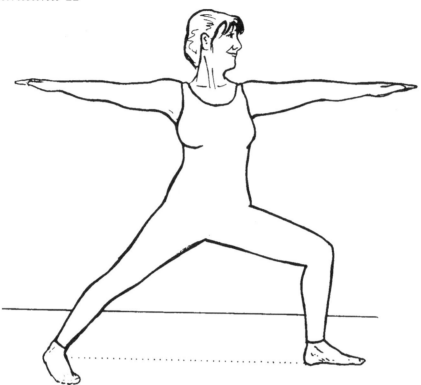

This is the second variation of the Warrior shown on page 198.

INSTRUCTIONS

Begin in Mountain Pose. Step to the side, opening your feet 3 1/2 feet apart. Turn your right foot out 90 degrees, to 3 o'clock position. Turn your left foot inward to 45 degrees, to 2 o'clock position. Keep your torso facing forward.

Inhale, as you lift your arms parallel to the floor, with your palms down. The extension goes through your wrists into your extended fingers, with your thumbs opened.

Exhale, bending your right knee until your shin is perpendicular to the floor (knee directly above ankle).

Inhale, lifting your chest and making sure your shoulders are directly above your pelvis. Keep your shoulders back and down.

Exhale, turning your head to direct your gaze at your right thumb. Keep your right knee aligned above your ankle, while maintaining a feeling of solidity in your left straight leg. Stay for a minimum of 6 breaths.

Inhale, straightening your right knee and turning your feet to the front. Repeat on the other side.

VARIATION

A more challenging variation is to gradually move your forward thigh to be parallel with the floor. As you strengthen your external hip rotators, and stretch your adductors, this becomes more possible. Remember, as always, to keep your shin perpendicular to the floor as you challenge your hip mobility.

FOCAL MOVEMENTS

External hip rotation with abduction, ankle dorsiflexion with the outer foot, and adduction of the shoulder blades. This pose is an open-hip pose as it tones the outer thighs and stretches the inner thighs. Feel the strength of your deep hip rotators and the adjacent hip abductors (gluteus medius) on the extended leg. Strengthen both quadriceps to stabilize knee alignment. Focus the stretch to your inner thighs (adductors) and your extended leg's outer calf and ankle (gastrocnemius and soleus).

PRECAUTIONS AND COMMON ERRORS

Aligning the feet in standing is given for slender, posturally aligned bodies only. Most other people may need to position their feet with an increased side-to-side width for stability. A misalignment of the bent knee is common. To avoid this, keep your shin perpendicular to the floor. Only with full freedom of your hips will your thighs come parallel to the floor. The back knee is frequently locked or bent, rather than extended and lengthened. It is normal for your pelvis to rotate away from your straight leg yet exert an effort to minimize this twist. Adjust your pelvis so your waistline remains parallel to the floor. Pelvic thrust may be difficult to maintain, due to a restriction in your inner thigh muscles. Weakness of the deltoids will cause your arms to drop, while weakness of the serratus anterior may cause your breath to be shallow.

BODY READING

All the standing poses reveal ankle stiffness or fallen arches. This pose particularly challenges the back ankle's capacity to lift, and maintain a natural arch. Scoliosis may prevent your pelvis from being level, thus a lack of symmetry in hip and shoulder height will become apparent. The challenge of knock-knees will be felt as shortness in your adductors anywhere along the inner thigh.

BENEFITS

Warrior II is a challenge to both physical and emotional stamina, but, with persistence, your endurance will increase. Many students find the Warrior Poses exhilarating, and use them instead of coffee breaks to recharge themselves in midafternoon. The openness of the groin region releases compression of the lower back and is a necessary part of a complete back rehabilitation program.

DOWNWARD FACING DOG

Adho Mukha Svanasana

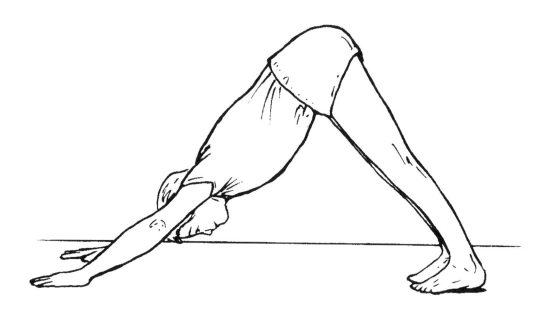

Adho *means "down,"* mukha *means "face,"* and svan *is the Sanskrit word for dog. This exquisite pose resembles the motion of a dog extending its spine and legs.*

INSTRUCTIONS

Begin in Cat Lift Pose, on your hands and knees, with your spine pulled downward between your shoulders and your head lifted. Move your hands forward one hand length from the natural Cat Pose. Place your knees and feet hip-width apart, then pull your toes forward.

Inhale, pressing downward on your upper back between your shoulder blades.

Exhale, lifting your hips up and back, while reaching your chest backward toward your knees. Slowly straighten your legs. Stay in the posture with full rhythmic breathing. Continue to press your chest backward, toward your feet, until your arms are even with your ears. Emphasize lifting your hips to narrow your waist, then slowly press your heels downward, without them touching the floor. Stay there with a steady upward lift for a minimum of 6 breaths.

Exhale, coming out of the pose. Return to Cat Pose.

FOCAL MOVEMENTS

Hip and shoulder flexion and ankle dorsiflexion. Feel the strength of your lower back as it pulls toward your thighs due to the strength of your psoas muscle. Work the tops of your shoulders (deltoids) and between your shoulder blades (trapezius) as you move your chest toward your knees. Focus upon the powerful firmness of your thighs (quadriceps) used in holding your legs straight, and drawing the thigh muscles up to help increase the strength of your uppermost quadricep, which is a hip flexor (rectus femoris). Focus awareness on the stretch of the back of your legs and the sensation of extending your spine toward the ceiling (erector spinae).

PRECAUTIONS AND COMMON ERRORS

The shoulders are overworked if there is not a straight line from hips to shoulders to wrists, and your head is in front of your arms. Your heels should not touch the floor. If they do, your hands are too close to your feet. In this event, your middle or lower back will tend to round, making it difficult to fully extend your thoracic spine and achieve full shoulder flexion. Another possible explanation for having your heels on the floor is that your ankle joints have excessive mobility in dorsiflexion. Check yourself in the Joint-Freeing Series to re-evaluate this motion. To correct your knee alignment, focus upon developing strength in the lowest segment of the quadriceps and the tibialis anterior muscles in the front of your shins by lifting your toes.

Students with sciatica should bend their knees or avoid this pose if they feel nerve pain (tingling or burning) down the back of their legs or buttocks.

BODY READING

Downward Facing Dog Pose extends the spine fully and tends to straighten excessive spinal curvatures. Those portions of the spine with curvature that may be willing to change become apparent when we watch the difference between relaxing the effort in the pose and making a strong effort to extend the pelvis and lumbar spine upward. Stiffness (weakness of the shoulders) results in the rounded upper back, forming less than a straight line.

BENEFITS

The pose strengthens your upper back and arms, improving upper back posture and openness of your chest. The internal organs are inverted and receive an opportunity to become repositioned, which may improve digestion. The quadriceps are strengthened, while the hamstrings are fully stretched.

In Structural Yoga, there are four poses in which the body is in the same anatomical position. These poses are the Downward Facing Dog, Complete Boat, Stick, and Upward Extended Legs. (One can also add the Plow Pose, Halasana, to this list). In all these poses, the spine and legs are extended, with the torso at a right angle to the thighs. This motion is a primary position of sitting and getting up from sitting. These asana variations allow your body to benefit from the motion being done in a variety of gravitational variations.

BRIDGE

Setubandhasana

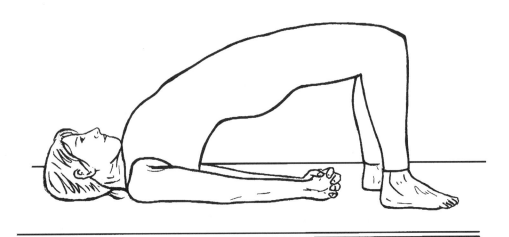

Setu means "bridge" and bandha means "a lock," implying a solid, stable construction.

INSTRUCTIONS

Begin lying on your back, palms upward beside your hips.

Exhale, bending your knees, and placing your feet close to your hips. Separate your feet and knees to hip-width.

Inhale, expanding your chest and pulling your shoulders close, as you lift your hips up to form a smooth arching bridge from shoulders to knees.

Exhale, then

Inhale, rotating your arms outward from the tops of your shoulders.

Exhale, holding your weight on the outer shoulders.

Inhale, lifting your chest. Then steady the pose with full deep breathing for 6 to 12 breaths.

Exhale, lowering your hips, while thrusting your lower pelvis upward to bring your spine down one vertebra at a time. This snake-like motion decompresses any tendency to overarch your spine.

VARIATION

In this more elevated pose, lift your chest fully and, after externally rotating your arms, join your hands together. This shoulder rotation with hand-lock position, or Karmasana (Pose of Karma), creates the necessary preparatory strength for Shoulderstand. When you can stay here comfortably for twenty-four breaths, you can safely begin to be trained for the Full Shoulderstand. Ideally, the cervical and thoracic spine are both lifted from the floor. Come down from the pose as before.

FOCAL MOVEMENTS

Hip extension, knee flexion, with scapula adduction and depression. Focus strength to your buttocks (gluteus maximus) and back of your thighs (hamstrings). The power of the upper back is directed to the squeezing and lowering of the shoulder blades (middle and lower trapezius). There is a stretch in the front of the upper thighs (hip flexors) and upper chest (pectorals).

PRECAUTIONS AND COMMON ERRORS

If you have a stiff or weak neck, over-lifting your chest or prolonged holding of the pose can aggravate your condition. Instead, go into the pose on an inhale, pause, then come out on an exhale. Repeat 6 to 12 times to relieve your neck, as this increases circulation through your tissues. Keep your knees directly above your ankles to avoid pressing your knees toward each other while your feet are apart, as this may strain the delicate inner knee ligaments and tendons.

It may be necessary to lift your chin to allow free breathing and neck comfort. In proper alignment, the position will retain the natural curve in the back of your neck so that it is off the ground. With persistence, the spine between the shoulder blades can also be free of the floor, enabling the body's weight to be supported by the contact of the triceps (back of the upper arms) without any portion of the spine on the floor.

Only when this is achieved should the full shoulderstand be attempted. A lack of strength in the triceps will put undue pressure on your neck, causing potential strain to discs, nerves, or blood supply. Pads or props will not correct the weakness, but rather serve to compensate for it. A better practice is to develop triceps strength in Cat Bows first, rather than risking stress to your neck. When well-trained students have their hands on their backs for the Full Bridge Pose, or Supported Shoulderstand, their forearms will remain parallel to each other and no part of their spine will be on the ground.

BODY READING

Weakness of the adductors will splay your knees to open wider than your ankles. If your hips cannot be lifted level to the slant of knee to shoulder alignment, the hip extensors (gluteus maximus and hamstrings) are weak. Weakness of the buttocks and hamstrings and/or tightness of the hip flexors will prevent your pelvis from coming to full height. Weakness of the middle trapezius and/or tightness of the lower pectoralis clavicular and the anterior serratus muscles will prevent your hands from joining.

BENEFITS

This pose is the primary preparation for the Shoulderstand. The internal organs and vascular supply are benefited, as they are in the Shoulderstand. The head and neck receive a vascular flush that may benefit head and neck aches. The entire back is strengthened, from the shoulders to the buttocks and thighs.

UPWARD STRETCHED LEGS

Urdhva Prasarita Padasana

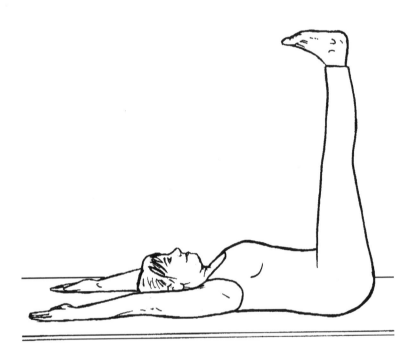

Urdhva *means "upright" or "above."* Prasarita, *like* Uttana, *means "extended" or "stretched fully."* Pada *means "foot," or "leg." Sometimes this is called the "L Pose," due to its shape when viewed from the left side.*

INSTRUCTIONS

Begin lying on the floor with your feet together, hands beside your hips, palms downward.

Exhale, bending your knees toward your chest, coming into Energy Freeing Pose (Apanasana).

Inhale, raising your legs to a fully extended position, legs together, with your heels reaching upward, directly above your hips.

Exhale, pulling your abdominal muscles backward and pressing the small of your back to the floor.

Inhale, raising your arms overhead, palm upward along the floor, while keeping your shoulders down and away from your neck. Sustain the pose with steady full breathing for a minimum of 6 breaths.

Exhale, bending your knees to your chest, and then lower your legs to the floor.

FOCAL MOVEMENTS

Hip flexion is the major motion, with knee extension and shoulder flexion. Feel the strength of your quadriceps, and the muscles crossing the tops of your thighs to your pelvis (hip flexors), as well as the uppermost section of your arms (deltoids). There may be a great effort on the part of your abdominals to steady the pose. Lessen the intensity of stress there to give your hip flexors more challenge. Focus your attention on a comfortable, yet steady, stretch of the calves and hamstrings, so your heel cords are lengthened. Your feet will be aligned as they are in the Mountain Pose.

PRECAUTIONS AND COMMON ERRORS

If your lower back arches during the pose, do not hold it for long. Shift the focus to pulling your abdomen backward. It may be helpful to place your hands under your hips to assist your abdominal strength. A mild arching of your lumbar spine during the lift and lowering of your legs is normal due to the contraction of the psoas muscles.

If your legs tremble, relax the effort to straighten your knees, and allow them to bend to a level where shaking is minimized. The trembling can be due to a weakness of your hip flexors or a tightness in your hamstrings. If you squeeze your legs together, which strengthens your adductors, this will produce a stronger hip flexion and will help end the shaking. An alternative is to bend your knees and continue bringing your thighs more gradually to a right angle with the floor. After some time in this variation, your hip flexors will develop more stamina and your legs will fully extend. With sciatica, keep your knees bent or, if it is acute, avoid the pose entirely.

BODY READING

Lack of flexibility of the hamstrings and/or weakness of the quadriceps forces the knees to bend and may keep your legs from reaching a right angle to the torso. Tightness of the pectoral clavicular section and/or weakness of the deltoids and trapezius keep the shoulders and arms from lying flat. Weakness of the triceps and/or tightness of the biceps will prevent the elbow from straightening. Overuse of the psoas muscle and/or weakness of the abdominals will arch the lower back from the floor.

BENEFITS

This pose prepares the body for inverted poses. It teaches the proper way to use the abdominal muscles in harmony with the lower back. The pose can train you to distribute effort throughout your back, thus avoiding straining any region.

SUPPORTED SHOULDERSTAND

Ardha Salamba Sarvangasana

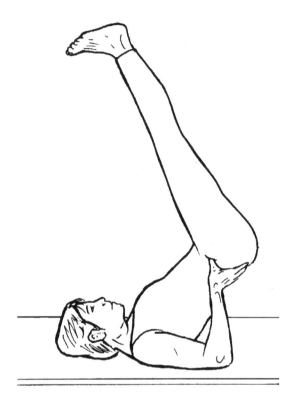

Ardha means "half," Salamba means "supported," and Sarvang means "the entire body," or, more literally, "all the limbs." The variation given is a mild version of Supported Shoulderstand, that is safe for most people, while the full version often needs to be modified to the individual. This position is also called Viparita Karani Mudra, or the Inverted Action Seal. As a Tantrikasana, this movement is claimed to reverse the solar (abdomen) and lunar (forehead) regions, producing a balance of opposite forces that leads to serenity.

INSTRUCTIONS

Begin lying on the floor with your knees bent, feet resting close to your buttocks.

Exhale, bringing your knees toward your chest; press your palms into the floor beside your hips.

Inhale, deeply.

Exhale, straightening your legs upward and backward, reaching them behind your head. Simultaneously push the floor with your hands to assist making the movement smooth.

Inhale, externally rotate your shoulders while pulling your elbows closer. Then apply pressure into the floor with upper arms from elbows to shoulders, emphasizing shoulder extension strength.

Exhale, bending your elbows, then lower your pelvis into your hands for support.

Inhale, adjusting the height of your legs to a comfortable level, with your knees above your head. Stay for a minimum of 10 deep breaths.

Exhale, bending your knees close to your head and lower your arms to the floor.

Inhale, as you pause there and adjust to get comfortable.

Exhale, as you roll your spine to the floor and allow your head to come off the floor to lessen the pressure in your back. Pause in Energy Freeing Pose.

Inhale, straightening your legs to Upward Extended Leg Pose.

Exhale, lowering your legs to the floor, with your heels extended. Rest in Relaxation of a Corpse.

FOCAL MOVEMENTS

Thoracic and shoulder extension, hip and elbow flexion, and scapular adduction. Focus on the strength of your upper back to arch forward (thoracic extension) and pull your shoulders narrow (trapezius) to lift your chest, while pressing your elbows firmly into the floor (latissimus and triceps). Encourage yourself to relax your neck and swallow.

PRECAUTIONS AND COMMON ERRORS

This pose should not be done if you have a neck injury, diabetes, or glaucoma. Menstruating women should refrain until cycle is ended. For students with unregulated high or low blood pressure, a pranayama sequence called "Tank Sealing" (Tataka Mudra) can be learned from a teacher to alleviate these difficulties.

Students who cannot hold the Bridge Pose with elbows close and hands clasped have not developed sufficient strength in their upper back and/or stretch in their chest to do this pose without a potential strain to the neck. Among the problems associated with inadequate preparation are headaches, nausea, soreness of neck and shoulders, and dizziness or lightheadedness as blood pressure is lowered from being in this pose. Other problems include poor posture, such as increase of forward head, rounding of the shoulders, caving in of the chest, and diminished respiratory function.

When the ideal preparations have been mastered, the Shoulderstand can be done with the entire spinal column off the floor. The outer arms and shoulders hold the weight of the pose.

BODY READING

The tightness of the chest (pectorals) and weakness of the upper back (trapezius) that you may have discovered during Bridge Pose are exaggerated here. The elbows may spread (due to weakness of the middle trapezius and inflexibility of the serratus anterior) as the body is raised. They will continue to spread the longer the pose is held. The upper back may round due to weakness of the erector spinae. Weakness of the biceps and brachioradialis lessens stamina in keeping the lift of the chest during this pose.

I distinguish three levels of the pose. For the beginner, the thoracic spine is rounded and the elbows splayed apart. This level is difficult to hold, as it causes much strain on the arms and back, so it should only be held briefly, less than 10 breaths. The second level is achieved with a straightening of the thoracic region and bringing the elbows closer. The length of stay can be prolonged to 2 minutes. The third level is achieved by adducting the scapula and externally rotating the shoulders. In this complete version, the weight is fully held by the shoulders with the spine off the floor. At this level, there is such a degree of comfort that the student can stay fairly long, 5 minutes or more.

BENEFITS

The Shoulderstand is called the "Mother of all the asanas." As a mother provides nurturing to the entire family, so the Shoulderstand is named "entire body pose" (Sarvangasana). In spite of a lack of sound research on specific yoga asanas, this pose is considered by yoga masters to provide the greatest benefits to many physiological systems. It is especially considered to benefit the thyroid gland and the endocrine system in general, as well as the digestive system. It is soothing to the nervous system and calms anxiety and fear.

ABDOMINAL TWIST

Jathara Parivartanasana

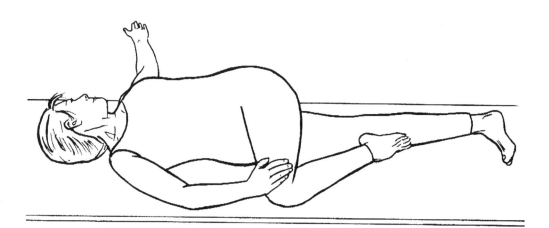

Jathara *means "stomach" or "abdomen," and* Parivartan *means "revolving," "turning," or "rolling about." This motion rotates the lower abdomen away from the upper abdomen, often increasing peristalsis.*

INSTRUCTIONS

Begin lying supine, with your legs together and your arms extended straight out from your shoulders, palms up.

Exhale, placing your left foot on your right knee.

Inhale, lifting your hips from the floor.

Exhale, sliding your hips six inches backward to your left, twisting onto your outer right hip, while gently pulling your left knee toward the floor with the aid of your right hand.

Inhale, lengthening the posture, making one line from heel to head.

Exhale, turn your head and look toward your left hand. Stay for a minimum of 6 breaths.

Inhale, returning to center position and extending your legs, aligned. Reverse sides.

FOCAL MOVEMENT

Hip adduction and spinal rotation. Feel a contraction of your inner bent thigh as it moves toward the floor. Strengthen the lower lateral abdomen (abdominus oblique) by pulling your belly backward as you stretch the same region on the opposite side, and your outer hip region (gluteus maximus and latissimus) by pulling your knee down toward the floor.

PRECAUTIONS AND COMMON ERRORS

With sciatica or sacroiliac strain, care should be taken to minimize the effect in the sacral region of the lower back. It is ideal to feel the pose in your outer hips and thighs, *not* your posterior central pelvis (sacral region). Keep both shoulders and arms flat on the floor throughout the pose. Your body should remain in a "T" position.

Maintain a feeling of alignment with your extended leg, through your spine, to your head. If you feel uncomfortable, have your teacher check your alignment and give additional verbal and physical adjustments.

BODY READING

Tightness of the pectorals will result in the shoulder lifting from the floor during the pose. This can also be due to excessive pulling to get the bent knee to the floor. Due to an asymmetry of the outer hips (abductors), the pose may feel quite different from side to side.

BENEFITS

A great stress reliever, this pose promotes a deep relaxation, in addition to opening the lower lungs. A focus upon fully breathing promotes flexibility in the mid back and lower rib cage. It is of great benefit to asthmatics, who often find they can breathe more easily as it opens the upper abdomen and lower lungs. Twisting the bent knee to the right side opens the lower left rib cage, freeing up blood flow to the stomach, pancreas, and splenic flexure of the colon. Twisting the knee to the left side opens the region of the liver, gall bladder, and hepatic flexure of the colon. Holding the pose for some time often produces a gastric release, indicated by peristaltic sounds as nutrients move their way down your digestive tract. It may also correct misaligned vertebrae, so an adjustment sound should not alarm you. Do not attempt to adjust your vertebral column, but rather emphasize lengthening your spine as you encourage rotation.

This pose, when sustained, counteracts the effects of the Supported Shoulderstand. The most common choice of a counter-pose is the Fish (Matsyasana), as it reverses the full neck flexion of the Shoulderstand. But in the case of the modified Shoulderstand, as presented with an emphasis on back-bending, the Abdominal Twist is a more complete counter-pose.

ENERGY FREEING POSE

Apanasana

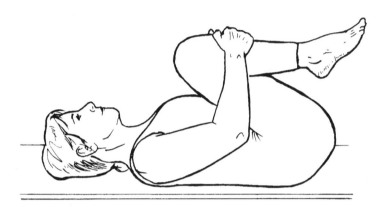

Apana *is one of the five types of prana energy. It is a force that moves down and out of the lower body. It is the force behind the elimination of feces, urine, orgasm, birthing a baby, and menstruation. When apana is healthy and balanced, these functions are regular and without discomfort. Correct practice of this pose can restore apana prana's functions in the channels of elimination.*

INSTRUCTIONS

Begin in a supine pose, with your hands at your sides.

Exhale, drawing your knees toward your chest.

Inhale, reaching out to hold your mid-shin region with your hands.

Exhale, compressing your lower abdomen away from the tops of your thighs.

Inhale, relaxing the pull of your arms, without losing your grip on your shins.

Exhale, increasing the pulling of your arms, drawing your thighs closer to your rib cage. Repeat the rhythmic coordination of alternate pulling and relaxing six times. Then hold the pull steadily for an additional 12 breaths.

VARIATIONS

The pose can be practiced in three ways:

- Rhythmically, pulling your knees toward your chest on exhalation, releasing the pull on inhalation;
- Tightly and strongly, with your knees together; or
- Mildly, with the knees separated and drawn toward your shoulders.

FOCAL MOVEMENTS

Spine, hip, and knee flexion; with shoulder adduction to create a lower abdominal compression. Feel the strength of your abdominals and hip flexors, where your thighs meet your pelvis, contracting during the exhale movements. Use a mild force to keep your shoulders back using the latissimus and triceps, while using your pectorals to draw your elbows to your sides. Encourage a stretch of your buttocks (gluteus maximus) and lower back (lumbar erector spinae).

PRECAUTIONS AND COMMON ERRORS

Perhaps the most common error in this pose is underestimating its value. Most students do not hold the pose long enough for it to do its duty. It is named Apanasana because it stimulates the expulsion of excessive or irregular wind energy from the lower body. When the pose is held to duration, it will release tensions of the lower digestive system, stimulate peristalsis, release back pain, or produce a general sense of openness in the body.

For some people, this pull may bother the knee. An alternative is to hold your hands behind your knees so the exertion is applied to your hamstrings. If your neck feels strained or your chin is pulled up, place a pillow under your head. There may also be discomfort in the inguinal region, where the thigh connects to the pelvis. This may be relieved by strong mindful relaxation of the site. Or you may need to modify the pose by allowing your knees to open wider than your torso with your feet together.

BODY READING

An inability to keep your legs together indicates weakness of your adductors and/or tightness of your abductors. Inability to bring your thighs to within two inches of your ribs indicates tightness of the hamstrings and lumbar erector spinae and/or weakness of the rectus abdominis and hip flexors. If your chin is pulled up or your head is lifted from the floor, this indicates tightness of the trapezius, thoracic erector spinae, and sternocleidomastoid.

BENEFITS

This pose is deceptive as it has a vast array of potential benefits when practiced thoroughly. It can relieve stiffness and pain due to vertebral compression or misalignment in the lower back. A prolonged stay of 10 to 30 minutes is renowned for its ability to release back spasms. In this case, you may need to have an assistant support your legs to maintain comfortable pressure while you discharge, or the pose can be done with your feet held in position against a wall. This is also effective in many cases for releasing menstrual cramps. Holding the posture may relieve abdominal gas and promote sufficient peristaltic motion, ending constipation. It frees up stagnant abdominal circulation and promotes vitality, hence its name. The key ingredient is patience and using variations for optimal benefits.

STICK POSE

Dandasana

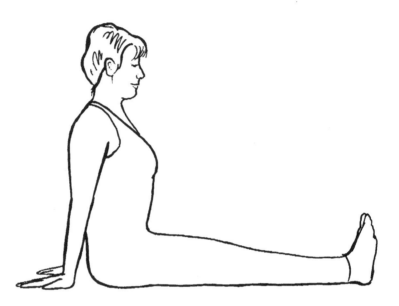

Danda *means "stick" or "staff." It refers to the spinal column, and to the staff of power and sovereignty. This staff is wielded by Vishnu to preserve the universe, according to Hindu iconography.*[3]

INSTRUCTIONS

Begin sitting erect, with your legs together, extended in front. Place your palms flat, with your fingers pointed backward, adjusting your arms until your shoulders and wrists are comfortable. Your personalized arm placement will bring you to your maximum erect height.

Inhale, lifting your chest, while reaching through your heels.

Exhale, pulling your shoulders backward and downward. Stay steadily, with full breathing, for a minimum of 6 breaths.

---

[3] Margaret Stutley, *The Illustrated Dictionary of Hindu Iconography* (Boston: Routledge & Kegan Paul, 1985), p. 35.

FOCAL MOVEMENTS

Hip flexion and thoracic extension. Feel the strength of the top of your thighs (quadriceps and hip flexors) and your entire back, both your surface muscles (latissimus and trapezius), and the deep muscles (erector spinae). Encourage a mild stretch of your wrist flexors and hamstrings.

PRECAUTIONS AND COMMON ERRORS

While in some teaching styles, the fingers are turned forward in this pose, this placement stretches the wrist joints beyond normal range of motion, which can aggravate Carpal Tunnel Syndrome. Hence your wrists will be safer from overstretching their ligaments with fingers pointing backward. Avoid locking your elbows (hyperextending) in this pose, and in all weight-bearing straight-arm poses. Remember to engage your triceps muscles, rather than your elbow joint. In general, allow your back to do twice the effort of your arms.

For someone in acute sciatica pain, this pose may be more comfortable with knees bent. If this doesn't help, avoid the pose and concentrate on strengthening your back-bending poses, especially with Cobra and Locust.

BODY READING

Curvature of your legs—either knock-knees or bowed legs—will not allow the knees or ankles to come together at the same time. With short arms, your hands may need to be placed behind your hips, so that the lift can be achieved in your chest. This adjustment of hand placement should also be made when the pelvis tilts backward, causing a rounded lumbar spine.

BENEFITS

This pose strengthens the group of muscles supporting the "stick"—the spine. Thus, it promotes ease in all sitting postures by toning the hip flexors, abdominals, and back muscles. By the art of relaxation and following the procedure described in *Yoga Sutras*, a meditative state can be achieved here (see chapter 2).[4] When practiced on an energy level as a Tantrasutra, this pose increases the flow of vitality throughout the subtle body.

---

[4] Stiles, *Yoga Sutras of Patanjali*, chap. II, sutras 46–55.

HEAD-TO-KNEE POSE

Janu Sirsasana

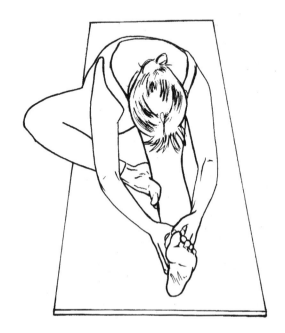

Janu *means "knee," and* sirs *means "head." This posture of humility bows the head over the knee.*

INSTRUCTIONS

Begin in Stick Pose and, without the assistance of your arms, bring your right foot up your left thigh, resting your sole against the inner surface of your leg. Your outer right thigh will remain stationary against the floor.

Inhale, raising your arms to upward salute, with the palms together.

Exhale, extending your torso forward, leading with your chest, lowering your hands to a comfortable place along your left shin.

Inhale, raising your chest, and arching your mid back as you pull your shoulders backward.

Exhale, extending forward, lowering your head between your arms.

Repeat the inhale, lift, exhale, forward-bending sequence several times, until your torso is fully extended over your left leg, with your forehead close to your shin. Pull your shoulders back and down to allow your chest to fully lift. Hold the pose for a minimum of 6 deep rhythmic breaths.

Inhale, lifting up to upward salute.

Exhale, lowering your arms and return your legs to Stick Pose. Repeat on the opposite side.

FOCAL MOVEMENTS

Hip flexion with abduction and external rotation. Focus attention to the strength of the upper thigh (rectus femoris and psoas) of your extended leg, while pulling back and down on your bent knee (gluteus medius and external hip rotators). Relax your groin (adductors) and the back of your extended leg (hamstrings), as you allow your middle- and low-back muscles (latissimus) to stretch.

PRECAUTIONS AND COMMON ERRORS

Avoid using your arms to place your bent leg into position. If you pull the foot of your flexed leg into the groin region, you are more likely to twist your pelvis and spinal column. This, in turn, will twist your spine, making your shoulders uneven in the full pose. Activate your upper thighs as you sit upright. The forward-bending motion should originate from the hip flexors (psoas) and abdominal muscles. Do not use the strength of your arms to create a pull on your backside.

If there is a back injury or excessive tightness in your back, bend your knee to the point where you feel an even distribution of the stretch throughout your back and hamstrings. If the pose is set up asymmetrically, with your hips twisted, or if there is a lateral spinal curve (scoliosis), your shoulders and elbows will be uneven relative to the floor. For scoliosis, it may be helpful to stay in one side longer to lengthen the shortened segment of your spine. Scoliosis often manifests as one hamstring being tighter than the other.

BODY READING

Scoliosis creates an asymmetry of the back during the pose, one side being higher than the other. While difficult to detect from inside the pose, look to your elbows for height asymmetry as a sign of misalignment. Other signs of scoliosis include high pelvic crest, which may alter the shape of your lateral abdomen about the waist. One side may be like an hourglass and the other a smooth curve, or even a straight line. There can also be a distortion in the shape of your ribs seen from the front or back, with one side of your chest being forward. For women, this can give the appearance of one breast being larger than the other (see chapter 11).

Bending your knees in forward bends will isolate the hip flexion function of those hip flexors, which also cross the knee. This optimizes their strength and effectiveness at creating a hip-joint-focused forward bend. By bending your knees and strongly pulling the top of your pelvis forward to maximize the hip flexors, your spine can extend more. You can take advantage of this by slowly moving forward with your upper torso and, over several breath spans, slowly begin to straighten your knees and draw your chest toward your lower thigh.

BENEFITS

Head-to-Knee Pose opens the hips and tends to create a deeper release in the hamstrings than do double leg-forward bends. Like all forward bends, this pose is calming to the mind, as it stimulates the "relaxation reflex," lowering blood pressure and heart rate.

Forward-bending poses are ideal to train the posterior intercostal muscles. By directing respiration to create movement in the back of the rib cage, these muscles are toned. The entire spinal column will also be made more mobile. Hence, this focus is particularly beneficial for stiff backs or scoliosis. Forward bends also tone your patience muscles.

WESTSIDE BACK STRETCH

Paschimottanasana

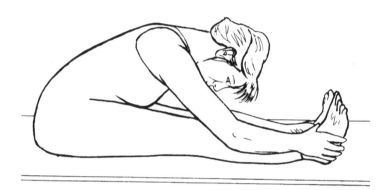

Paschima means "west," implying a stretch of the entire backside from the heels to the occipital ridge at the base of the skull. It is traditional to face east while doing yogasanas, hence the front body is called the east side and the back, the west.

INSTRUCTIONS

Begin, seated in Stick Pose (Dandasana) with your hands beside your hips to support your back.

Inhale, stretching your arms overhead into the Palm Salute (Namaste gesture).

Exhale, bending forward gently to test the sensitivity of stretching your back and legs. Take hold of your legs where it is easy to reach. If your back is tight, lift your chest, being certain to maintain an alignment of your legs, with knees and ankles together.

Inhale, lifting your chest to the point where your arms are straight.

Exhale, bending forward by flexing your elbows, to allow your head to drop between them. Repeat, testing your limit of comfort, until a full stretch is felt evenly throughout your legs and back. When your limit is reached, relax, holding the posture steadily, with deep ujjaye breathing for 12 breaths.

Inhale, coming up with your chest extended upward and your arms raised, palms together in Upward Palm Salute (Namaste gesture). Lift your chest, while relaxing your shoulders. Stay for 3 wave breaths.

Exhale, lowering your arms, returning to the Stick Pose.

FOCAL MOVEMENT

Hip and spine flexion. In the upward extension phase, focus upon the strength of your middle back (latissimus) and hip flexors (psoas). The latissimus can only be contracted when your arms are actively pulling your chest up and your shoulders back and down. After coming out of the pose, encourage an upward lift from your waist to counter-stretch your upper back.

PRECAUTIONS AND COMMON ERRORS

If you have lower-back problems, follow the suggested instructions carefully, so that the effects of the stretch are maximized in your legs and minimized in your back. This guideline helps all students extend their forward-bending capacity, while protecting the deeper and more sensitive back muscles from being overstretched.

This pose is not recommended for students with sciatica or disc problems. Stretching of the hamstrings is beneficial for these conditions, but should be done under supervision to minimize the stress to the lumbar region. In the case of people whose middle back is stiff or who are overweight, the diaphragm is not free to move. As a result, there can be a spasm of the diaphragm. In this case, they will grasp their upper abdomen and gasp for air. The spasm can be instantly relieved by arching backward in Stick Pose, lifting your chest out of the upper abdomen. To prevent this from occurring, students should work only in the upward extension phase until the mid-back musculature and the posterior section of the diaphragm is freed.

The legs should remain together throughout the stretch, as in Stick Pose. If the legs are bowed, the knees will stay separate, although it is helpful to try to narrow the distance between the knees. The lower back should share the effects of the pose with the hamstrings. If the pose is felt predominantly in the lumbar region, the knees should be bent. This will transfer the strain off the back and intensify the stretch of the hamstrings. Often, bending the knees intensifies the stretch of the hamstrings to such an extent that the muscles release and lengthen. This is especially the case in students with tight ligaments and tendons that do not stretch with the Head-to-Knee pose. The neck should extend evenly with the rest of the spine.

BODY READING

Forward bend reveals the flexibility of the long muscles (hamstrings and erector spinae), as well as the flexibility of the spinal column. The pose is one of surrender and, with the proper attitude, this becomes humility, not humiliation. When the chin goes up, so does the ego. Lowering the chin increases humility.

BENEFITS

Forward bends are sedative. This pose is particularly sedative as you learn to relax during the exertion of the forward-bending motion. Increasing the duration of the pose is especially beneficial for hypertensive students. Students for whom muscle tone was developed by running may suffer through the tightness of their hamstrings for some time before they limber up. With persistence, they will uncover a tremendous energy storehouse.

SPINAL TWIST

Marichyasana

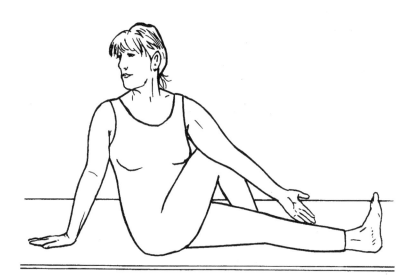

According to B. K. S. Iyengar, Marichi was a sage in Indian mythology. He was the son of Brahma, the Creator, and the grandfather of Surya, the Sun. His name means literally "the Lord of the Dawn." In the Bhagavad Gita, *chapter 10, sutra 6, he is one of the original seven great soul teachers (Maharishis). In sutra 21, Marichi is identified as the chief of the forty-nine winds, the source of prana.*

INSTRUCTIONS

Begin in Stick Pose (Dandasana).

Exhale, bending your right knee to place your foot to the outer side of your left knee. (Men, pause to adjust yourself.)

Inhale, arching your back, while lifting your chest.

Exhale, twisting your upper body to the right, placing your right hand, centered, about 12 inches behind your sacrum. Bring your left elbow to the outer side of your right knee.

Inhale, pulling both shoulders back and down as you expand and lift your chest.

Exhale, pulling your right knee over until it is centered above your foot. If possible, straighten your left arm to take hold of your left shin.

Inhale, extending your spine farther.

Exhale, rotating your head and upper body to the right. Maintain the lift with deep breathing and a steady effort from your upper back muscles. Stay in the pose a minimum of 12 breaths.

Repeat the sequence on the other side.

VARIATIONS

- A gentler method is to hold your outer right knee with your left hand, keeping your forearm parallel with the floor. This is particularly beneficial to increase hip adduction strength and abductor stretch.
- Bend your left knee, placing your foot outside your right buttock. Your left hand holds your right ankle. This creates the Half Matsyendrasana. This is the pose named after the first yoga teacher, whose story was told in the Introduction to Part One (see page 3).

FOCAL MOVEMENTS

Spinal rotation with hip adduction, shoulder extension, and scapular adduction. Focus attention to the strength of your mid back (latissimus) to lift your chest and extend your shoulder. Contract your inner thighs (adductors), then pull your flexed knee to the side. Feel the stretch of your outer hip (gluteus maximus/medius) and your lateral rib cage (serratus anterior).

PRECAUTIONS AND COMMON ERRORS

Twists should be entirely avoided in the case of sacroiliac pain or instability, as they can further destabilize the joint.

This pose has two forces. The initial force is a vertical lifting of the spine and chest. The secondary force is a lateral spinal rotation. If the forces are not applied sequentially, the spinal column will be compressed and/or misaligned. Insufficient lift compresses the abdominal organs and can overwork the arms at the expense of the back muscles. The rotation force comes from the shoulders both pulling backward, thus widening the chest.

Encourage your chest to lift first before twisting. Consider the pose, first, as a backbend that is followed by a twist.

While twists can snap a misaligned vertebra into place with a pop sound, they should not be used for that purpose. When you emphasize lifting your chest and back during twists, misalignments will be corrected, not by joint manipulation, but rather by reinforcing deep erector spinae muscle strength. Over time, this process will help to stabilize vertebral alignment. Regions of the spinal column that require frequent adjustments are weak. This method will develop stamina, bringing less need for manipulation therapy.

Twists are often not held long enough. They should stimulate a relaxation reflex. The release can occur as yawning, sighing, peristalsis moving the intestines, a call to the toilet, gastric reflux burps, a release of pelvic gas, or even an emotional release. Yogis encourage natural reflexes to occur. Suppressing natural reflexes tends to cause physical repercussions.

BODY READING

Twists will reveal scoliosis. Look especially for ease on one side and difficulty on the opposite. The chest will often collapse on the concave side of the spinal curvature. Twists can be therapeutic when done differently to compensate for postural imbalances.

BENEFITS

The spinal rotation strengthens the deep muscles of the erector spinae group and sends more blood to the spinal discs and other deep tissues. In addition, it tones the abdominus obliques, producing firmness at the waist area. Holding the posture strengthens the diaphragm, which, in turn, moves in a massagelike manner into the digestive organs. This often stimulates peristaltic action, which results in gastric sounds while the pose is held.

COMPLETE BOAT

Paripurna Navasana

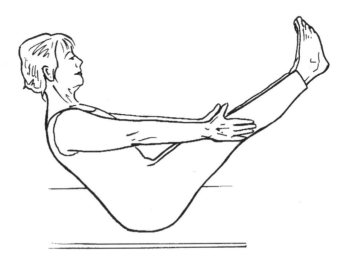

Paripurna *means "complete" or "whole," nava means "boat" or "vessel." An analogy is made of the body being like a boat crossing the sea of worldliness (samsara), leaving the port of ignorance (avidya) of our true nature and sailing toward the final destination of Self-knowledge and spiritual liberation (kaivalya).*

INSTRUCTIONS

Begin in Stick Pose.

Exhale, bending your knees, bringing your palms to the floor beside your knees.

Inhale, lifting your chest.

Exhale, lifting your legs and balancing on your hips with the aid of your hands on the floor.

Inhale, lifting your chest and arms parallel to the floor, with your palms facing each other. Slowly extend your legs, with your knees together.

Exhale, steadying the pose and staying for 6 to 12 full breaths.

Inhale, becoming taller.

Exhale, lowering your legs to the floor, returning to Stick Pose.

VARIATIONS

Each of these phases represents an increased tone of both the hip flexors and lower abdominals. Stay at each level, until it is mastered for 6 steady breaths, before proceeding to the next phase.

- Begin in Stick Pose and bend your knees, balancing on your hips. Then place your hands on the floor in front of your hips. Keep your legs together.
- Repeat the steps above, then lift your feet to the height of your knees.
- Continue by straightening your legs. Keep your hands on the floor beside you for support.

FOCAL MOVEMENTS

Hip flexion with spine and knee extension. Encourage the strength of the upper thigh to the pelvic region (hip flexors), as well as the abdominals (rectus abdominis). Balance their efforts to the straightening of the back and lifting of the chest from the erector spinae. Feel a passive stretch throughout the back of the legs (hamstrings and gastrocnemius) as you lengthen through your heels.

PRECAUTIONS AND COMMON ERRORS

Be cautious if you have a posterior coccyx (vertical) tailbone. Sitting on a cushion may stabilize your balance. This is a good pose to develop your overall stamina. Encourage yourself to extend your stay in this challenging pose beyond what is normally recommended, especially students with lower-back conditions.

BODY READING

Weakness of the psoas and lumbar erectors will keep your lower back rounded. A lack of strength in your quadriceps will make it difficult to straighten your knees and maintain balance. In this case, bend your knees and round your lower back. If there is lower-back pain in the pose, try to release it by bending your knees. Should an instability result, place your hands behind your back, fingers pointed away, and use your shoulder muscles (latissimus, trapezius, and triceps) to support you.

BENEFITS

The pose is beneficial for a number of abdominal and back conditions, including sciatica, lumbago, colitis, constipation, irregular menstrual cycle, and lethargy. A sturdy vessel can weather any storm. Navasana is a great pose for creating physical sturdiness and stamina. The muscles of the lower body are evenly developed with regular practice and better sitting posture is achieved.

COBRA

Bhujangasana

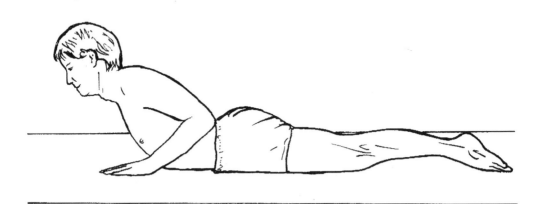

Bhujanga means "cobra." This is sometimes called Sarpasana, meaning "serpent." In the story of Adam and Eve, the serpent possessed the knowledge of discrimination between good and evil. This pose promotes our capacity for discrimination as we evolve to a higher level.

INSTRUCTIONS

Begin lying prone on your abdomen with your legs together. Men should adjust themselves for comfort. Center your head, with your chin on the floor, then place your hands beside your chest. Keep your elbows upward, then pull your shoulders back and down so your upper arms are parallel.

Inhale, raising your head and chest with just the strength of your back muscles.

Exhale, holding the pose so that only your back feels the effort. Bend your elbows back, keeping your arms close to your body. Stay steady, lengthening your spinal column for 12 breaths.

Exhale, lengthening your chest forward as you come down. Relax, resting your hands next to your hips with your head to one side.

FOCAL MOVEMENTS

Upper-back extension. Focus strength to the long erector spinae muscles. Feel the forward stretch of your chest at the sternum, creating an elongation of your abdomen.

PRECAUTIONS AND COMMON ERRORS

Avoid lifting to a height where your lower back feels the effort. Lengthen your spine in the pose so that the effort is spread over a greater length of your back. The most common error is to overuse your arm strength to lift your chest. The ideal is to keep your body in one extended line, thus resembling a cobra. Imagine that your upper arms are an extension of your spine. Since cobras don't have arms, don't use them in this pose.

BODY READING

An inability to lift the entire rib cage from the floor is due to weakness in the erector spinae muscles. If the legs splay apart during the lift, it may be due to weakness in the adductors or a tight psoas muscle. The feet will not come together in the case of knock-knees. Should the feet come off the floor, it may be due to lordosis (swayback), tightness in the hip flexors, or both. When the elbows cannot be held in alignment with the wrists and shoulders, there is tightness in the pectorals and weakness in the middle trapezius. The neck should remain long and neutral. Scrunching of the back of the neck is due to weakness in the sternocleidomastoid and overexertion of the upper trapezius.

BENEFITS

Cobra strengthens the deep muscles of the spine, the erector spinae, and may be of relief to sciatica sufferers. The stretch opens the upper abdominal region, relieving compression of the diaphragm and promoting a fuller breathing pattern. It can often release gas trapped in the upper digestive tract.

LOCUST

Salabhasana

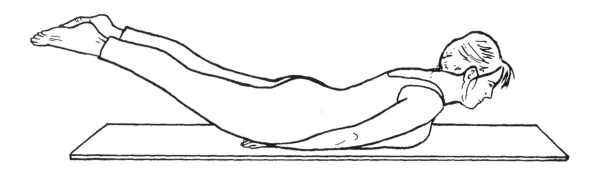

Salabha *means "locust." Grasshoppers are vegetarians. In mimicking its qualities, the pose promotes power to our digestion.*

INSTRUCTIONS

Begin lying prone, chin on the ground, with your arms palm upward beside or beneath your thighs.

Inhale, extending your legs as you lift them off the floor. Your upper body can be moderately lifted to counterbalance your weight. Stay steadily with your feet hip-width apart. Continue to lengthen your neck and spine throughout the stay. Remain for 6 to 12 breaths.

Exhale, lowering your legs and relaxing with your head to one side. Maintain full, natural breathing.

VARIATIONS

- The posture can be done lifting one leg at a time. This is called Half Locust—Ardha Salabhasana.
- The pose can also be done with the arms lifted behind the back. This variation, in some yoga circles, is called the Boat Pose (Navasana).
- Pressing your hands firmly against the floor can bring your legs higher. This transfers the tone to the middle back (latissimus dorsi) and back of the arms (triceps). For the purpose of strengthening your hips, it is recommended to do the pose as given.

FOCAL MOVEMENTS

The primary motion is hip extension, with a secondary focus on spine and knee extension. Direct strength, especially to the buttocks (gluteus maximus) and hamstrings. Then extend your legs to tone your knees (quadriceps) and upper back (trapezius and erector spinae of the deep back). Feel an elongation of your pelvis and legs away from your abdomen to tone your abdominals.

PRECAUTIONS AND COMMON ERRORS

The effort should be spread over the length of your back, including your hips and shoulders. In all backbends, avoid overexertion of your lumbar region. Stay in the pose only as long as you can maintain full breathing. Shallow and/or rapid breathing is a preliminary sign of strain that may not be felt until after the pose's effort is over.

BODY READING

An inability to lift your feet above 12 inches is due to loss of tone of the hip extensors, the hamstrings, and the gluteus maximus. Another sign of this imbalance is that one knee may be extended, while the other is slightly bent. Uneven leg length, due to rotation of the iliac pelvis, may be revealed by an uneven lift of the legs.

BENEFITS

This is an invaluable pose to a complete yoga routine, though it is often neglected. For many people, this is a more challenging pose than the Cobra, as this posture tones the entire backside. It can relieve nerve strains, like sciatica, if their source is an anterior nerve-root compression. In this type of pain due to compression, symptoms are often exaggerated by forward bending, which further compresses the anterior nerve roots of the spinal nerves.

This motion creates a springing action within the spinal column, allowing it to lengthen more easily during both backward and forward bending poses.

HERO

Virasana

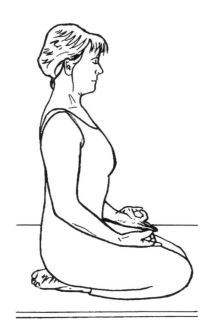

Vira *means "hero." A variation, in which the full length of the legs are strongly contracted together, is called the Thunderbolt, or Vajrasana. Vajra refers to a channel of consciousness within the Sushumna Nadi, the central subtle nerve. The spiritual force called Shakti Kundalini travels through Sushumna, hence this channel is experienced on a subtle dimension after spiritual awakening. Yogis are considered to be spiritual heros.*

INSTRUCTIONS

Inhale, as you begin in Cat Pose, with your head up and your spine arched downward.

Exhale, bringing your legs and inner ankles together. Press your hips backward, as in Fetal Pose (Garbhasana).

Inhale, as you slowly lift your upper body to an erect posture. If there is no strain at the knees or ankles, come fully erect with a natural lumbar curve, shoulders back and down, and hands palm up, resting on your thighs. Join the tips of your thumbs with the tips of your forefingers in the Gesture of Wisdom (Jnana Mudra). Remain inwardly focused for 1 to 5 minutes before releasing the pose.

FOCAL MOVEMENTS

Hip and knee flexion, ankle plantar flexion. Encourage a feeling of strength in your spine to become erect and tall (psoas and erector spinae). Relax into any stretch of the muscles of the front thighs (quadriceps), shins (tibialis anterior) or ankles.

PRECAUTIONS AND COMMON ERRORS

This pose requires more than normal range of joint mobility for the knee and ankle joints. It is the only pose I give that asks joints to go beyond their normal range. I find its benefits outweigh the possibility of strains, if you are sensible about progressing gently to your limitations. However, some students will persist at stretching through painful tightness. If you are making a face when you do this pose, you are straining. Learn to recognize strain as a sign to stop. Come forward and take the weight on your hands, instead of your knees.

The pose should not be held if there is a strain in your knees. Instead, lean your torso forward and do the pose as a partial Cat Pose by taking some of your weight on your hands. If a strain is felt in the ankles only, a pad can be placed under the lower shin up to the top of your ankle. The pad should not extend to the end of your foot.

If strain is felt in your knees, place a pad behind your knees to lessen the weight on your ankles and diminish the stretch of your quadriceps. A wooden meditation bench may be advisable for more prolonged sitting.

BODY READING

When viewed from the front, the pose may reveal lateral spinal curvatures. Viewed from the side, it can reveal tight hip flexors, creating an excessive lumbar arch, a rounded thoracic spine, or a forward head. Inability to bring your hips to your heels is due to either tight quadriceps or ankles.

BENEFITS

Here the upper body is beautifully aligned, uplifted in a proud heroic gesture of self-confidence. Often asanas benefit the psyche more than the physical body. This is one in which the attitude of being heroic is both physically and energetically felt. By opening yourself to a spiritual mood, the pose can generate a techniqueless state of meditation. When using a meditation cushion or bench, the pose affords an erect posture for pranayama and meditation. The primary physical benefits are in toning the thighs and ankles, which promotes flexibility of the lower back. Hero pose also improves digestion and is the only pose I find helpful immediately following a meal.

CAMEL

Ustrasana

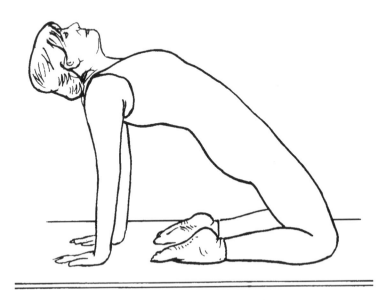

Ustra *means "camel." In Hindu mythology, the camel is dear to the ancient teacher Rizhi Sukra, who personifies the planet Venus, the preserver of virility.*[5] *The pose is believed to enhance vitality and sexual pleasure.*

INSTRUCTIONS

Begin in Hero Pose, then place your hands on the floor 6 inches behind and to the side of your feet, with your fingers pointing backward.

Inhale, lifting your chest fully, expanding it, then leaning your head backward to look at the ceiling.

Exhale, maintaining the lift of your chest for 6 breaths.

Inhale, lifting your pelvis up and forward, until your torso comes into a straight line from your knees to your shoulders. Stay in the pose for 6 breaths.

Exhale, releasing the pose by lowering your hips to Hero Pose.

---

5 Stutley, *The Illustrated Dictionary of Hindu Iconography,* pp. 136 and 149.

VARIATIONS

- If sitting on your shins in the Hero Pose is not possible, the same back-bending motion can be achieved using Stick or Bound Angle Pose as the foundation for your legs.
- The pose can be partially done by lifting only your hips without expanding your chest or lifting only your chest without lifting your hips.

FOCAL MOVEMENTS

Hip, thoracic, and shoulder extension, with neck flexion gradually moving backward toward neutral. Focus upon strengthening your entire back—gluteus maximus, latissimus, and erector spinae. Holding your head to look forward will tone your sternocleidomastoid muscle. A strong pelvic thrust will stretch your hip flexors (psoas) and front of your thighs (quadriceps). Lifting your chest will stretch the side of your rib cage, serratus anterior, and the central abdomen (rectus abdominis).

PRECAUTIONS AND COMMON ERRORS

If you have a weak neck, don't let your head hang backward in the pose, as your neck could be strained due to the challenge to the sternocleidomastoid. Doing this shortens your spine. Concentrate instead on the entire spinal column lengthening. The effect of the pose should not strain your lower back. If it does, thrust your pelvis forward by tightening your buttocks and/or bringing your hips back to lessen the stretch of your quadriceps. If your quadriceps feel tight, open your thighs beyond hip width to allow your adductors to release their grip on the quadriceps.

BODY READING

Avoid overworking one part of your body and underworking another. The ideal is to challenge the strength of your hips evenly as you challenge your shoulders, thus producing a stretch of your chest that is equal to the stretch of your quadriceps.

BENEFITS

Camel Pose fully opens the chest and is beneficial for respiratory conditions such as asthma or emphysema, in that it can create a vacuum inside the chest cavity. The stretch of the quadriceps is important for runners, in that it can free the hip joint, thus increasing the length of the stride. The stretch of the quadriceps and hip flexors is also important for its progressive effect at relieving back conditions, especially sciatica.

FACE OF LIGHT

Gomukhasana

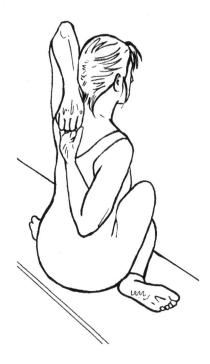

Go *means "cow" or "light."* Mukh *means "face." The pose is usually translated as the Face of a Cow. However, I prefer Face of Light, as the pose promotes an expression of radiant serenity.*

INSTRUCTIONS

Begin by sitting in Hero Pose.

Exhale, sitting to the left side of your feet.

Inhale, as you come erect.

Exhale, folding your right leg over the top of your left, bringing your feet to the sides of your hips, with your knees nearly on top of each other.

Inhale, stretching your left arm over your head, folding it so that the palm of your hand reaches down your spine.

Exhale, reaching your right hand across the back of your waist as far as possible. Then flex your elbow so your hand reaches toward your left hand. If possible, grip fingers together. Keep the back of your hand toward your spine.

Inhale, expanding your chest as you firm the grip of your hands. Breathe steadily for 6 to 12 rhythmic breaths.

Exhale, releasing your arms.

Inhale, stretching your legs out to Stick Pose. Then reverse the pose.

FOCAL MOVEMENTS

Hips are in adduction with external rotation. The knees are in flexion, upper shoulder and elbows are in flexion. The lower shoulder is in extension and internal rotation. Continue to squeeze your thighs firmly in adduction. By keeping an erect spinal column, you are more likely to be able to flex your upper shoulder enough to bring your hands together.

PRECAUTIONS AND COMMON ERRORS

Avoid sitting on your feet, rather keep them to the sides of your hips. It is more important to maintain an erect posture than to join hands. If you do not touch hands, hold a tie with your upper hand and grip it with your lower hand. After a few breaths, you can slowly inch your hands closer together to deepen the opening of your shoulders. Avoid stressing your lower shoulder, as it is in a delicate position that could stretch ligaments rather than muscles.

BODY READING

Unevenness of the hips indicates tightness in the external hip rotators, gluteus maximus, or abductors. An inability to cross the legs, if not due to the size of the thighs, is usually due to tightness in the hip abductors. If the upper arm does not come even with the ear, there is shortness in the triceps, pectorals, and/or latissimus. An inability to raise the lower hand up the back is due to restrictions in the shoulder internal rotators and/or biceps brachii.

　　While this pose is beneficial for sciatica, it is only helpful if your abductors are free. An ability to have the knees close together indicates the sciatic nerve is free enough to be able to benefit from the pose. Thus those with sciatica who cannot bring their knees together may be aggravating their condition. The stretch ideally is felt in your outer hips rather than the center of your buttocks.

BENEFITS

This is a wonderful pose for its combination of deep release of the hips and shoulders simultaneously. It releases hidden tensions in joints, nerves, and muscles. Staying in the pose may stimulate the digestive fire, agni, helping to improve elimination. Over time, the pose produces serenity, the natural state of a cow at pasture. Eventually, that serenity unfolds into a radiant spiritual light. Then the pose can be said to have given its full benefits.

RELAXATION OF A CORPSE

Savasana

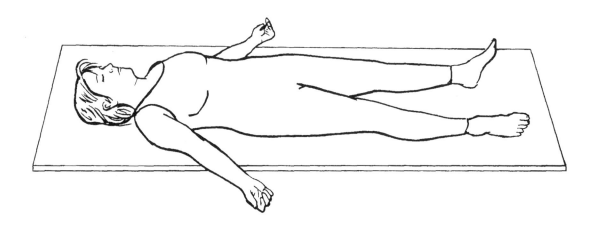

Sava means "corpse." In this deep relaxation posture, you lie motionless, appearing outwardly as still as a corpse. The relaxation deepens into meditation upon the constancy of duality, the nature of activity (Shakti) within stillness (Siva) can be directly perceived.

INSTRUCTIONS

Inhale, in Stick Pose.

Exhale, then bend your knees toward your head, and roll your spine downward using a strong pelvic thrust as you go into the floor. Once your lower back is flat, rest your upper-body weight on your forearms.

Inhale, extend your legs, spreading them hip-width apart as you bring them to the floor.

Exhale, reach your arms down and outward from your shoulders.

Inhale, tuck your shoulder blades down while rolling your arms outward to leave your chest lifted and full.

Exhale, lengthen your head away from your shoulders, adjusting it so it feels level.

Take a few breaths with your mouth open to release the air that was held in the sinus, mouth, and tracheal passageways. Continue with mouth breathing as long as you feel tense or fatigued. This is the only purpose for which mouth breathing is appropriate. When you feel a reflex of relaxation progressing over your body, gently close your mouth, breathing with ujjaya pranayama for some time, while completely relaxing your body in a motion-free posture.

Concentrate your mind upon your breath's wave-like motions, then scan your body from head to feet, feeling and listening to each part's messages in turn. Allow your body scan to take from 2 to 5 minutes. Next, consciously slow your breathing. After some time with this, encourage your thoughts to move more slowly. To deepen the relaxation reflex, concentrate on the rising and subsiding patterns within your body, regardless of where you experience them. Remain mentally alert, yet physically passive, for a minimum of 5 to 10 minutes. When you are finished, roll onto your left side and curl up for a few moments of deep breathing before you transition to sitting.

VARIATIONS

• If your shoulders or neck are uncomfortable, a variation is to allow your hands to rest on your abdomen. For some people, their shoulders will relax more completely with their hands beside their head, elbows bent out to a right angle. This latter adjustment is particularly restful for persons with well-developed shoulder muscles.

• If your lower back is uncomfortable, an alternative is to bend your knees, letting them rest together, with your feet slightly apart. Or you can place a rolled towel behind your knees to release tension in your lower back.

• If lying on your back is uncomfortable and you are unable to lie still, an alternative is to lie on your abdomen. In this event, lie with your feet apart, toes inward, and your arms crossed to support your head. This posture is called the Crocodile, or Makarasana.

• For ladies who are pregnant, relaxation can be accomplished by lying on the right side, knees bent, with a pillow beneath the head and a second pillow between your knees.

• If you are not comfortable and cannot adjust yourself so that relaxation becomes an automatic event, ask your instructor for a manipulation. In this case, become limp as they move your limbs or head to provide better support and an opportunity for improved circulation. Allow the adjustments time to take effect. You may not be comfortable for 30 to 60 seconds. If discomfort persists beyond this point, adjust again. Continue to reposition yourself until you find the optimal placement for your body to surrender to the pull of gravity and your innate "relaxation reflex."

GUIDED MENTAL IMAGERY

There is a wide variety of mental instructions that help to deepen the effects of yoga. Any of the following three questions may be utilized for a portion, or the whole, of the relaxation period.

1. Where am I feeling my body reactions?

2. What am I feeling?

3. Is the feeling emotional or physical in nature?

These questions can be answered in depth, or simply left as questions to be repeated in a mantra-like fashion. The latter method serves to strengthen the path of self-inquiry and may be utilized during seated contemplative meditation practice.

By staying conscious during relaxation, you improve the strength of your mind. At first, relaxation training may put you to sleep or bring about an unconscious emptiness. These reactions are quite normal and are indicative of neurological reprogramming to your parasympathetic nervous system. These are the anatomical structures of your "relaxation reflex." Should you go unconscious, relax and make the transition from stillness slowly, gradually, moving with deliberate anticipated motions.

One special variation is called the Yogic Sleep or Yoga Nidra. In this procedure, students remain alert for up to an hour, feeling a detailed multidimensional awareness through their physical body, organs, subtle-body chakras, subtle nerves, to your spiritual body of light. This is a powerful method of uncovering the innate life-force energy within you—an energy that transcends death. By direct experience, yoga students can come to know that force, as they disengage all physical, sensory—and to some degree, mental—activities. The body is dropped fully. What is left can only be known by experience.

FOCAL MOVEMENTS

Passive hip and shoulder external rotation. Remain in an attitude of attentive relaxation.

BODY READING

The feet should remain about two feet apart. Less than this indicates constriction in the groin muscles or adductors. Without this width, the hips are not able to achieve their full turn-out position. The angle of the feet will indicate balance or lack of it in the hip rotators. The anatomical norm is for both feet to be turned out 45 degrees. Less than this indicates that the external hip rotators are weak on that side, and that the internal hip rotators are tight.

The shoulder blades will lie flat, unless the pectoral muscles are tight. Observe the location of the hands. In full relaxation, the palms will be upward, with the fingers slightly curled. The head will be level from chin to forehead, making swallowing an easy and natural event. If the chin is up, then a pillow should be placed beneath it to compensate for the shortness of the upper chest (pectoralis major), tightness in the upper back (trapezius), and weakness of the neck flexors (sternocleidomastoid).

If the body reading results obtained from the standing evaluation cited in this book are compared with those felt, but not seen, during lying relaxation, intriguing correlates may be discovered. The standing posture reveals vertical (that is, top-to-bottom) misalignments. The Relaxation Pose reveals horizontal, or front-to-back, misalignments. When the same findings are revealed in both postures, this is significant. The imbalances so uncovered need particular attention to alleviate the postural changes and to strengthen their underlying muscular weaknesses. There are only four muscles in the body that are both horizontal and vertical. The two most important ones are the psoas and the diaphragm. All body misalignments will affect a change in their positioning, as well as their functioning. They are particularly involved in spinal changes or distortions, such as scoliosis, or uneven pelvis or shoulder. The other muscles in this pattern are the sartorius and the sternocleidomastoid. The sartorius is involved in stress at the knee, hip, and sacroiliac joint, while the sternocleidomastoid is usually weak in students with temporomandibular (jaw) and neck tensions.

BENEFITS

This is the classical pose for relaxing the body/mind to fully absorb the benefits of yoga practices. The deep relaxation that this pose promotes helps, over time, to restore and rejuvenate the student. During Corpse Pose, the body rests steadily and becomes a place for us to enter deeply. We become explorers who can travel ever deeper into ourselves, through layers of consciousness, to encounter the treasure that we are.

A longer Corpse Pose, from 20 to 60 minutes, is recommended as a "fatigue fighter," or to recover from summer heat exhaustion. The Corpse Pose is highly regarded as a treatment for hypertension. There are numerous physiological studies of Hatha Yoga practices for lowering blood pressure. The most graphic of these studies involves the use of Corpse Pose for a group of forty-seven hypertensive patients whose average age was 46.[6] The original blood pressure averaged 186 mm. Hg. for systolic and 115 mm. Hg. for diastolic, with the mean being 134. Their mental exercise was to pay attention to the sensations of breathing at the nostrils, specifically to feel the warmth of the expired air and the coolness of the inspired air. Following three weeks of practice, the subjects showed a change in mean blood pressure from 134 to 107. Drug requirements decreased an average of 68 percent. Other studies of students with normal blood pressure showed no significant change to blood pressure following the same exercise.[7]

Relaxation processes have been used as an adjunct for treating substance abuse and for lessening addictive behaviors. It should be noted that in these circumstances, the client needs to learn not only how to relax but how to replace abusive behaviors with positive affirmative activities.

In Tantrik Yoga, Savasana is used as a contemplation of the ephemeral nature of life and the significance of acting responsibly for the positive fulfillment of your destiny to help others. There are many ways death can come. By reflecting on its inevitability, we build tremendous courage, fortitude, and confidence.

---

[6] Dr. K. Datey et al., "Shavasana: A Yogic Exercise in the Management of Hypertension," *Angiology* (1969): 20, pp. 325–333.
[7] James Funderburk, *Science Studies Yoga: A Review of Physiological Data* (Honesdale, PA.: Himalayan International Institute, 1977), pp. 36–38.

BOUND ANGLE

Baddha Konasana

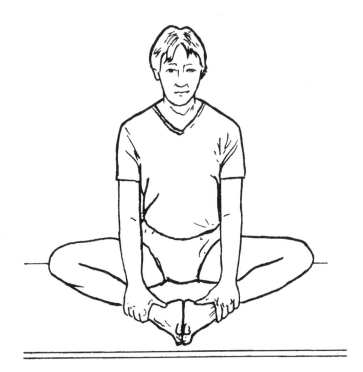

Baddha means "restrained" or "bound." Kon refers to an "angle." This pose is called Bhadrasana, or the auspicious pose, in the classic text, Hatha Yoga Pradipika *(chapter 1, sutras 53–54). It is given at the end of the yogasana sequence to indicate that pranayama and meditation practices should be done at this point of the series. When practiced as a yoga pose for physical benefits, it is sequenced following Face of Light Pose and prior to Relaxation of a Corpse Pose.*

INSTRUCTIONS

Begin in Stick Pose.

Inhale, sitting tall.

Exhale, drawing your feet soles together with a minimum of arm effort, then holding above your ankles.

Inhale, sitting erect, chest expanded, with your arms straight. Breathe steadily, adjusting your feet forward until your lower back is straight. Adapt the pose so that the effort to remain erect comes predominantly from your back and not your arms. Tense your outer hip muscles to pull your knees closer to the floor. Remain in the pose as long as you can sustain steady and comfortable breathing.

VARIATION

- Yogacharya B. K. S. Iyengar does the pose with his hands encircling the ends of his feet. This variation can be used, provided there is no effort at pulling the toes from the floor.

After the pose becomes comfortable, it can become a meditation pose, which is the intention in the classical method of Bhadrasana. In the completed pose, the arms are extended with the fingers in Wisdom Seal (Jnana Mudra), the thumb and forefinger joined, the other fingers extended toward the floor. This pose makes an energetic pyramid of your entire body with four lines—one from each knee, one from the feet, and one from the base of the spine—converging at the head.

FOCAL MOVEMENTS

Hip flexion with abduction and external rotation. Direct strength to your hip flexors (psoas) and outer hips (gluteus medius and external rotator group). Create a release in your groin to stretch your inner thighs (adductors).

PRECAUTIONS AND COMMON ERRORS

Be careful not to strain your knees. Pay particular attention not to have stress at your inner knee area adjacent to your kneecaps. Taking the upper thigh flesh and turning it outward from the groin may relieve your knees. Another method is to grip the inner knee tendons of the tripod muscles (hamstrings, gracilis, and sartorius) and turn their flesh outward. Maximizing the external rotation from your hips often releases pressure from your knees or groin.

The ideal posture is with the lumbar spine unchanged from Stick Pose and the knees as close to the floor as possible. If, in bringing your feet closer to the perineum, either is diminished, keep your feet farther forward of your pelvis.

BODY READING

If your lower back cannot come forward to an erect spinal posture, place a pad beneath your hips. The pad should be thick enough to correct this alignment. The need for this adjustment indicates tight adductors and/or weak hip flexors (most likely the psoas muscle). One knee higher than the other is often accompanied with a spinal curvature or mild scoliosis.

BENEFITS

Like Stick Pose, this pose trains the spine and hip muscles for prolonged sitting meditation and pranayama practices. Because of its open-hip stance, this pose also releases restrictions on the lower spine, thus helping it to elongate. In essence, freeing the hips liberates the spine and allows the back to become independent of the pelvis and legs.

Chapter 21

ASANA
KINESIOLOGY

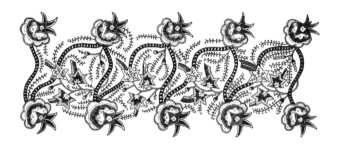

Many students want to know if what they are feeling is correct. This is an excellent question and the answer varies. In the Structural Yoga™ approach to Classical Yoga, the student is directed to hold the pose so that attention is focused upon the specific sites feeling the sensations of stretch and strength. The beginner often reports feeling the poses all over. This is normally a sign of lack of sensitivity training. When there is too much sensation, the student may be overwhelmed and unable to determine where or what is being felt.

It takes time to understand anatomy and yet remain detached enough from that intellectual knowledge to gain somatic knowledge of your feeling mind/body. Many regular students cannot distinguish the feeling of stretch from those of strengthening. While this may seem to be an astonishing statement, it is quite true nonetheless. Even yoga students of many years fail to think clearly about their experience of practice, especially in intricate asanas where the body is doing several joint motions simultaneously. For instance, in simple cross-legged sitting, it is not easy to determine what one feels in the musculature. The knees are flexed, the hips are flexed, and they are externally rotated. This combination of joint motions requires discrimination to perceive kinesthetically and to understand intellectually what is occurring in the musculature. With anatomical mindfulness and detachment as core to their training, students will be able to give details on the specific areas reacting to a posture.

A beautiful practice of yogasana is a work of art—or, more accurately, it is a combination of a work of art and a work of diligent persistent effort guided by discrimination. As you continue to practice yogasanas, you may find yourself wondering if you are doing the poses properly or feeling the poses in the right places. This is a good question to continue to ask yourself.

Where Should I Feel the Pose?

For students on the beginning level, there is a right and wrong way to do the yoga poses. There is a correct appearance and correct feel for the postures. The right way will alleviate the sources of your stress and physical tension. The right way just plain feels good. Where you feel the poses will vary according to your postural imbalances, your strength, and your flexibility. Figure 20 on pages 250 through 253 illustrates the 24 poses of the Structural Yoga Therapy™ routine and indicates the ideal muscles that will be strengthened and stretched.

This summary is misleading, however, unless you remember your specific postural imbalances. Muscles will not stretch or strengthen normally when there are postural imbalances. The shape of your bones may be different from that shown in pictures in anatomy atlases. These two factors will give your body feelings in places that are different from other students.

I encourage students in my classes to tell me where they feel the poses for two reasons. First, I want them to be practicing self-observation as much as possible. By focusing your attention on yourself, you are more inclined to self-adjust and lessen your tension. Second, I want to protect them from hurting themselves or working in detrimental ways. Since I know anatomy and yoga better than most of my students, I know where the safe and unsafe places are in every yogasana.

For students who practice irregularly, but are not beginners, most of the previous considerations are also valid. For them, however, additional concern is needed to provide motivation for establishing regularity. The need is there to keep the practice at a level of intensity that is fresh, insightful, and stimulating, yet not overly aggressive.

For students on the committed level, yoga is a personal practice aimed at getting to know yourself. For them, there really is no wrong way to do the poses. Regular reading of the guidelines given in Patanjali's *Yoga Sutras* will definitely deepen the experiences available from yoga practice.

Figure 20 summarizes ideal places to focus your intention to strengthen and stretch. The movements and muscles cited are optimal for receiving the benefits of the poses. Be gentle and do not demand that your body feel the effects as cited. Persist, nonetheless, at consistently guiding yourself to find these places of your anatomy while in the yogasanas.

Figure 20 is based upon practices as described in this book and asanas from the text of B. K. S. Iyengar in his *Light on Yoga*.[1] As his method is well accepted for its precision of anatomical placement, it is the most readily usable method of Hatha Yoga for this study. Note that, while many different teachers may teach the Extended Triangle Pose, their placement of the body may vary tremendously from the method presented here. Hence, this chart is only accurate for the way the poses are presented here. To apply these

---

[1] B. K. S. Iyengar, *Light on Yoga* (New York: Schocken Books, 1979).

principles to other styles of yoga would require a separate study to determine the kine-siological effects of modified poses.

Table 5 on pages 254 through 255 lists the poses to strengthen and stretch the mus-cles indicated in the middle column. Three poses are given for each purpose, listed in order of their increasing effectiveness at working the complete combinations of actions of the muscle cited. When choosing poses from Table 5 to work on specific area, remem-ber to practice them in the sequence in which they are presented in Figure 20.

Gravity—An Additional Factor in Asana Kinesiology

The effects of gravity cannot be underemphasized. The same pose done in different body placements creates an extremely different benefit to the musculo-skeletal system. An astute student will notice in the Structural Yoga Therapy™ series that there are sev-eral postures in which the body is at a right angle (90 degrees) of hip flexion. These include Downward Facing Dog, Upward Stretched Legs, Supported Shoulderstand, Stick, and the Complete Boat. To this, one could add the preliminary motion of the Half-Forward Bend, and the more advanced Plow Pose (Halasana). In each instance, there is a contraction of the hip flexors (rectus femoris, psoas, tensor fascia lata, and sar-torius) and a stretch of the hip extensors (hamstrings and gluteus maximus). In each, the relationship of the body to gravity is changed, so the kinesiological effects are different. For instance, to compare the effects on the hamstrings in these poses, the pull is mildest in the Complete Boat and Inverted Action Poses and somewhat greater in Stick Pose. Yet most students do not feel these effects unless their hamstrings were extremely short. The effectiveness of stretching the hamstrings is more pronounced in Half-Forward Bend and a full stretch is usually experienced in Downward Facing Dog Pose.

Similarly, if we compare these poses for their effectiveness in strengthening the hip flexors, the effect is mild in the Inverted Action Pose, stronger in the Stick Pose, and most challenging in the Downward Facing Dog and Complete Boat Poses. By taking these factors into consideration, we can grade the level of difficulty more precisely when composing your personalized Structural Yoga Therapy™ program.

Designing your Personal Program

By summarizing the muscles you need to strengthen and muscles you need to stretch, you have created a thorough evaluation. The next step will be to find yoga poses that stretch and strengthen the specific muscles you want to change. The first line of Table 5 shows muscles strengthened, the second line the poses which stretch the muscle. The poses on each line are ranked for three levels of intensity. The first pose cited will pro-duce a mild effect, the second a moderate effect. The third pose presents the strongest challenge to the muscle. From this you can find the appropriate asana to practice for a personalized program.

To create the most effective practice, you will need to sequence the program prop-erly. This book gives the sequence in the progression of its writing. In chapter 33, you will see a list summarizing all the practices presented in the proper practice sequence. You can delete certain practices and still maintain the sequence.

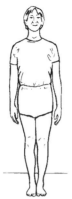

Mountain
Tadasana

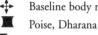 Baseline body reading

Poise, Dharana

Spine, sternum

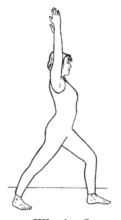

Warrior I
Virabhadrasana

Hip adduction; shoulder flexion

Hip adductors; tensor fascia lata and middle deltoids

Gastrocnemius, tensor fascia lata

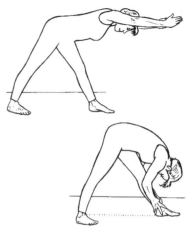

Side-of-Hip Stretch
Parsvottanasana

Hip flexion; with adduction

Psoas; hip adductors

Hamstrings; gluteus medius

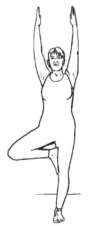

Balancing Tree
Vrksasana

Hip abduction; with external rotation

Straight leg adductors and external rotators

Lengthen spine

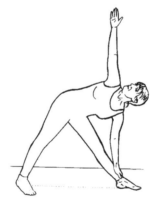

Extended Triangle
Utthita Trikonasana

Hip flexion; spinal lateral flexion

Rectus femoris; abdominis oblique, sternocleidomastoid

Hip adductors, hamstrings

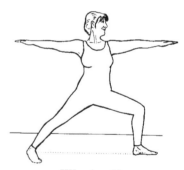

Warrior II
Virabhadrasana

Hip external rotation with abduction; ankle dorsiflexion; scapula abduction

Hip external rotators, abductors

Gastrocnemius, soleus; hip adductors

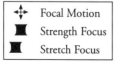 Focal Motion

Strength Focus

Stretch Focus

Figure 20. Structural Yoga™ Kinesiology.

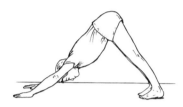

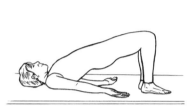

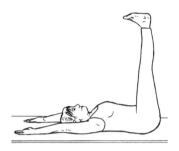

Downward Facing Dog
Adho Mukha Svanasana

⬌ Hip and shoulder flexion; ankle dorsiflexion

◼ Psoas; deltoid; tibialis anterior

◠ Gastrocnemius, hamstrings, lengthen spine upward

Bridge
Setubandhasana

⬌ Hip extension; knee flexion; scapula adduction with depression

◼ Gluteus maximus; hamstrings; middle and lower trapezius

◠ Hip flexors, pectorals

Upward Stretched Legs
Urdhva Prasarita Padasana

⬌ Hip and shoulder flexion; knee extension

◼ Psoas, rectus femoris; deltoids; quadriceps

◠ Passive hamstrings, gastrocnemius

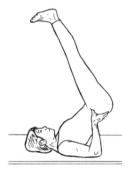

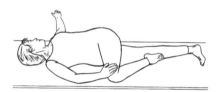

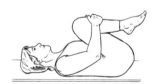

Supported Shoulderstand
Salamba Sarvangasana

⬌ Thoracic and shoulder extension; hip and elbow flexion; scapula adduction

◼ Latissimus, triceps; psoas; biceps; middle trapezius

◠ Pectorals, upper trapezius

Abdominal Twist
Jathara Parivartanasana

⬌ Hip adduction, spinal rotation

◼ Hip adductors, abdominis oblique

◠ Gluteus medius, latissimus

Energy Freeing
Apanasana

⬌ Spine, hip, and knee flexion; shoulder adduction

◼ Rectus abdominis, hip flexors; latissimus, triceps; pectorals

◠ Gluteus maximus, lumbar erector spinae

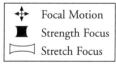

⬌ Focal Motion
◼ Strength Focus
◠ Stretch Focus

Figure 20. Structural Yoga™ Kinesiology (continued).

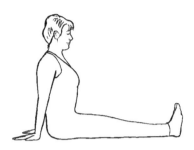

Stick
Dandasana

↔ Hip flexion, thoracic extension

▮ Psoas, rectus femoris, latissimus

▮ Passive hamstrings, wrist flexors

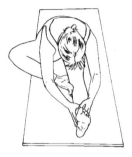

Head to Knee
Janu Sirsasana

↔ Hip flexion with abduction and external rotation

▮ Psoas, rectus femoris; gluteus medius; external rotators

▮ Adductors, hamstrings, latissimus

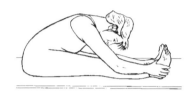

Westside Back Stretch
Paschimottanasana

↔ Hip and spine flexion

▮ Psoas, latissimus

▮ Hamstrings, erector spinae, latissimus

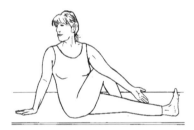

Spinal Twist
Marichyasana

↔ Hip adduction, spine rotation, shoulder extension

▮ Adductors; abdominis oblique, sternocleidomastoid; latissimus, triceps

▮ Gluteus medius

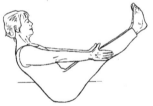

Complete Boat
Paripurna Navasana

↔ Hip flexion, knee and spine extension

▮ Psoas, rectus femoris; Rectus abdominis, erector spinae

▮ Passive hamstrings

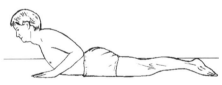

Cobra
Bhujangasana

↔ Thoracic and shoulder extension; scapula adduction

▮ Erector spinae, triceps, lower and middle trapezius

▮ Pectorals, Rectus abdominis

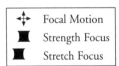

↔ Focal Motion
▮ Strength Focus
▮ Stretch Focus

Figure 20. Structural Yoga™ Kinesiology (continued).

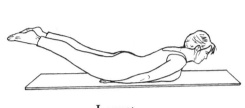

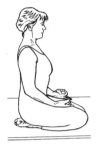

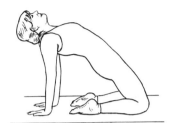

Locust
Salabhasana

⬄ Hip, spine, knee extension

◼ Hamstrings, gluteus maximus; erector spinae; quadriceps

⊏⊐ Passive hip flexors, rectus abdominis

Hero
Virasana

⬄ Hip and knee flexion; ankle plantar flexion

◼ Psoas, erector spinae

⊏⊐ Quadriceps; tibialis anterior

Camel
Ustrasana

⬄ Hip; spine; shoulder extension; neck flexion

◼ Gluteus maximus; erectors, latissimus, triceps; sternocleidomastoid

⊏⊐ Psoas, quadriceps

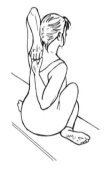

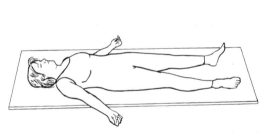

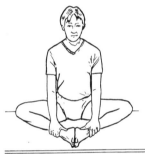

Face of Light
Gomukhasana

⬄ Hip adduction and external rotation; shoulder internal rotation

◼ Psoas, adductors, lower trapezius

⊏⊐ Gluteus maximus, gluteus medius, triceps, anterior deltoid

Relaxation of a Corpse
Savasana

⬄ Passive hip and shoulder external rotation

Attentive relaxation

Bound Angle
Baddha Konasana

⬄ Hip flexion; abduction with external rotation

◼ Psoas, sartorius; gluteus medius; external rotators

⊏⊐ Hip adductors

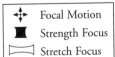

⬄ Focal Motion
◼ Strength Focus
⊏⊐ Stretch Focus

Figure 20. Structural Yoga™ Kinesiology (continued).

Table 5. The Kinesiology of Yogasanas.

BODY REGION	MUSCLES AFFECTED	YOGA POSES TO STRENGTHEN AND STRETCH
NECK	Sternocleidomastoid Flexion, lateral rotation	*Strengthen*: Spinal Twist, Extended Triangle, Camel *Stretch*: Twisting poses
	Upper Trapezius Extension	*Strengthen*: Camel, Cobra, Locust *Stretch*: Bridge, Shoulderstand, Plow
SHOULDER	Middle Deltoid/Supraspinatus Abduction to 90 degrees	*Strengthen*: Extended Triangle, Warrior II, Side Body Support *Stretch*: Seated Spinal Twist, Face of Light, Eagle
	Anterior Deltoid Flexion to 90 degrees, internal rotation	*Strengthen*: Balancing Tree, Downward Facing Dog, Eagle *Stretch*: Stick, Camel, Plow
	Posterior Deltoid Extension, external rotation	*Strengthen*: Cobra, Bow, Supported Shoulderstand *Stretch*: Down Dog, Face of Light, Reverse Namaste
	Pectoralis Major Flexion, adduction, internal rotation	*Strengthen*: Stick, Energy-Freeing Pose, Spinal Twist *Stretch*: Cobra, Camel, Downward Facing Dog
	Teres Major Extension, adduction, internal rotation	*Strengthen*: Camel, Cobra, Plow *Stretch*: Downward Dog, Spinal Twist, Face of Light
	Teres Minor/Infraspinatus Adduction, external rotation	*Strengthen*: Camel, Supported Shoulderstand, Bow *Stretch*: Cat, Spinal Twist, Face of Light

	Biceps Brachii
	    Shoulder and elbow flexion
	    Supination of the forearm
		Strengthen: Cobra, Stick, Supported Shoulderstand
		Stretch: Reverse Namaste, Revolving Head-to-Knee, Face of Light

	Latissimus Dorsi
	    Extension, adduction, internal rotation
	    Lateral flexion and rotation of spine
		Strengthen: Camel, Spinal Twist, Shoulderstand
		Stretch: Energy Freeing, Abdominal Twist, Westside Back Stretch

SCAPULA	Middle and Lower Trapezius Adduction, depression	*Strengthen*: Bridge, Camel, Cat Bows *Stretch*: Cat (back up), Head-to-Knee, Westside Back Stretch
	Serratus Anterior Abduction, elevation	*Strengthen*: Energy Freeing, Crow, Head-to-Knee Pose *Stretch*: Cobra, Camel, Spinal Twist
	Rhomboids Adduction, elevation	*Strengthen*: Cobra, Camel, Reverse Namaste *Stretch*: Cat (back down), Stick, Spinal Twist
SPINE	Erector Spinae Extension, lateral flexion, rotation	*Strengthen*: Cobra, Extended Triangle, Locust *Stretch*: Extended Triangle, Side Angle Pose, Westside Back Stretch

	Rectus Abdominis
	    Flexion, lateral flexion, rotation,
	    Pelvic thrust
		Strengthen: Upward Stretch Legs, Boat, Nauli
		Stretch: Cobra, Locust, Bow

	Abdominis Oblique Lateral flexion, rotation	*Strengthen*: Extended Triangle, Spinal Twist, Abdominal Twist *Stretch*: Same poses on the opposite side of muscles

Table 5. The Kinesiology of Yogasanas *(continued)*.

BODY REGION	MUSCLES AFFECTED	YOGA POSES TO STRENGTHEN AND STRETCH
HIP	Psoas Flexion, external rotation	*Strengthen*: Energy Freeing, Stick, Westside Back Stretch *Stretch*: Camel, Bow, Reclining Hero
	Gluteus Maximus Extension, external rotation	*Strengthen*: Bridge, Camel, Locust *Stretch*: Energy Freeing, Westside Back Stretch, Squat Pose
	Gluteus Medius Abduction, internal and external rotation	*Strengthen*: Balancing Tree, Extended Triangle, Locust *Stretch*: Side of Hip Stretch, Spinal Twist, Head to Knee
	External Rotators External rotation	*Strengthen*: Balancing Tree, Head-to-Knee, Bound Angle *Stretch*: Side of Hip Stretch, Eagle, Face of Light
	Hamstrings Extension, knee flexion	*Strengthen*: Bridge, Locust, Camel Pose *Stretch*: Side of Hip Stretch, Extended Triangle, Westside Back Stretch
	Tensor Fascia Lata Abduction, flexion, internal rotation	*Strengthen*: Energy Freeing, Side Angle, Spread Leg Stretch *Stretch*: Spinal Twist, Joint Freeing Series #7, Face of Light
	Sartorius Flexion, abduction, external rotation with knee flexion	*Strengthen*: Side of Hip Stretch, Warrior I, Bound Angle *Stretch*: Camel, Bow, Runner's Stretch
	Rectus Femoris Flexion of hip, knee extension	*Strengthen*: Warrior II, Upward Stretched Legs, Boat *Stretch*: Bridge, Runner's Stretch, Camel
	Adductors Adduction, hip flexion	*Strengthen*: Cobra, Warrior I, Side of Hip Stretch *Stretch*: Triangle, Bound Angle, Spread Leg Stretch
	Gracilis Adduction, hip and knee flexion	*Strengthen*: Side of Hip Stretch, Bridge, Bow *Stretch*: Head to Knee, Bound Angle, Spread Leg Stretch
KNEE	Quadriceps/Tensor Fascia Lata Knee extension	*Strengthen*: Warrior I and II, Squat *Stretch*: Energy Freeing, Hero, Camel
	Gastrocnemius Knee flexion, ankle plantar flexion	*Strengthen*: Mountain on toes, Eagle, Squat on toes *Stretch*: Extended Triangle, Warrior I, Downward Dog
ANKLE	Anterior Tibialis Dorsiflexion, inversion	*Strengthen*: Extended Triangle, Downward Dog, Squat *Stretch*: Stick, Hero, Fetal
	Posterior Tibialis Plantar flexion, inversion	*Strengthen*: Hero, Camel, Hero with knees lifted *Stretch*: Warrior I, Downward Dog, Squat
	Soleus Plantar flexion	*Strengthen and stretch*: Same as Posterior Tibialis
	Peroneous (Fibularis) Longus and Brevis Plantar flexion, eversion	*Strengthen*: Extended Triangle, Spread Leg Stretch with toes outward *Stretch*: Lotus, Hero, Reclining Hero with toes inward

Where Shouldn't I Feel the Pose?

This is an important issue to keep in mind during any form of exercise. There are two areas of the body where one should never feel a reaction from any activity, and most certainly not as a result of a yoga pose. These areas are the inner knees and the sacroiliac joints. Neither of these areas is covered by muscles or contractile tissue. They possess only ligaments for stability. Since ligaments do not stretch, these areas are particularly vulnerable to pain from activities that place stress upon them. These two areas of the body lack muscles to provide stability and resilience.

The region of the inner knees lies between the kneecap (patella) and the tripod tendons that form the lower ends (insertion points) for three muscles—the gracilis (an adductor), sartorius (the longest muscle in the body, an external hip rotator), and the semimembranosis (the most medial hamstring). In addition, all three muscles flex the knee joint. In the inner knee space, there are only ligaments and cartilage to provide stability and mobility to the knee. The most familiar of these structures are the anterior cruciate ligament and the medial meniscus (cartilage). The knee does not allow the twisting or lateral movements that are commonly required of activities like skiing, tennis, or golf. Some martial arts warm up with knee circles, which are potentially harmful to this region. In yoga poses, pay particular attention to bent-knee poses with hip rotation, such as cross-legged sitting, as in the Lotus position, or forward-bending poses like the Head-to-Knee Pose and its variations.

This area is vulnerable to postures in which the foot is planted and the knee is not aligned to the foot. This sometimes occurs during practice of the Warrior poses for students who do not keep a back leg firmly extended. Another pose in which the knee is vulnerable is sitting between the feet with the feet turned outward, an uncommon variation of the Hero Pose (Virasana).

The sacroiliac is located at the base of the spine, where the sacrum, composed of five fused vertebrae, joins the iliac pelvic bones on its left and right sides. In men, the joint is more stable as three sacral vertebrae join the iliac, while in women, only two connect to the iliac. They may be seen on some slender individuals as dimples above the buttocks. The sacroiliac joints should have a subtle mobility, but should never be stretched, as they possess only ligaments to maintain their integrity. Ligaments do not stretch. It is common in my experience with some long-term women yoga teachers that they have chronic pain in this area, caused from stretching this joint. This often comes about during spinal twisting motions, and extremes of forward-bending poses. These should be done so that the stretch is felt in the deep buttock or hip-joint area.

The sacral area is vulnerable to forward bends, most especially those seated poses done with the knees straight. This is the case in the Head-to-Knee Pose and the Westside Back Stretch Pose. If this area is felt, adjust the pose so that the stretch is felt in the middle or lower back, or into the hamstring muscles. By following instructions carefully, there is no danger in yoga poses. Above all, you must learn to be sensitive to your body as the home of your inner teacher and allow your intuition to guide you. After all, yoga is a journey that can take you back home, so don't get sidetracked by the scenery along the way.

Another important feature to watch for during yogasanas is excessive mobility. If you know you have hyperextended knees or elbows, or in general are simply naturally flexible, be cautious of where you feel your poses. This is especially true when you are holding the poses a long time, and when you find yourself repeating the same postures for relieving your stress. Hypermobile joints tend to become overused. The surrounding muscle tissue will often lack muscle tone, firmness, and stamina. A locked joint, while providing stability, lacks mobility and the ability to adapt to change. Personality and joints are living in the same body/mind, so they may resemble each other.

When doing yoga poses with straight arms or legs, such as Warrior poses, standing forward bends, Downward Facing Dog, Stick Pose, and Spinal Twists, be cautious that you are not locked into position. Rather, keep the ability to change your flexibility every time you do these poses. See if you can focus your awareness on strongly contracting specific muscles within these poses. If you can, chances are you are not locking your joints.

For standing poses, as a test of locked knees, I often encourage students to lift their toes and see if the posture remains the same or changes. If your knees are locked, you'll move. Locking the joints blocks the flow of mindfulness, making you unable to experience other parts of yourself. It's important to be able to move your awareness to any part of your body at will.

It is fascinating to note that advanced students report feeling the pose all over. This is because their mind/body has been refined from focusing on a gross physical body, to one of sensing energy and sensation (subtle emotion). In this case, the energy body of prana has been trained to flow evenly throughout the system, and the mind has been trained to witness these subtle emotions and energy patterns. Over time, the irregularities in each body have been worked through. The student becomes stable, and peaceful in situations that formerly would have proved stressful.

Since most people have postural imbalances and resulting muscle imbalances, the places where the pose is felt will vary. This is evident in Table 3 (see page 103). In an aligned body, the effect of the pose is indicated in figure 20.

By taking the time for a postural analysis, you will identify which muscles to stretch and which ones to strengthen to achieve better alignment. Next, referring to Table 5, you will locate the poses to practice for your specific muscle stretching and strengthening needs. Studying anatomy will enable you to greatly amplify the efficiency of yoga asanas, which will, in turn, promote a balance between your muscles' capacity for strength and stability, and for flexibility and openness.

The short-run benefit of attention to anatomy is a strengthening of areas of weakness and a stretching of specific areas of tightness. In this way, your body functions more efficiently. Less effort is required to perform your daily activities. In the long run, especially if you receive personal guidance from an experienced instructor, your posture will improve, the residual effects of injuries will diminish, and your performance of athletic activities will be enhanced.

Principles for Good Practice

There are several other elements that will enhance the benefits of your yoga practice. It is most important that you begin with and maintain throughout practice an open mind and receptivity allowing the yoga to benefit you in any way. It is also very important that you let go of expectations. I say to new students, "Leave your expectations at the door with your shoes."

We are all multidimensional beings. The experiences of yoga affect us on all levels—body, mind, and Spirit. The body region where the predominant effect is found or felt will also vary from day to day. So, even if you come to yoga to relieve your chronic back-ache, along the way you may become aware of your physically held emotions. The variety of inner work accompanying yoga is as unique as the students who come to it. While there is a right place to feel the pose for you as an individual, there is no right time or place for your emotional and mental issues to come into the light of awareness.

As you practice these structural yoga asanas, you will discover that your body begins to change. The postural changes may not be apparent at first. You may find changes on the level of increased flexibility, or in the ease of holding a pose, indicative of increased strength. Over time, these changes will affect your body segment alignment and, thus, your posture as a whole. Aligning ankles to knees, knees to hips, hips to shoulders, shoulders to head, in this order, will progressively stabilize your new posture. In practicing the postures, always correct your alignment from the lower joints to the upper.

THE BASE OF SUPPORT

One important concept of the inner work with structural yoga asanas is called the base of support. This refers to the idea that each segment of the body is supported from below. If the segment below is misaligned, the segment above will tend to become misaligned, unstable, and uncomfortable. Hence, an awareness of discomfort is heightened, because the body part below where you feel the stress is not providing support. While instability is felt in the segment that is out of alignment, the cause is often from its base of support being misaligned.

In correcting postural misalignments, therefore, it is recommended that you work from the ground up. In standing postures, correct the ankles, then knees, and so on, up to the neck. For instance, if there has been chronic neck pain, it is not recommended to put much effort into realigning the neck until much work has been placed into correcting the shoulders and upper back.

In terms of aligning within an asana, do not correct for your neck until you have corrected misalignments from your ankles up to knees, to hips, to back, then to the neck. Often, when adjusting your body in this manner, the base of support is re-established for each segment and this will alleviate discomfort in the more superior joints. Hence, your neck will adapt to the lower segments and become much more comfortable, without directly correcting its position.

In all postures, the progression for correcting alignment is to start from the base of support—that is, from the ground—and proceed upward, one joint at a time. In so doing, the upper body will automatically align itself around a more stable, comfortable, aligned base of support.

To get the most from your practice, it is important to keep in mind the overview of yoga. A common pitfall in practicing yoga is forgetting yoga principles to achieve competence in Hatha Yoga. To avoid this and stay on track, I suggest you read and reread the opening chapters of this book. I also highly recommend reading *The Crown of Life* by Kirpal Singh, a wonderful book that puts the entire range of human development into a yogic perspective.[2]

Sequence for Mastery

There is a progression I recommend in order to thoroughly learn the practices of Structural Yoga Therapy™.

1. Learn the position from the "how to" portion of the instructions.

2. Study the major muscle and joint actions cited, so that you can develop clarity of the focal motions recommended for the posture.

3. Train yourself to follow the experiential sequence cited in the *Yoga Sutras* (II, 46), learning to become steady and comfortable in the posture and in the movements leading into and out of the posture. To deepen the practice, the next sutra recommends that yoga posture be perfected through "relaxation of effort, lessening the tendency for restlessness, and identification with the Infinite stream of life." This is, of course, a never-ending story, revealing the intention of yoga to be a method of attaining reintegration with our True Selves.

---

[2] Kirpal Singh, *The Crown of Life* (Delhi, India: Ruhani Satsang, 1971).

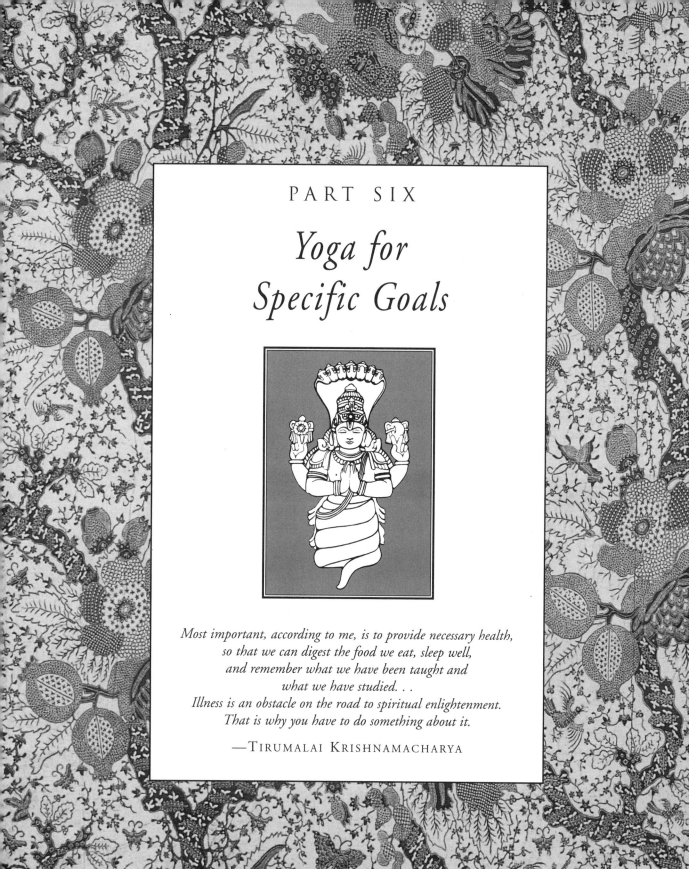

PART SIX

Yoga for Specific Goals

Most important, according to me, is to provide necessary health,
so that we can digest the food we eat, sleep well,
and remember what we have been taught and
what we have studied. . .
Illness is an obstacle on the road to spiritual enlightenment.
That is why you have to do something about it.

—TIRUMALAI KRISHNAMACHARYA

INTRODUCTION

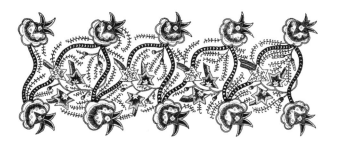

Goals are the steps you take to manifesting your dreams. In Part Three, I discussed the common goals that students bring to yoga class and individual sessions. They include improving posture, enhancing body awareness, increasing strength, increasing joint freedom/flexibility, managing stress, cardiovascular fitness, digestive health, relief from pain, awareness and meditation training, and developing a spiritual practice to connect with a Power Higher than your self.

Part Six contains general suggestions for accomplishing these major goals through Structural Yoga Therapy™. I have refrained from giving specific routines to allow for your creativity and self-study. I encourage you to ask your teacher for help. Teachers are crucial to developing a successful yoga practice. Make good use of your teachers without leaning on them. Teachers can share their experiences, so you can learn from their mistakes. In this way, much misdirected work can be avoided. If you expend great amounts of time and energy in your practice, but are without guidance, these efforts may be wasted. Be open to learning a different way. You are always invited to correspond with the author should you desire assistance.[1]

---

[1] See page 344 for contact information.

Chapter 22

IMPROVING POSTURE

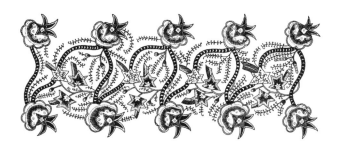

To perfect your posture and poise, the following muscles need to be strengthened regularly: the psoas, gluteus maximus, latissimus dorsi, erector spinae, trapezius, and rectus abdominis. The psoas supports the spine and balances the pelvic girdle upon the thighs. The gluteus maximus is responsible for the power of the pelvis and legs, and also supports the spinal column at the lumbar region. The latissimus dorsi makes up two-thirds of the back and, together with the deeper erector spinae muscles, keeps the trunk erect. The trapezius opens the chest and maintains neck and shoulder posture. The rectus abdominis is antagonistic to the psoas. They need to work harmoniously to maintain the posture of the abdominal and lower back regions.

If these muscles are regularly exercised, your posture will improve. Postural strength is greatly enhanced by understanding how these muscles work and learning to utilize them in daily movements. Specific postural imbalances can be improved by following the recommendations in Table 6 on page 266.

For a more detailed approach, follow the guidelines given earlier for body reading and utilize those insights for your unique features. The individual poses of your customized routine should be progressively developed for up to twelve breaths each to maximize your stamina.

Scoliosis

Of all the postural changes that one might have to deal with, scoliosis is perhaps the most challenging. The father of modern medicine, Hippocrates, "applied the term 'skoliosis' (crooked) to any curvature of the spine and developed methods to treat it. . . .

Table 6. Structural Yoga Therapy™ Recommendations for Postural Imbalances.

POSTURAL CHANGE	THERAPEUTIC YOGASANAS
Body leans forward	Hero, Energy Freeing, Camel
Body leans backward	Extended Triangle, Downward Facing Dog, Squat
Forward head	Cobra, Extended Triangle, Camel
Tilted head	Extended Triangle, Abdominal Twist, Spinal Twist
High shoulder	Same as above—adjust scapula downward, contracting lower trapezius, latissimus
Round shoulders	Warrior I, Downward Facing Dog, Camel
Arm turned out	Upward Extended Legs, Stick, Westside Back Stretch
Arm turned in	Bridge, Spinal Twist, Camel
Arm out from hip	Stick, Camel, Bound Angle
Winging scapula	Bridge, Supported Shoulderstand, Cobra
Flat back	Side-of-Hip Stretch, Head-to-Knee, Back Stretch
Lordosis (excessive lumbar curve)	Upward Legs, Boat, Reclining Hero
Scoliosis (lateral curve)	Side-of-Hip Stretch, Extended Triangle, Head-to-Knee
Khyphosis (hunchback)	Downward Facing Dog, Bridge, Camel
High hip	Side-of-Hip Stretch, Head-to-Knee, Half Locust
Hip twisted	Warrior I, Abdominal Twist, Spinal Twist
Hyperextended knee	Warrior II, Bridge, Camel
Knock-knees	Balancing Tree, Warrior II, Head to Knee
Bowed legs	Warrior I, Side-of-Hip Stretch, Face of Light
Leg outward	Warrior I, Side-of-Hip Stretch, Boat
Leg inward	Balancing Tree, Extended Triangle, Face of Light
Fallen arch/Flat foot	Mountain (balance on toes), Hero, Fetal

Scoliosis is a complicated deformity characterized by lateral curvature and vertebral rotation. As the disease progresses, the vertebrae and spinous processes in the area of the major curve rotate toward the concavity of the curve. . . . The disc spaces become narrower on the concave side of the curve and wider on the convex side. . . . Forms of spinal deformity can be broadly classified into structural and nonstructural types. In nonstructural scoliosis, the curve is flexible and corrects on side bending toward the convex side; in structural scoliosis, the curve fails to correct on side bending."[1]

Nonstructural scoliosis is sometimes developed as a result of a specific activity done for a long period of time. This is also called functional scoliosis. Any one-sided activity can produce this type of curvature. Examples are playing golf, bowling, tennis, racket ball, or carrying a heavy weight on just one side. This often occurs in mothers carrying their infants on the same hip, or from being a waitress and carrying a heavy tray on the same shoulder. In this type, the body's muscular and skeletal structures have been temporarily distorted to accommodate the requirements of the functional task at hand. There are usually marked differences, not only in posture (one shoulder or hip being higher), but also changes in strength and stamina from one side of the body to the other. I have seen clients with this type of curvature make dramatic changes in a relatively short period of time. When the activity causing the curvature was habitual for less than a year, the body can resume its original shape within about two to four months of personally mentored Structural Yoga Therapy™.

There are four varieties of curvatures. The right thoracic curve is the most common. A second is a thoracolumbar curve, characterized by a long major C curve to the right, through both the lower and upper regions of the back, in which there is only one long change of direction. The other two types are double curves of the shape of an S. These may be right upper thoracic and lower thoracic, or right thoracic and lumbar curves.

In America, children are screened by their school nurse to determine the likelihood of scoliosis. Signs of structural scoliosis are detectable in preteen and pubescent years. Curves over 30 degrees are closely watched, while those over 45 degrees are candidates for metal bracing or surgery to prevent further degeneration.

CASE STUDY—JANE

Jane came to me on a referral from another yoga teacher I had trained. She is 27 years old, married, and works for an on-line publishing firm. Her school nurse had diagnosed her with scoliosis at age 8. Throughout grammar school, she received yearly orthopedic consultations to monitor the progression of her curvature. When she reached her teenage years, she was placed in a Milwaukee Brace, a rigid, full-torso device designed to check the curvature. She wore this all day for two and a half years, until she turned 16. Her scoliosis had never caused her pain, but wearing the brace was a major cause for her feeling lonely and set apart from other teenagers.

Her intention in coming for Structural Yoga Therapy™ was to see if she could lessen the curvature or stop it from progressing. She had remained physically active, was going to a gym two to three times per week, and had taken yoga for the past two years. In spite of being fit, however, she was beginning to develop increased tension in her back and also wanted to find out how this tension might be related to her curvature. I told her of a case I had treated about ten years previously, in which a woman in her late 30s want-

---

[1] Hugo Keim and Robert Hensinger, *Spinal Deformities—Scoliosis and Khyphosis,* Clinical Symposia, vol. 41, no. 4 (Summit, NJ: CIBA-GEIGY Corp., 1989), pp. 3–24. They also say that an adult with a mild curve of less than 30 degrees is generally not in danger of progression; that patients with scoliosis who become pregnant do not necessarily have a marked increase in their curve due to the pregnancy, but they usually have an increase in associated low back pain; and that in severe deformities, premature death is usually caused by respiratory disease and superimposed pneumonia.

ed to change her previous experience in childbirth. She had a 45-degree curvature that seemed to worsen in the later stages of pregnancy for both her deliveries, which occurred while she was in her 20s. I gave her a program and she kept up with it. She had no trouble with her back during or following her next pregnancy. In fact, her spinal curve diminished to less than 25 degrees within a year of beginning the specialized program.

Jane's examination revealed a double curve. The right thoracic portion extended from C6 to T10 and, at its apex, was 43 degrees. A left lumbar curve of 18 degrees was accompanied by a forward right iliac crest and a nearly immobile left sacroiliac joint. Her joint mobility was average for all motions, with the exception of external hip rotation. This motion, on both sides, was increased from the average of 45 degrees to 55. Muscle testing revealed tightness in the hamstrings, external shoulder rotators, and right cervical rotators. I also uncovered weakness in both sides of her middle trapezius, left adductors, right external hip rotators, left quadratus lumborum, and both gluteus maximus muscles. In addition, I measured the mobility of her lower rib cage during full respiratory inhalation and exhalation. The difference averaged one and a half inches.

I explained all these findings to her using my anatomy atlas as a reference. She was particularly intrigued and pleased to learn that the tension she was experiencing was all in weakened muscles. I told her that I often find that clients with similar symptoms get relief from tension in a remarkably short period of time, usually within six to eight weeks of following regular yoga therapy prescriptions.

The initial program I gave her consisted of doing Cat Pose half pushups (Cat Bow) for middle trapezius strength, Sunbird Pose for gluteus strength, Cobra for realigning the lumbar region, Locust with single leg variations for gluteal strength and lumbar alignment, and Warrior I and Side Stretch (Parsvottanasana) for adductor tone and pelvic/lumbar realignment. All exercises were given in the form of repetitions, inhaling into the posture and exhaling out. This method promotes flexibility, which I wanted to optimize to see how adaptable her body was at this point in life.

She was faithful in following the unusual variations to standard poses that I found necessary for her. On her third appointment, she remarked that her lumbar discomfort, which was the worst of her tensions, was improved and, while her neck tension remained, it had lessened. Since she was in a positive mode about her yoga practice and saw that she could clearly make changes to it, I increased the duration of her program. I doubled the repetitions of her program from six to twelve, continuing to emphasize suppleness. I gave her additional work to increase the tone of her intercostal muscles and diaphragm. I have found that strengthening these major respiratory muscles is crucial for cases of spinal curvature. So often the symptoms of asthma or allergies seen in clients with scoliosis are also treated successfully with the same intercostal breathing methods. This exercise proved to be her least favorite and she found it easy to forget. In spite of this, her costal expansion continued to increase as time went on. After three months, her measurement increased to nearly double its initial state—from one-and-a-half to two-and-a-half inches. Her curves were measured at 38 degrees right thoracic and 15 degrees left lumbar. She has continued for over a year and her curves are still diminishing. Now they are 32 and 15 degrees respectively. Her program is adjusted once a month to account for her changing body posture.

Chapter 23

ENHANCING BODY AWARENESS

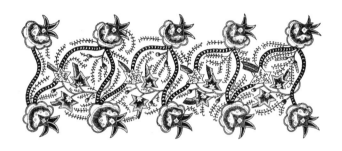

In our fast-paced culture, fitness has become a necessary component to surviving the challenges of society. It is estimated that about half our population exercises regularly in some form or another. Often, these exercises promote health and a degree of stress relief. Yoga has also been touted as an ideal form of fitness exercise, a holistic method of training, not only the body, but the mind as well. The mental training of yoga challenges students to be aware and self-conscious, and to learn to appreciate the messages the body is constantly sending. This portion of the training is especially important. It forms the portion of Classical Yoga in its transition from Hatha to Raja Yoga.

While Hatha Yoga emphasizes physical discipline and isolates the components of the body, Raja Yoga is for training the mind. The often-neglected intermediate step is to detach from the body's signals and learn to be still, to deepen perception of mental, physical, or sensory input. The momentary stillness, not intended to be long enough to be called mediation per se, teaches yoga students to listen to their innate biofeedback. On a theoretical level, students learn about the subtle body and its composition of nadis and chakras. On the practical level, they learn to experience subtle signs of energy and emotions as precursors of an array of experiences—getting sick, angry, excited, or spiritual. During this type of training, students are encouraged to stay in the yogasanas for 30 to 120 seconds or longer, to rest in relaxation pose for ten, or even fifteen, minutes in silence, and to focus deeply upon the naturally arising "currents of sensation." This is indeed a training in listening, watching, waiting, and being patient.

Patience is a virtue of which we can never have too much. One major recommendation I have to develop patience is to make a commitment to practice for a specific amount of time daily for a given number of weeks. Making a commitment prevents us from being influenced by the natural changes of life's cycles, or by our own emotional and mental instability.

A practical way to approach mastery of the Structural Yoga Therapy™ asana program is to rotate through the entire program in a given manner. For developing self-awareness and body feedback, I recommend following this sequence of all 24 poses summarized in Figure 20 (page 250–253).

Day 1—Standing poses, sitting poses, relaxation (on pages 250 and 253)

Day 2—Joint-Freeing Series, inverted poses (on page 251)

Day 3—Forward- and back-bending poses and ujjaye breathing (on page 252)

CASE STUDY—BOB

Bob came to yoga as do many others, out of pure unadulterated curiosity. He worked in the neighborhood of the Yoga Therapy Center in Boston as a psychologist. After seeing the business sign for several years he decided to check out individual sessions for his lumbar and hip pain. He had developed the pain following participation in a three-week tennis camp. He didn't identify it as being the result of any specific incident, but felt that the tennis camp program was more vigorous than he had been used to.

His pain had been consistent over the past six years, though it had varied from extreme to mild. At its worst, he had spent six to eight weeks in bed before getting relief. A complete medical examination revealed no disc degeneration or neurological conditions that would have been responsive to medical care. He had seen a chiropractor for some time, but was unstable following spinal adjustments. Over the course of the past six years, he had also gone to physical therapy, acupuncture, and tried Iyengar Yoga for a season. He was inspired enough by the yoga to continue, twice a week, on his own. Despite the fact that the initial cause of pain had been tennis, he continued to play an average of five days a week for about an hour and a half. He found that tennis gave him the change he needed from sitting in therapy all day. His goal for coming to Structural Yoga Therapy™ was to get a stretching program that would enable him to be relieved of pain and prepare him for tennis.

In the initial session, it became clear to me how his body had compensated for playing tennis. Being right-handed, he had developed a left thoracic curvature of nearly 20 degrees, ranging from C6 to T6. The curve also elevated his left shoulder. The curve brought with it an elevation of the left rib cage. There was also a shortening of the left leg of approximately three-eighths of an inch. The joint examination found knee flexion limited to 118 degrees, hip flexion of 78 degrees, internal hip rotation of 10 degrees on the right and 30 degrees on the left, and right cervical rotation of 30 degrees. The muscle exam revealed tightness on the following muscles related to the previous findings: both quadriceps, right psoas, right abductors, left sternocleidomastoid, and upper trapezius. The weak muscles included both gluteus maximus, left adductors, latissimus, and right sternocleidomastoid.

The postures I chose for him to address these issues were Side Stretch Pose for stretching the abductors; Cat Pose, done with the right knee forward of the left for balancing leg length and releasing the rigidity of the spinal curves; Wall Hang, for stretching the hamstrings and erector spinae; Stick Pose, lifting the chest with the aid of the arms for strengthening the latissimus dorsi and triceps; Table Pose (Chatush Padapitham), for the same benefits; and Runner's Stretch, with the back knee pressed down to stretch the quadriceps. By giving emphasis to strength for the middle and upper back and shoulder region, I intended to develop sufficient stamina so that, in later sessions, he could apply that strength to reverse the curvature resulting from tennis.

Following the examination, I recommended he take a break from tennis until the yoga therapy had had a chance to take effect. I gave him a challenging program consisting of yogasanas alternating with deep Ujjaye Pranayama. The breathing exercises were to emphasize the intercostal motions. For the first month, this deep breathing was painful, as there was chronic restriction in the intercostal tissues. After the first four weeks, he was able to expand his rib cage two and a half inches up from his initial reading of one and a half. The measurement was made at the lower border of the sternum to compare the expansion of normal full inhalation with normal full exhalation. My rationale was that, for his body to release the pain that had accumulated, he would need to mobilize, not only the deep back musculature of the erector spinae, but also the intercostal musculature and costal articulations as well.

Changes on this level require also a change in consciousness. By this, I mean a shift away from listening to mental considerations about fitness and vitality to listening to the body's more subtle messages of depth of breath, nasal versus oral respiration, relaxing into muscular tension rather than pushing through resistance to force more endurance, and feeling emotional precursors like warmth in the head or chest, or tension in the hands and feet.

Much of my emphasis in Bob's yoga therapy program was not simply about releasing the tight muscles and strengthening his weak muscles. It was more about reframing the way he thought while exercising. I found that the best progress for him was in those sessions in which I guided him and gave him a specific awareness on which to focus. We tape-recorded the sessions, so that he could listen to the new body consciousness that I gave him. As many exercises he did were held for a duration of 30 to 60 seconds, there was plenty of time for his mind to wander into old patterns. By giving him specific imagery and focused awareness, he could both achieve the physical goals and change the way he looked at himself.[1]

A month after beginning his program, Bob felt ready to try a mild set of tennis. He had been faithful to practice, spending no less than five days a week doing his 30-minute routine, so I agreed. It turned out that he began to enjoy the feelings his body was producing with yoga more than the results he was getting from tennis. So he devoted more of his extra time to yoga. As time went on, we spent more time developing intercostal

---

[1] The source of these mental exercises and positive body imagery is from "The Body," in Louise Hay, *You Can Heal Your Life* (Carlsbad, CA: Hay House, 1987), pp. 124–144.

breathing during the poses and getting feedback from the imagery he was receiving while holding the poses.

Bob began to speak more about his feelings of frustration and anxiety of being cooped up in his life-style. It seemed that, the more he deep-breathed, the more he wanted out of his trap. He sometimes became emotional during the poses that released the intercostal region around the upper back and chest. During one particularly powerful session, he felt energy rushing out of his shoulders and into his hands. He described it as "electric flashes coming out of my fingers." By releasing the musculature of the back, he was able to release the weight that had held him bound. He made some changes in his life-style, deciding to work independently instead of for a community health plan provider. He was then able to specialize in seeing the type of clientele he chose. Bob felt freer in many ways, not only more supple and in touch with his body. He shared that he was often able to listen to body messages while seeing clients, and that this helped him to reveal how to go deeper and stay focused on the truth. Bob felt that he had learned how to carry his yoga practice into the rest of his life. He felt well served by yoga and its ability to heighten his self-awareness.

Chapter 24

INCREASING STRENGTH

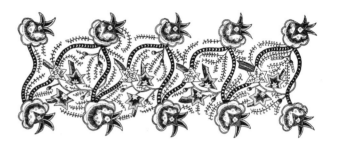

A thorough body-reading assessment may have revealed that you have specific muscle weaknesses. You might, for instance, have found that high shoulders revealed that your lower trapezius, latissimus dorsi, and pectoralis sternal muscles were weak. If you marked four postural imbalances, this may have given you a list of perhaps as many as a dozen muscles that are weak. It may seem too formidable a task to spend the time required to strengthen all these muscles. Instead, I suggest that you take one muscle from each group of postural imbalances and do the most effective toning exercise for that muscle. In this way, you will have four exercises to do that focus your attention on feeling the challenge to the strength of each of these four muscles.

In addition, the isolation exercises and the individual poses of a Structural Yoga Therapy™ program will reveal weakened muscles. The insights that you derive from noticing that your attention does not go to the muscles indicated reveals a lesser degree of weakness than that indicated from the postural analysis. Once the postural muscles are stronger, you can then consider redirecting your attention during asana practice to repositioning your body to effect more toning to the muscles indicated. '

You will progress in your asana practice if you gradually increase your holding time from 3 breaths as a beginner, to 6 breaths during regular practice, then to 12 breaths once you have reached a committed level of practice. This increased holding time will enhance your stamina, as well as your will power. Willpower is a fascinating feature of the mind. It reveals itself in exercise as a determination to continue to use a muscle's strength in spite of the mind's wavering nature.

*Giving yourself the challenge to work a weakened muscle
amounts to strengthening the physical locations of your mind.*

Where else does your mind live but in the body? And where else does it manifest its formless nature into form but through musculo-skeletal activity? To be skilled at any physical activity is to be able to control your thoughts and emotions. To direct your attention is the process of yoga meditation (dharana) as it applies to daily life.

CASE STUDY—BETTY

Betty worked as a pediatric nurse for a major Boston hospital. She had nearly lost her right leg following an automobile accident a year before at age 54. She had lost circulation to the right lower leg and was told that she might need knee-replacement surgery later. Before the accident, she had knock-knees. Following surgery to rebuild the shattered middle left leg and lower right leg, her knees were bowed outward. The right tibia was put back together with eight metal pins. In addition, she had been diagnosed as having osteoporosis in both knees. She also had fractured her 6th thoracic vertebra and was having moderate pain in the mid-scapular region as a result. Betty was constantly in mild to moderate pain.

Her daily routine was to walk two miles every other day and to do weight training recommended by her physical therapist on the alternate days. These consisted of straight-leg lifting (hip flexion) with a 20-pound weight and hip extension (Locust Pose) toning with a 5-pound weight. She had been introduced to yoga previously, and was also doing four daily repetitions of the Sun Salutation.

My examination revealed that her right ankle was limited to 50 percent of normal mobility, her right knee's flexion was 110 degrees (normal being 150), and her hip flexion was 75 degrees on both sides (normal is 90). The right leg bowed out from straight to 10 degrees, and the left bowed 7 degrees. As a result, the hamstrings were both found to be tight, as well as the right quadriceps. Her major need, however. was for strength. The weakened muscles included the right psoas, the gluteus medius and tensor fascia lata on both sides, the left sartorius, the gluteus maximus on both sides, and the middle trapezius.

I told her that a commitment would be needed to make progress with the difficulties she was suffering. She agreed to daily at-home practice and individual sessions twice a month for six months. With this in mind, I created a program for her to begin Structural Yoga Therapy™. The routine started off with polishing her four rounds of Sun Salutation. I had her do all sets of the Runner Pose with the right leg back, so that we could work through the tightness of the quadriceps. I also had her emphasize both Downward Facing Dog and Cobra Poses to expand the middle back forward, thus strengthening the musculature around the fractured T6 vertebrae. At first, this was painful, but with concentration, she learned how to initiate the motion from the front by lifting the sternum rather than squeezing the shoulder blades. This made all the difference in alleviating her pain.

As she had been so brutally damaged in the auto accident, I knew there would be more pain coming up as she released the trauma. Whenever there is a trauma, there is the likelihood of its being too intense to be fully experienced. In such cases, the body armors itself to defend its limited capacity to both experience and release pain. Hence, much of my work with Betty was in learning how to re-experience the painful memories, the tissue-held trauma, and not associate it with the idea that more pain would result. She needed to learn the concept of GIGO, Garbage In—Garbage Out. When we take in something that is unpleasant, we must later, no matter how much later, expel it.

The major method I use for this is a combination of conscious awareness with mindfulness—staying in the here-and-now moment—and a discharge breathing technique. When trauma is experienced, an untrained mind seeks to go anywhere but into the experience of suffering and pain. With training, the mind can be present to all emotional sensations with no residual reactions—no GI, therefore no GO. The discharge breathing method directs the breath to specific areas of the body. Exhalation and a release of previously unexperienced emotions occurs from that specific point. This training leads quickly to learning true pranayama.

By this, I mean that yoga breathing is the preliminary stage in which the student directs the breath to physically open those areas on inhalation and discharge stress on exhalation. For instance, you can measure the expansion of the rib cage and determine that you are doing intercostal breathing. In the same way, you can see the abdomen constrict during exhalation and slightly expand during inhalation.

As contrasted with this, one aspect of pranayama is the capacity to direct the feeling of energy as heat, as a wave-like sensation, as vitality, or as emotional positivity to a specific physical or subtle-body structure. Prana-yama literally means "to regulate the flow of life-force." To directly feel a discharge of physical or emotional pain while you breathe is the most obvious sign of success in pranayama. Betty needed to learn, first, how to do yoga breathing. Only then could we would progress to learning pranayama for pain control.

The next portion of Betty's routine consisted of individual poses focusing on feeling the development of strength to the specific muscles I had found to be weak during the initial consultation. For this, I frequently referred her to the anatomy atlas for detailed visualization. I also had her look at the muscle involved and watch how its contraction revealed changes under her skin. The word *muscle* comes from a Greek word meaning "mouse." Apparently, the ancient Greeks imagined there were mice moving beneath the skin causing ripples when we move.

During the practice of Extended Triangle Pose, Betty focused on the stretch of the hamstrings, while consciously tensing her gluteus maximus on both sides to increase her hip external rotation. She also practiced the bent-knee version of Locust Pose, lifting one leg at a time to tone these same muscles. Locust Pose, with straight legs, was also given to strengthen her hamstrings. She also did Sunbird Pose for hamstrings and gluteal strength. To tone the sartorius muscle, I had her sit in the Bound Angle Pose and lift one foot at a time. At first, this was extremely difficult to do on the left side, but she was able to get a lift of 12 inches after about two weeks. To polish the motion, I had her try not to lift the knee, but rather to focus the lift from the foot. Try it! It's a challenge, even for well-toned bodies. The final pose of her routine was to practice the Fetal Pose (Darnikasana) with her legs in three different widths. This was for the purpose of releasing the upper-hamstring, adductors, and gluteal tightness, as well as to help make her knees and thighs more supple.

In developing her strength, I had Betty begin by doing the poses to her capacity, as determined by how long she could hold the pose and feel the strengthening effect in the desired muscle. As soon as her awareness shifted to working another region, she was to relax and release the pose. Within four weeks, by counting the number of full complete breaths, she was able to stabilize her exercises to a holding time of six breaths. At first, her body was so imbalanced that she often found a great difference in the comparative tone of the two sides. This was especially true for her hip muscles.

In her first month of yoga therapy, Betty missed nearly one week of practice because of a boat trip that made doing yoga impossible for her. When she returned for the follow-up sessions, I did Yoga Bodywork, taking advantage of the poses she had been practicing to deepen their effectiveness. By contrasting an extension of her musculature with pressing at the origins and insertions of the muscles to strengthen specific muscles, she was able to get a more effective workout. In holding her in the poses, she could relax extraneous stress and concentrate on developing the muscle tone more precisely where she wanted.

This type of hands-on yoga therapy enabled me to deepen Betty's capacity to direct her breathing. I now directed her to a releasing pranayama method. By inhaling through the nostrils and exhaling through the mouth, a more sedative effect could be realized. This breathing method has been shown to lower blood pressure and heart rate when done for short periods of time. Over a period longer than two to three minutes without adequate training, students tend to hyperventilate. By providing hands-on training, I intended to show Betty how to direct her ability to release both emotional and physical tension. I put my hand where I wanted her to send the breath. By having my hand there, I could press during the exhale phase and encourage her capacity to direct awareness and muscle tone.

We spent much time learning to direct the breath to the center of the abdomen and, gradually, to the posterior wall of the abdomen, wherein lies the psoas muscle. At first, her breathing was irregular. Then she learned to consistently contract her abdomen with each exhalation. A few moments later, she experienced an emotional release of her pelvic girdle, which she described as the image of her pelvis and legs falling from her body. She felt light and enjoyed a sense of freedom from the heavy metal that clamped her legs together. As the session reached its end, she learned to direct the feeling of subtle energy through her pelvis and down each leg. This calmed her and brought her to a feeling of tremendous peace. She rested for about ten minutes, which she described as being timeless. Enough progress was made in the first month that she was able to receive a more challenging series for the second month.

A reassessment session later revealed a need for hip flexor strength, especially in the long flexors, which also cross the knee and hence flex it. I modified her initial weight-training program by giving focus to the sartorius, tensor fascia lata, and rectus femoris with alternating lifts. In so doing, Betty learned how to isolate the component elements of hip flexion and knee extension. At this point, she added psoas isolations with two variations, supine leg lifts with knee bent and then straight with a five-pound ankle weight.

The Fetal Pose had done its work, so we were able to drop it from the routine and add Bound Angle and the Groin Stretch for increasing the hip external rotation (turn-out) and toning the five adductors in their interactions with the four quadriceps. These new poses were done with varying distance between the pelvis and heels to alter the effect over the nine muscles involved.

After the completion of the second month, Betty was able to do Camel Pose to complement the Bound Angle Pose variations. Her ability to tolerate the extremes of these two poses revealed a balance of tone with suppleness between the musculature of the anterior and posterior thigh. Betty was pleased with the marked improvement in her strength and body balance. She moved on from individual sessions to coming for group lessons after the fourth month. She continues to benefit from both individual and group sessions.

Chapter 25

INCREASING JOINT
FREEDOM AND FLEXIBILITY

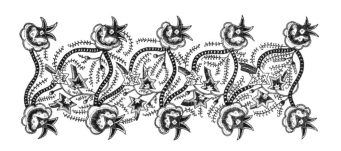

While, for many people, the terms yoga and flexibility are synonymous, for me they are not. Initially, I, like many others, thought that yoga would greatly improve flexibility. There are even scientific studies that have documented the improvement in flexibility. I cannot dispute their findings, but I can say that my experience differs.

What I find is that yoga does help people maintain their natural suppleness and regain any lost flexibility due to injuries or the aging process. But I do not see that structural yoga, as my way of teaching an aspect of Classical Yoga, increases students' constitutional flexibility.

Regular practice of the entire Joint-Freeing Series (Pavanmuktasana) will create more flexibility in a general manner. This series is especially beneficial for those persons with morning stiffness or osteo-arthritis. If the mobility you are seeking is in one joint, I recommend doing the entire series and adding variations of motions for the stiff joint. For example, if you have stiffness in your right shoulder, upon completing the series for the shoulder, repeat the shoulder movements while standing or in half-forward bend. I also recommend that you practice the wrist motions simultaneously.

If you are seeking increased mobility for a specific motion, like touching your toes, or for a sporting activity, I recommend that you practice the entire isolation exercises immediately following the Joint-Freeing Series. To emphasize forward-bending motions, do the Wall Hang and Half-Forward Bend at least three times each. On alternate days, weave them together, alternating one with the other.

A secret of increasing joint freedom is to do small variations of the motion desired—micro-motions—a minimum of six times. The motions should be made in a forward and backward movement. Raise one side as you lower the other, making a crescent motion like a clock's pendulum, clockwise circles, counterclockwise circles, figure eights then reversed, and infinity symbols then reversed. These motions are particularly effective for freeing the hips. By following this pattern, you will definitely loosen up the joint. This method was given to me by a master teacher in a creative system called Standing Wave Yoga.

A common reason why people come in for yoga is for relief from lower back pain and as an alternative treatment program to a diagnosis for herniated or slipped vertebral discs. This is another opportunity for me to bring out my anatomy atlases and reveal some of our body's secrets. There are many misconceptions around these anatomical structures. The discs are not a jelly-like fluid in a cartilaginous sack between the vertebrae. According to *Gray's Anatomy* (considered in medical schools as the Bible of anatomy), the gel center of the disc becomes fibrocartilage after age 10. This material is extremely durable, compared by one author to prestressed concrete! "Moreover, the fibrocartilage in discs is surrounded by hyaline cartilage, a substance as friction-free as Teflon™ that prevents the vertebrae and discs from touching—and makes wear and tear on the disc virtually impossible."[1]

"In the 1950s," Griner relates, "researchers performed postmortems on a group of people who had been diagnosed with 'ruptured' discs. Only one-tenth of 1 percent of the sample actually had ruptured discs."[2] What caused the compression that was misdiagnosed as a ruptured disc? One possible culprit is tight muscles. In the case of lumbar discs, the most-suspect muscles are the psoas and the quadratus lumborum. For cervical discs, the suspect muscles are the scalenes, levator scapulae, splenius capitis, and upper trapezius.

CASE STUDY—CYNTHIA

Cynthia came on a referral from the co-director of the Beth Israel Deaconess Hospital's Mind/Body Medical Institute in Boston, where I had offered a yoga class to the staff and their patients for five years. She agreed, nine years later, to fill me in on some of the inner life changes that yoga therapy has afforded her.

> The Mind/Body program had done much to help me deal with back pain but little or nothing to relieve the pain itself. In coming to see you I had no expectations for full recovery. I was at home full-time, with a nanny full-time. Another piece I want to tell you is about my temperament. I had always been extremely driven and impatient. When I went into labor, my office had a pool on how long it would be before I returned to work: one week was the outside guess, even though I had said from the

---

[1] Thomas Griner, *What's Really Wrong with You—A Revolutionary Look at How Muscles Affect Your Health* (Garden City, NY: Avery, 1996), p. 78.
[2] Griner, *What's Really Wrong with You*, p. 29

beginning I would be home a year. While the ecstasy of Madeleine, then and now, has helped me a lot with patience, even staying home with her was a function of my needing to do everything to perfection.

Cynthia had been experiencing chronic lower-back and neck pain for seven or eight years. She described the onset of the currently acute neck pain as following a backpacking adventure when her baby was 10 months old. Now the pain had gotten worse, especially when lifting the now 1-½ year old child. Cynthia was 32 years old. She had found some relief through chiropractic care, though she seemed to have reached a plateau, receiving no further benefit from it for the past nine weeks. She had been doing yoga as a result of the Mind/Body program, but was upset at herself for repeatedly falling asleep during the lying relaxation exercise, with which every yoga class ends. "I did not consider myself the 'yoga type,' but I was desperate," she said.

My evaluation revealed a straight cervical region with left thoracic curvature from C7 to T4 of approximately 12 degrees, and a right lower thoracic curvature from T8 to L2 of 22 degrees. She had dislocated her right hip in 1982. Muscle testing and body reading revealed weakness in both sides of the latissimus dorsi, lower abdominals, hip flexors on both sides, and the left gluteus maximus. The only tight muscle revealed was the right psoas. This finding is often correlated, as it was in this case, with a right lumbar scoliosis.

In her situation, because of the need to care for her child constantly, I gave an initial program that was a mixture of yogasanas and isolated-muscle strengthening exercises. In this manner, optimal toning can be achieved in a minimal period of time. My strategy was to alleviate her pain as quickly as possible. Then stamina will be built over time, as we gradually progress into more complex motions that will challenge the strength of the currently weakened and posturally distorted areas of her body.

The initial series of practices included isolation exercises to tone the hip flexors one side at a time. These consisted of leg lifting from a supine position and holding the leg at three heights for four breaths each. Then we isolated the psoas muscle from the other hip flexors by doing a right leg lift 2 feet out from center, with the thigh externally rotated. By slowly moving through the range of motion and minimizing the compensatory rotation of the pelvis, the muscle can be toned. The left gluteus maximus was also isolated and toned by doing a variation of Locust Pose (Salabhasana), with the left knee bent and the thigh externally rotated. When the posture is done in this manner, the gluteus maximus is separated from the hamstrings, and stamina is built more quickly than in the standard Locust Pose. The pose was given only on the left side for the first phase of yoga therapy.

The lower abdominals and latissimus dorsi were toned by the practice of Locust and Cobra Poses. An extra emphasis was placed upon the shoulder position, with them being brought backward and downward to accentuate the challenge to the latissimus. Initially, the Cobra increased the pain in her upper back, but this effect was short-lived, releasing once the pose was relaxed. All exercises were given for four repetitions, with an initial hold of two rounds of Ujjaye Pranayama. Whenever there is pain, the importance of learning and deepening the correct practice of this energetic breathing practice cannot be overemphasized. Without proper breathing, pain tends to persist, or at best becomes irregular.

Two weeks later, for our follow-up session, the poses were polished and some improvements in muscle tone noted. The sequence was adjusted to the next level of challenge, increasing most to 6 repetitions. In addition, the Bridge Pose was added, as the tone of her left gluteus maximus had improved. Today, this is still Cynthia's favorite movement. The muscular isolation version of Locust was eliminated from her routine. Follow-up muscle testing revealed a loss of tone in the left tensor fascia lata and internal hip rotator. An isolation exercise was given to this muscle in a supine leg lift, with the hip turned inward.

This response is common when working to tone the postural muscles of scoliosis. I often find that the gluteus medius, tensor fascia lata, sartorius, and gluteus maximus need to be reassessed from week to week. These muscles act as stabilizers for the pelvis and prevent pelvic rotation and hip elevation, which in turn changes the angle of scoliosis at the vertebral column.

Following the end of the first month, Cynthia mentioned an unexpected benefit. She had her first-ever pain-free menstruation. I was delighted to hear this, in spite of the fact that she never mentioned to me that she had painful menstruation. This is not an uncommon side effect of scoliosis, when looked at from the Ayurvedic perspective. This view would call her condition a Vata imbalance. The remedy is often toning both the internal and external hip rotators, rhythmic ujjaye breathing exercises with variations, meditation and life-style changes to establish regularity in daily habits.

At this point, Cynthia began to meditate and guidance in developing a spiritual practice was also given. She remarked in the second month that "I had only thought of meditation as relaxation until I read the book you recommended, *Meditate,* by Swami Muktananda.[3] I cried from reading this book and felt the longing for something previously unnamed. I felt that I was coming home to a spiritual part of myself." We chanted the meditation mantra my spiritual teacher had recommended and she began to sit for meditation for twenty-five minutes instead of lying down. Cynthia claims,

> The evolution of my meditation practice astonished me. When we first started at the Mind/Body program I found it strange and embarrassing. Then, when I came to your Yoga Therapy Center, I felt that your place and your calmness unnerved me for a long time. I only tried it because I was absolutely desperate. And I couldn't sit up for it for many months—my back couldn't hold me up. Some time into our practice, I began experiencing what I thought were strange *physical* reactions. The most notable, and we talked about it afterward, was completely losing sense of my physical self/size. I felt almost as if I got very large, then very small, then had absolutely no sense of a boundary (like skin or shape) between the world and me. Strangest of all, it wasn't unsettling. Also, I began eating better. I just didn't feel like eating crap anymore and started to follow a few of your Ayurvedic diet recommendations.

---

[3] Swami Muktananda, *Meditate* (South Fallsburg, NY: SYDA Foundation, 1980).

We continued to meet for regular sessions for the next seven months. Her inquiry into meditation deepened and she began to spend as much time on meditation as yogasanas. The curvature of her spine diminished to nearly half of the initial reading. In the sixth month, the curvatures were read as 6 degrees upper left thoracic and 14 degrees lower right thoracic. She was free of shoulder and back pain and reported being much stronger in general. Nine years later, I received this letter:

Dear Mukunda,

I had been pain free for some months before I left your practice and moved back to Maine. I remember when one day I realized I was pain free. It was nearly overwhelming—I hadn't been completely pain free in seven or eight years. I have had a couple of bouts with "normal" back pain/fatigue since—too much gardening improperly, for example—and they make me panic a little. Still, I have been pain free all but for occasional days for nine years. I'm building a house with my partner and we've done it all on our own, with no pain or problems.

Whenever I experience stress, I feel it in my back. For all intents and purposes, that is the only back pain I experience—stress pain. I consider it a service provided by my body (or something greater?) to remind me that I am screwing up and need to stop. . . . At some point, I lost a fair amount of weight, about twenty pounds. It was very gradual, over a year or two, and I don't know exactly what to attribute it to. I'm glad though, I certainly haven't evolved beyond vanity! While much less of a perfectionist, I'm still a money-grubbing capitalist, an impatient one at that. There is a major change, however. When things don't go as planned, I don't really get upset about it. I don't mean the outward manifestation, I mean I don't feel that horrible gut feeling. I believe I may just well have cultivated some detachment.

When I reviewed this case study, I wasn't sure where to place it in the book. Cynthia had experienced improvements in some unpredictable multi-dimensional ways. I asked her to evaluate which area had had the most impact for her. "For me," she replied, "the relief from pain was the best—somewhat to my surprise I got to the rest of the areas in this sequence—increased strength, improved flexibility, improved posture, enhanced body awareness, stress management, and meditation training." Cynthia was a remarkable client, in that she was so available. As she put it, "she was desperate," so all areas of her life were affected positively by Structural Yoga Therapy™ done in a Classical Yoga context.

Chapter 26

CARDIOVASCULAR

FITNESS

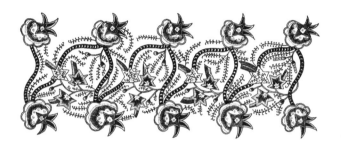

In general, the complete structural yoga asana routine will be beneficial to health, but it is not an aerobic program. It is a good place to begin, however, until you feel ready for a more specific program targeted at cardiovascular health. The best yoga routine for cardiovascular fitness is the Sun Salutation. A gradual increase in the total number of rounds of practice should be the goal. There are four stages of mastery of the Sun Salutation. The first is to memorize the twelve positions and go through them in sequence. The number of rounds to practice at this stage is two to four. The second stage is to regulate your breathing pace. Coordinating your body movements to your breath may not come too quickly, so be patient with this phase of training. At this phase of training, increase the number of rounds to six, and continue until you build up to twelve nonstop cycles. Do not be in a hurry to increase the cycles. It is safer to check your heart and respiratory rate following a cycle to be certain you're working your body at a safe level.

Monitor your breath rate following the rounds in Relaxation Pose. Time how long it takes to return to relaxation breath (two-thirds your normal rate). When recovery is made within two minutes, the routine may be increased to give a more aerobic benefit to your cardiovascular system. Increase the rounds at an interval of two, no sooner than every third day. At this rate, someone in good health may be up to twelve rounds within one month. This will create a cardiovascular routine of over ten minutes. The practice of an average cycle of the Sun Salutation's 12 motions takes one minute, done at 12 breaths per minute.

To move to phase three, increase to twenty cycles. Once you can sustain this level for one week, practice the routine at a faster pace, timing yourself. The twenty-minute routine can then be reduced to fifteen minutes and gradually to even less. Keep your breath paced to your body motions, regardless of your speed. Pacing the progression sensibly creates an excellent cardiovascular routine.

After a student reaches level three of the Sun Salutation, I also recommend regular practice of the Cleansing Breath (Kapalabhati) of at least three rounds of 30 breaths. This practice tones the musculature covering the internal organs and provides a vitality exercise to the heart.

Phase four is achieved by maintaining a 20-minute program at any desirable pace. Ideally, students train to be able to do the pace progressively faster than the traditional slow and fluid manner. During this phase of training, disregard the coordination of breath to body motions. Allow your breath to flow in a natural, unobstructed manner. This level is optimal for cardiovascular health. Teachers and teenagers are often given more for their training. It is common to expect them to practice up to 100 cycles regularly.

Thomas Griner tells us that our blood pressure can become "abnormally and dangerously elevated" for several reasons. One reason is a spastic muscle. A major blood vessel that brings blood to the head and neck is the carotid artery. If we apply pressure above the carotid body (which is located on the internal carotid artery, just above its separation from the common carotid artery on either side of the neck), a pressure point on the artery, we can decrease our blood pressure. The sternocleidomastoid muscle is positioned along the carotid body, and when the sternocleidomastoid is spastic, blood pressure can rise. By releasing spasticity in this muscle, we can help to lower some types of high blood pressure.[1]

The yogic technique of Jalandhara Bandha (Neck Lock) takes advantage of this parasympathetic reflex by applying pressure here during yoga pranayama exercises. When taught correctly, this method can also help prevent high blood pressure by bringing the chin down toward the jugular notch during the pause between inhalation and exhalation. Its full use needs to be regulated by a teacher trained in pranayama variations.

CASE STUDY—JEFF

Jeff was a highly stressed man in his mid 40s when he was hit by a heart attack. In the last two years, he has benefited greatly by being introduced to Dr. Dean Ornish's program for reversing heart disease, sponsored by Beth Israel Hospital in Boston. Through this program, he learned a series of gentle yoga practices, changed to a much healthier vegetarian diet, and learned to express his emotions more effectively. One of my apprentice teachers, Laurie, who had been teaching for this program, began to work with Jeff. She frequently asked questions about how to supplement and personalize the work given in this program. I gave Laurie my advice, yet I feel that her own yoga practice gave her intuitive insights into how to be with people, in spite of her lack of medical background. I'll let Jeff tell his story in his own words:

---

[1] Thomas Griner, *What's Really Wrong with You—A Revolutionary Look at How Muscles Affect Your Health* (Garden City, NY: Avery, 1996), p. 133.

In many, many ways yoga has greatly enriched my everyday life. It has and continues to be somewhat of a struggle to maintain the discipline to take the time for my morning asanas and evening deep relaxation and meditation. It has helped so much to have a group of recovering heart patients to work with in this regard, and having Laurie as a teacher has been a godsend.

I believe that my life very much depends on my consistency with my yoga practice and the other areas of my heart reversal program. Daily deep relaxation, visualization and meditation sessions relieve the day's stress to such an extent that I do not feel like the same person when I rise from my mat to cook my evening meal. Music sounds more intimate to me. I feel more present for other people. I have more patience, and ultimately go to sleep easily after my brief nightly reading.

When I awaken it is often just a few minutes prior to the alarm and I get out of bed calmly and turn it off. On days after I have missed my evening relaxation session, I leap from my bed in a tense panic to turn off the alarm. On those off days, I tend not to sleep soundly and may even have nightmares.

I begin my day with prayers, followed by a shower. I cook my breakfast cereal with fruit and make my lunch. Then I do some brief inspirational readings and begin my yoga. I primarily listen to a yoga tape that incorporates relaxation and gentle movement with Sun Salutation asanas. The half-hour that I take to do my morning asanas reward me with much lower stress at work, which is a demanding customer service job. I enjoy the 20-minute walk to work on the same route every day.

After I walk home in the evening, I listen to a deep relaxation tape for half an hour that incorporates breathing, pranayama, yoga, meditation and visualization. Twice a month my cohorts from the Dean Ornish program get together for a 2-hour yoga class with Laurie and group support session.

My yoga practice has helped me to keep my total cholesterol below 100 points. I firmly believe that my cholesterol count would not be as remarkable without doing my daily Yoga practice. At the time of my heart attack, my total cholesterol was over 280. I have to keep taking medication, I've tried hard not to, but my body just manufactures the stuff no matter what.

My blood pressure has always been pretty good, even before my heart attack when I was a heavy smoker. Yoga and meditation have been particularly good for my emotional sobriety. The proof lies in the days when I somehow rationalize away the necessity of doing my asanas and have to go through a day feeling tension. Then my temper is on more of a hair trigger, though this is not always obvious to others. So it becomes all the more imperative to do my asanas and deep relaxation techniques in order to have the quality of life that I have come to enjoy.

My community with fellow Quakers and my fellow heart patients has been intensified by my commitment to both fellowships. Yoga has given me a great deal of confidence and faith that the future holds terrific possibilities and serenity for life in the present. I just started back to school and intend to get my law degree, hopefully by the time I am 50.

I have become ever more confident of my health and I do not fear a heart attack. My stress tests have revealed that there is almost no evidence of scarring on the outer wall of my heart, only a slight shadow remains. My stamina has been very good. I can ride my bicycle up to 60 miles in an afternoon and have no soreness the next day. I do not fear back trouble, because I keep my spine flexible. My glands, muscles, and organs feel invigorated by my yoga practice.

I intend to continue my yoga practice for the rest of my life, one day at a time. It gives me such a wonderful platform for engaging in my daily life. My daily practice is such a beautiful discipline to have incorporated into my life.

Chapter 27

DIGESTIVE HEALTH

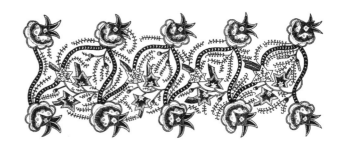

Many of the digestive organs, namely the esophagus, stomach, small intestine, and large intestine, are hollow to permit the free passage of food mixed with water. The accessory organs of the liver, kidneys, spleen, and pancreas are solid. This mixture of textures creates a diverse reaction when they press against each other during yogasanas. The inverted poses, twists, and forward-bending poses reposition the digestive organs. Holding these poses longer and deepening your breath is most beneficial to digestion. It is wonderful to know yourself so well that you are able to breathe into each individual organ. It is common that this repositioning creates peristaltic motion and accompanying sounds during these poses. This is especially true during Supported Shoulderstand. (Often my class sounds like a frog serenade following a rainstorm!) Encourage these sounds when practicing on your own. Whatever motion brought it up, repeat it, going into and out of the motion several times until the internal serenade is complete.

Constipation and irregular bowel movements are aggravated by irregular life-styles. The most effective therapy to address this immediately is to regulate eating and sleeping habits. The next step is to heighten your sensitivity to increase your self-observation skills. As a result, you will be able to detect foods that are indigestible to your system. These may include leftovers held over 24 hours that lose their life-force, overcooked foods, processed foods, and sugar. The third step is to develop humility and reverence for the process of growing, gathering, harvesting, and preparing food. Cultivate thankfulness for each person and the forces of nature that created the blessing of the food that will soon become your body. By blessing your food, you will find yourself drawn to eating foods that want to become your body. Review the Guidelines for Practice, chapter 4, and read the section "What Should I Eat?" beginning on page 32.

CASE STUDY—MATTHEW

Matthew, a 37-year-old radiology technician, came in the spring of 1990, recommended by a friend, initially seeking relief from chronic back pain. His situation was remarkably easy to work with, as he was highly motivated and compliant with all the recommendations I gave him. He had sought help from over ten professionals, including orthopedic surgeons, chiropractors, and massage therapists—all to no avail. I found that, while his treatments gave him temporary relief, the exercises he did were misdirected and too strong for the specific problem he had. With personalized attention, he was free of back pain within three months. He was a tremendous pleasure to work with, as he was so willing to learn, was disciplined in following instructions, and asked many insightful questions about the changes that occurred in his body from yoga.

One particularly remarkable event was when his back strengthening resulted in the loosening of the costal cartilage near the sternum. Matthew came in that week with an excited expression and said "I don't know what's happening, but my chest is cracking. Am I doing something wrong?" I explained to him, in the calm manner I use when confronted with a startled client, that it is normal for the sternum to move forward as a development of greater thoracic mobility and increased lung capacity. After all, he was making many changes, not only in his back, but also in his internal organs.

Given the success of his yoga practice at relieving back pain, he mentioned that he had colitis and had been taking medication for it for about six years. He asked me whether I had suggestions to help him lessen or eliminate his medication. I was delighted to have him continue to seek ways of changing his own physiology with yoga, and eagerly agreed to show him a rarely taught sequence of Classical Yoga practices.

I gave him a progression of abdominal exercises for the internal organs, beginning with pumping the stomach muscles (Agnisar Dhouti). This pranayama consists of pulling the abdomen back and forth while holding your breath. He practiced this faithfully twice a day, doing three sets of thirty pumps. It took him a couple of weeks to grasp the difference between the normal toning of his abdominal muscles and using his abdominal muscles to exercise his digestive organs. Once he got the feeling, he was hooked. Matthew progressed to the next level, which was the introduction of Stomach Lock (Uddiyana Bandha). This is a strong continuous pull, back and upward, that hollows the abdomen following an exhalation. He tended to overdo practices, as he was so well developed, and continued to be mildly overaggressive. For a few weeks, I had to continuously caution him about finding the right amount of effort to apply, so that he wouldn't get a racy heart or become short of breath from holding his breath too forcibly. These personality issues are directly related to colitis in the Ayurvedic and yogic view. In this perspective, colitis is more likely to occur in personalities that are fiery, aggressive, or misdirected.

About six weeks after he began to work on his digestion, I taught him an advanced Purification Exercise (Kriya) called Nauli. The word Nauli has no direct translation, but means roughly "a boat tossed about in a churning sea." In this practice, the student learns to isolate the rectus abdominis muscle that lies vertically in the center of the abdomen. The initial training consists of isolating the two sides of the muscle thus creating the appearance of a large vertical rope in the central abdomen. Nauli's benefits include restoring the digestive fire (agni) to its home site for vitality and increasing energy and sexual stamina. It is well known as a key to the sexual component of Tantrik Yoga.

Over the next month, Matthew began to isolate the two sides of the muscle. Later, he learned to move control from one side to the other. The resulting motion in turn tones and massages the underlying muscles that make up walls of the small and large intestines. It is this final variation that earns the purification exercise its Sanskrit name of Nauli. Matthew was quite faithful and devoted to his practice and developed this technique to be able to create the full practice in a relatively short period of time. Within two months of mastering the isolation of the rectus abdominus, he was able to come completely off his medication with his physician's blessings.

RELIEF FROM PAIN

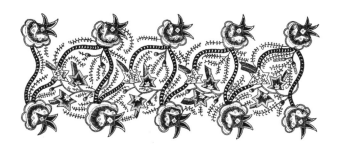

Structural Yoga Therapy™ is not appropriate for clients in acute pain. In this situation, yoga therapies of pranayama, stress management, counseling, and meditation training can provide the best support when provided by qualified yoga therapists.

*Tension is your body's way
of getting attention.*

Since I firmly believe the above statement to be true, I encourage you to listen to your tension and find what message it is sending to you. With regards to creating your personal yoga therapy program, I highly recommend you focus first on opening up the lines of communication around any area of pain, stress, or chronic discomfort. When you have a willingness to learn from the messages of your tension, they will speak to you. When their messages have gone unheard for a long time, they will often require that you take initiative to release the insensitivity that comes with chronic tension. Thus, to release pain, you must be with it. I do not mean to come to a confrontational stance, but rather to come to a stance of curiosity, one of wanting to learn and one of willingness to change old habits. With a stance of openness to life, anything is possible.

The challenge of assessing pain is to determine its source based on the symptoms of its manifestation. Situations of physical pain are always accompanied by muscular weakness and lack of joint mobility. Improvements in strength and flexibility often relieve pain.

Pain can also be present in the other dimensions of anatomy. As mentioned in chapter 6, there are five bodies in the yogic view of anatomy. Pain that is rooted in the ener-

293

getic or emotional subtle body is especially reflected in the breath. This pain will alter the location of the breath in the torso and in the nostril predominance. Pain that is rooted in the mental body is characterized by changes in the natural state of contentment. Thoughts of frustration or anxiety are mental pain, which is a suffering in reaction to changes in life—having an attachment to a particular outcome, wanting situations to be different than what they are, a nonacceptance of life being as it is. While psychotherapy is often utilized for emotional or mental pain. In the process of yoga, meditation and study of the true nature of your self is recommended. We are multidimensional beings, so the ideal yoga therapy program will incorporate physical poses, pranayama, and mental training. For the scope of this book, we will focus on lessening the physical imbalances and pay attention to how this will affect your other dimensions.

Changes in any factor will change the other factors. Increasing strength will improve joint mobility and tend to lessen pain. I find this approach has worked well for me. I do not have students in pain focus on stretching, as this rarely lessens the disease. It often hinders the body's ability to send messages to the mind. Often, with chronic back pain or other joint conditions, students will make great strides at lessening their pain by focusing only on strengthening the weakest muscle they've found in their body-reading analysis. This finding is surprising to both sufferers from chronic pain and their physical therapists and caretakers. Those in pain should focus their program on toning just one or two weak muscles and give themselves four weeks to determine the accuracy of my statement.

All too often, the pain of a chronic condition dissipates your capacity to concentrate on relaxation. Relaxation and meditation are often, but not always, quite effective for relief of chronic pain. In case studies where clients have tried these methods without success, I have found that Structural Yoga Therapy™ does make a difference. In some cases, a program combining the benefits of meditation and Structural Yoga Therapy™ is necessary, while in others, just specific strengthening programs make enough of a difference that other holistic approaches can then be applied.

If you don't have success in achieving relief from chronic pain by following this manual, contact the author. At the root of this therapy is an accurate Ayurvedic diagnosis of your constitution and the condition, which will be covered in a future book.

For regions of pain or chronic stress, I especially recommend that you develop strength in the areas inferior to the site of pain. Pay attention, as well, to stretching and relaxing the area directly opposite the pain. For instance, if you have pain in the posterior hip area, such as sciatica, strengthen the hamstrings and relax/stretch the upper quadriceps and hip flexors. Thus, back-bending poses like Cobra and Locust are recommended. Forward-bending poses are contraindicated. I have found that this procedure brings the greatest relief in the shortest amount of time. Later on, focus your attention to strengthening the painful area directly.

In working to overcome pain, I have found it critical to define the territory as accurately as possible. Once the specific imbalances in skeletal muscles have been defined, then yoga therapy can become more efficient. You need to uncover, not only what joints are restricted or hypermobile, but also which specific muscles responsible for those motions are tight or weak. In addition, you need to know the consequences of the imbalance or pain. Often, this is more than just the area of discomfort. This is especially true in chronic pain cases where the body has been adapting to avoid pain over some time.

Once this is uncovered, then the proper asanas can be chosen, based upon the summary found in Table 6 (page 266). In practicing the yogasanas, it is not enough to know how to perform them well. You must keep your attention on feeling the desired effect in the specific muscles. Keeping the feeling of the muscle strengthening or stretching is crucial to make the shift from simply practicing poses to doing poses therapeutically.

When you strengthen the weakest muscle, the pain level normally diminishes quickly. *In cases of recurring or chronic pain, the underlying difficulty is that the strength of the mind is weakened.* Pain is experienced as a sensation to be avoided, hence concentration is weakened. There is a natural loss of body consciousness that follows painful injuries.

When you strengthen specific muscles and maintain concentration about the physical location of the muscles involved, your mind gets stronger. This creates an anchor for the physical locations of the mind. Over time, your mind is able to know the difference between strengthening and stretching, and good pain versus bad pain. This mental training is the most crucial factor in overcoming pain. It is of prime importance that anyone working with pain in themselves, or as a therapist for others in pain and suffering, should practice meditation and prayer regularly. Since we are all subject to pain and suffering, why wait until your are faced with them again? Best to begin the practice of meditation and prayer immediately, and to commit to these beneficial practices for the rest of your life. Getting to know yourself is crucial to the relief of pain, and knowing your body is important. *Don't forget the "you" that lives in your body.*

As you will see in the case study to follow, skill in body reading through postural and range of motion analysis are essential in freeing pain. Body reading is not for the purpose of correcting the postural imbalance, but rather to use these as pointers toward alleviating muscular imbalances. As the muscles gain better functional symmetry, your will improve.

Remember, however, that your goal is not perfect posture, but freedom from the restrictions to the body that pain generates. In general, what I have found to be most effective is to strengthen the muscle immediately below the site of pain or injury. This provides a grounding support into which the painful tissues can relax. This is especially true in chronic pain. I find that working directly on the injury will either aggravate the pain or, at best, be of temporary relief. Long-term relief is often achieved with this procedure, especially in the case of chronic back conditions.

Contemplation of the experiential sequence of events is especially important in creating insight when working with pain. You will recall from the guidelines to practice (see chapter 4) that one unique factor of yoga is that we do not exert through pain. Yoga therapy for pain is focused on learning from the sensations that your mind labels as pain. This learning comes with a mental clarity obtained through sustained practice of contemplation (dharana). The process of working with pain through a mindful contemplation is to physically locate the spectrum of sensations that extends from pain and discomfort to ease and comfort. By finding the location of pain, you can learn to become mindful of what was previously subconscious. This contemplation allows you to sense where there are physical tensions that you can shift. By this shift, your subconscious tensions change in the terrain around the loci of the pain. This in turn induces the sympathetic nervous system's "relaxation reflex." Training in this manner makes a major shift, not only in muscle physiology, but also in your response to psychological stressors. For physiology does not know the difference between mind- and body-induced stress. All stress creates chemical, behavioral, musculo-skeletal, and postural changes.

An important aspect of working with pain is motivation. Motivation needs to arise from within you. The pain needs to be compelling enough to motivate you to do your homework. In my experience, if the motivation comes more from the teacher than the student, the beneficial results will be short lived. Without sufficient motivation, there will be a lack of compliance in fulfilling the recommendations given. Therefore, no matter how effective the program is, if it is not adhered to in a disciplined fashion, the problem will most likely recur. Sometimes the problem manifests in an unsuspecting fashion in another part of the body, or in a seemingly unrelated aspect of life.

From the yogic perspective of anatomy, pain has its roots in the three densest fields, or koshas. There is physical pain (in the annamayakosha) due to muscular or neurological disturbances. There is energetic or emotional pain (in the pranamayakosha) that manifests as irregular breathing and an unstable energy flow. And there is mental pain (in the manomayakosha) due to ignorance of the truth or negative thinking. A complete program will incorporate physical exercise, along with retraining of the breath and its underlying energy field, through positive attitude, reflection, life-style and meditation training. It is important for the yoga therapist to engage in discussions about the nature of pain and suffering. These are often the most productive lessons to be learned from injuries.

A yogi is someone whose energy does not leave the body.

Such a person has a high degree of presence, as they live fully in their body, energy, and mind, undistracted by physical sensations or disturbing thoughts. By practicing to be a yogi, you can learn to deepen your trust in yourself and find the lesson that life is presenting you now. Watch your energy and thoughts, and when this is not possible, watch your reactions. Over time your reaction time will speed up and you can become less reactive, more able to observe those inner situations that otherwise would knock you off-balance, and respond appropriately.

CASE STUDY—ERIC

Eric came to me on a referral from a massage therapist for his back pain. He is a 38-year-old physician doing medical research. Eric is 5 feet 11 inches tall, about 180 pounds, and appears to be in great physical shape. He rides his bike to work daily—a four-mile ride. He is married and has an 18 month-old daughter. A year before coming to see me, he went for a long hike with his daughter on his back. That night, he was up late with his daughter due to her restlessness. He finally put her to bed and he slept on a couchbed adjacent to her bed. He said that was a lousy bed.

He awoke with a mid-back spasm that continued for a year. At the time, his life was being subjected to many changes, bringing anxiety and a severe depression—he had just gotten a new job, they had purchased a new home, and his mother had moved close by. His current symptoms include constant pain in the lower thoracic and upper lumbar region, aggravated by forward bending or sitting. As his work involved sitting on a stool at a medical research laboratory, he was in discomfort during all of his working hours.

He had found that swimming increased the tone of his back, but did not diminish his pain. The most relief he had came from stretching with Iyengar Yoga poses that his wife had shown him. She had been taking classes and sought to give him some of her inspiration. He thought he'd try an individual session to see what personalized Structural Yoga Therapy™ could offer.

The initial session's body reading showed that he was in a constant "right-hand turn" from the lumbar spine. Joint-mobility testing revealed quite limited hip flexion in straight-leg tests. His left was 60 degrees and his right was 70 (normal is 90) during the initial visit, indicative of hamstring tightness. The antagonist muscle, the psoas (especially in the right iliacus portion of the muscle) showed acute tenderness when palpated. The most marked weakness was shown in his lower trapezius and latissimus muscles, both of which tested at diminished capacity of 50 percent. His shoulder external rotators tested at only 70 percent capacity.

The poses his wife had given him to do were insightful for a student untrained as a yoga teacher. They included Downward Facing Dog, Up Facing Dog, Abdominal Twist with both knees bent, and Head-to-Knee Pose.

I encouraged him to keep the poses, which he found most beneficial, and focused his personalized yoga session on three poses. The first two were a polishing of what he had previously been practicing. We did Up and Downward Facing Dog continuously, while I encouraged him to pull the shoulders back and down to engage the weakened trapezius and latissimus muscles. I kept this up until he began to show signs of fatigue and could no longer do the poses. Because of his size and physical development, I had him exert more than I would an average yoga student. This is a strategy not only to rapidly develop muscle strength, but also to reinforce neurological reflexes to gain better posture.

The third posture I gave him was the Spinal Twist (Marichyasana). A similar emphasis was placed upon the weakened muscles of the upper back, while rotating to his capacity to stretch the lateral hip muscles (abductors). During the initial session, I adjusted him by pulling both shoulders backward while standing behind him. My right knee was drawn inward and upward on the right side of his thoracic rib cage when he practiced the twist to the left side. This maneuver essentially reversed the position of his "right-hand turning torso" as seen during the body reading portion of the session. Eric reported an instantaneous release of the year-long tension in his mid back as this adjustment was applied. I told him I knew how to find his sweet spot.

Eric came back a week later for his first of three once-a-week follow-up visits. He reported a marked decrease in his pain. For the second session, we reviewed the three poses and I showed him a variation of the Spinal Twist, done while sitting in a chair. This allowed him to do some stretching at work and tone the weakened muscles of his mid back. I also began to do Yoga Bodywork to disengage the right iliacus muscle. At first, it was so tender it could hardly be touched. Then Eric learned how to do abdominal breathing to release the pain in his iliacus muscle. By directing his breath range to the lower right quadrant of his pelvis, he was gradually able to follow the instructions to "inhale into the pain and exhale to release it with the breath." With practice, he learned to tolerate more contact pressure and discharge the resulting sensations of discomfort.

At the beginning of our fourth session, he reported he had no pain for the first time in a year. He stated that he had learned how to be mindful of his posture, especially from the mid back to the sacrum, and maintain an erect extension in his back. Our work began to focus on posture, balance, and principles of maintaining symmetry in daily activities.

One year after his initial visit, Eric has continued coming for once-a-month individual yoga sessions and remains free of pain. In the last session, he told me that he continues because his practice is now a pleasure. It gets him high, especially when he pleasures himself with a slow and attentive 45-minute session once a week. He said, "My middle-aged body is more mobile than it has been and I am able to enjoy pleasure more than ever."

CASE STUDY—MELISSA

Melissa is a computer technician in her early 40s who came on a referral from a long-standing client who works with her. She is about 5 feet 4 inches tall, appearing very trim at 125 pounds. She has done yoga for two years, beginning with Kripalu Yoga. She is currently taking a once-a-week Iyengar Yoga class at her health club. She practices about "five minutes a day on her own."

Her symptoms are back pain, localized in the region of the upper right sacroiliac joint. This pain has gotten progressively worse over the past five years. It is accompanied with stiffness when she stands or walks for any length of time. Her doctors have ruled out pathology by tests and x-ray examinations. She is anxious to determine that her yoga practice has not aggravated the pain. In fact, she reports that she is fearful of several poses and doesn't want to do them. They include spinal twists and the standing Side-of-Hip Stretch (Parsvottanasana).

On examination of her doing the Wall Hang, this standing forward-bend position revealed a 10 degree left lumbar and lower thoracic curvature, ranging from L3 to T8. This was analyzed by a scoliometer placed on her back to reveal the rotation of the posterior rib cage. Her pelvis was level and her sacroiliac joints moved evenly when isolated with a standing waist-high hip flexion.

When I put her through the Joint-Freeing Series to test her range of motion, I discovered that all joints were normal. In spite of normal mobility, she did have pain in the right sacroiliac area with several motions—right hip adduction, right hip flexion, and left hip abduction. Thus her pelvis was doing a mild left-hand turn, which included a flaring of the right iliac crest from the sacrum.

In muscle testing, the left psoas had the most marked weakness, showing about 60 percent capacity, with a compensating rotation of the pelvis. Melissa was guarded and tender when I isolated the psoas muscles. When isolated, the sartorius muscles pulled the pelvis off line, causing an imbalance in leg length, making the left leg a half inch longer. An immediate test of its antagonist, the tensor fascia lata, balanced her pelvis resulting in symmetry in leg length. My strategy is to overdevelop the tensor fascia lata and internal hip rotators in general to restore balance in the pelvis. The erector spinae superficial layer test showed a weakness of about 50 percent. When isolated, they mildly corrected the spinal curvature, but the correction lacked stamina as it could not be sustained.

Because Melissa is in such good physical conditioning, she is capable of a normal yoga routine with minor adjustments in each posture to create strength or flexibility where she lacks it. First in her sequence was an exercise designed to rapidly improve the tone of the tensor fascia lata muscles at the outer pelvis by exercising them in isolation from their helpers. I had her do the fifth movement of the Joint-Freeing Series while lying on her side. In this manner, she was to go into internal hip rotation with the top leg pointed toes-down and heel-up. Then, keeping this position, she lifted the leg 12 times, slowly, up 24 inches, and then down.

The second of six poses was the Balancing Tree Pose, done normally, except that she held the inner thigh of the supporting leg extra taut to strengthen the adductors. When coming out of the posture, I had her remove the leg as slowly as possible, keeping the hip rotation as she lowered the leg. This action isolated the sartorius muscle and helped her maintain pelvic balance with the tensor fascia lata.

For the third posture, I had her practice Warrior I, with a focus on the internal hip rotator's strength. She needed to overcompensate for her pelvis' twist by emphasizing a twist forward of the left pelvis when the left leg was extended backward. Another way to put this is that I had her bring the tops of her thighs closer together, thus toning the adductors and stretching the left psoas. When her right leg was backward, I had her extend upward, lengthening her lumbar spine.

The fourth pose was the Extended Triangle, done with added external turn-out in the side toward which she was bending. This changed the standard position and brought the upper pelvic rim slightly forward of the "accepted Iyengar way" of teaching the pose. For her, this was needed to develop the weakened psoas muscles and give extra support from the gluteus maximus muscles.

Her next pose was Cobra, with a focus in sequence on strengthening the adductors, the buttocks, and the erectors. By moving her attention slowly up the body from the inner thighs to the back, and reversing the release, she could develop more foundational strength in the region below her pain. The last pose of her sequence was the Camel, emphasizing a forward pressure of the pelvis to stretch the quadriceps and psoas, while developing stamina of the hamstrings and gluteus maximus. The gluteus maximus is an important muscle providing stability to the sacroiliac joint. The stronger it becomes, the more secure the pelvis is in general.

Melissa left her private sessions feeling rejuvenated and inspired to continue her yoga practice, regardless of how her structural stress might change in the future. She seemed relieved to know that what happened to cause her pain was within the range of her ability to change and make a difference. She has continued to return for reassessments twice a year for the past five years.

Chapter 29

MANAGING STRESS

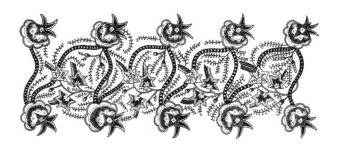

The main routines in yoga's repertoire for stress management are breathing exercises, guided imagery, and relaxation exercises. For persons with elevated blood pressure or hypertension controlled by medication, breathing exercises should be done in a reclining position, until a degree of breath control is gained. When you can willfully diminish your normal respiratory rate by one-third for two minutes, you can begin normal yoga pranayama exercises in a seated position. In other words, if your normal breath is fifteen cycles per minute, you must reduce it to ten cycles per minute for two minutes before seated practice is recommended. As Candance Pert, researcher into psychoendocrine immunology, points out:

> Conscious breathing, the technique employed by both the yogi and the woman in labor, is extremely powerful. There is a wealth of data showing that changes in the rate and depth of breathing produce changes in the quality and kind of peptides (chemical messengers also conveying subtle emotions) that are released from the brain stem. And vice versa! By bringing this process into consciousness and doing something to alter it—either holding your breath or breathing extra fast—you cause the peptides to diffuse rapidly throughout the cerebrospinal fluid, in an attempt to restore homeostasis, the body's feedback mechanism for restoring and maintaining balance. And since many of these peptides are endorphins, the body's natural opiates, as well as other kinds of pain-relieving substances you soon achieve a diminution of your pain. . . . The peptide-respiratory link is well documented: Virtually any peptide found anywhere else can be found in the respiratory center. This peptide

substrate may provide the scientific rationale for the powerful healing effects of consciously controlled breath patterns.[1]

Body relaxation exercise or progressive relaxation can be quite beneficial. In 1990, Howard Hall showed that the immune system could be consciously controlled. His studies at Case Western Reserve University in Ohio used relaxation and guided imagery to alter white blood cell physiology. Often, students learning such techniques need to be guided into the relaxation reflex, so recorded cassette tapes are useful. One of my yoga teacher apprentices who trains patients in Dean Ornish's program in Boston for reversing heart disease found patients reluctant to let go of their relaxation tapes. The comfort and security of letting go to a familiar voice allowed them to feel safe. I have discovered that the deeper levels of freedom from stress come from the unexpected. Even when students have used the same tape repeatedly, the unpredictable can still occur, if you allow it to. It is important to continue to reach for your intuition, your higher power or group consciousness, as a way to go beyond body and self-consciousness.

When we reach higher states of consciousness, it is natural to become unconscious or fall asleep. This is a normal reaction and no effort should be made on the part of a knowledgeable teacher to correct it. Over time, your own physiology, via the relaxation reflex, will make the necessary chemical and neurological changes to maintain an alert relaxation. If you ask for it, you can also be brought to insights about yourself that would support a more beneficial life-style. After your stress levels have been diminished through changes in breathing habits and life-style, you will be able to do the same exercises and remain fully alert. When relaxation can be done for 15 minutes without becoming unconscious, you can begin a practice of seated meditation if you have the desire for it. An ability to stay alert during supine relaxation shows the physiological readiness for meditation practice.

The process of relaxation often reveals previously hidden, specific subconscious tensions stuck in the emotional soup, the mixture we call stress. By the process of progressive relaxation and its spiritual relative, meditation, the dark side comes into light. "The angry person, energy concentrated in eyes, jaw, throat, arms, shoulders, and chest, is a self-destructive trigger waiting to be pulled. Breathing deeply into the belly relieves the tension in the upper body and starts to bring the deranged parts of the being into harmony, preventing verbal or physical violence to others—or to himself or herself. To be centered is to say yes to life."[2]

These often hidden emotions of our dark side have long been suspected of being beneath certain types of, if not all, disease. Candace Pert tells us that, in the 1980s, studies by Lydia Temoshok, who was a psychologist at UCSF, showed cancer patients who repressed anger as having slower recovery rates than people who were more expressive. Another trait common to cancer patients was self-denial, stemming from a lack of unawareness of basic emotional needs. The immune systems seemed to be stronger and the tumors were smaller for people in touch with emotions.[3]

---

[1] Candace Pert, *Molecules of Emotion: Why You Feel the Way You Feel* (New York: Scribner, 1997), p. 187.
[2] George Leonard, "Reflections on a Starry Night," *Yoga Journal* (July/August, 1999), p. 136.
[3] Pert, *Molecules of Emotion*, p. 192.

One of the most fascinating aspects of yoga is its reputation as a body/mind discipline, integrating mental and physical training into one event, and giving the experience of seemingly opposite paradigms unified. Science has recently been hot on the trail of this unified field theory. One major contributor has been Candace Pert. She said, "If we accept the idea that peptides and other informational substances are the biochemicals of emotion, their distribution in the body's nerves has all kinds of significance, which Sigmund Freud, were he alive today, would gleefully point out as the molecular confirmation of his theories. The body is the unconscious mind! Repressed traumas caused by overwhelming emotion can be stored in a body part, thereafter affecting our ability to feel that part or even move it."[4] This last statement had personal import for one of my recent clients.

CASE STUDY—ROBIN

Robin matches volunteers with elderly people because she enjoys relieving other people's loneliness. She works as a manager of volunteers who serve the state services for aging. Robin is an example of a client who was referred to me by one of my long-standing clients for back pain. Her supervisor, my client of ten years, had experienced working through his chronic pain with my supervision. However, I did not properly screen her in the initial telephone interview to discover that she was in acute pain. She arrived on a Tuesday following a traumatic episode of pain on Sunday that left her unable to work on Monday. She had first experienced back pain in 1985, following a weight-lifting routine at home, where she thinks she twisted her lower body inappropriately. Since then, she has experienced pain intermittently with occasional episodes of acute pain.

When Robin walked in the door of my office, I at once knew instinctively that her pain was not physical in nature. In spite of trusting my intuition, I have also learned to validate it by doing physical examination tests as well. She had acute pain on the right side, in the middle-to-upper thoracic region of her back. This was accompanied by pain in the middle region of the right inguinal ligament that connects the upper outer iliac pelvic bone to the lower central pubic bone. She also had recurring pain in the hip and lower back that was increased with hip flexion and external rotation. In taking her through the Joint-Freeing Series to test for range of motion and muscle strength, I found no irregularities. She also complained of pain in her left lower back and left elbow. Upon examination, the arm pain was found to be a localized sensitivity near the origin of the extensor carpi ulnaris. The right thoracic back pain was too acute to touch, so I left it alone.

My intuition told me not to give Robin any yoga exercise program, but to begin with gentle Yoga Bodywork massage on the forearm site of sensitivity. I taught her how to do slow abdominal breathing, contracting her muscles during exhalation. I also encouraged her to practice a mantra to help her detach from her pain. I massaged lightly for a few moments, gently guiding her into a relaxed state of mind. Within ten minutes, she began to cry. I encouraged her to relax, to allow any feelings to surface, and to

---

[4] Pert, *Molecules of Emotion*, p. 141.

share her thoughts or insights if she wanted to. As she cried, I guided her to allow her body to move spontaneously. The pressure I applied on a forearm vital point (marma) caused her to wiggle and arch her back. Her body twisted in unpredictable ways, often flexing and rotating at the hips and thighs. I sensed that she was releasing a pattern of postural tension in reaction to some stress. (She later reported not remembering any of these movements).

She began an enlivened story of the issues underlying her stress and pain. The most recent was a "recently failed romance that seemed to be the trigger for feelings of abandonment from losing both parents at a young age." She was filled with emotion as she spoke about the death of her father, which had occurred more than 20 years before. Her father had hidden the fact that he had cancer from his family. This was not revealed until after his death. I asked her to imagine being free of time and space, and just to put herself with her father, wherever he was at this time. We both felt his presence come into the room, and she quietly spoke to him of her feelings. She revealed that she suspected her father was gay and that he tried to hide it by having lots of children. She was the youngest of thirteen! She said that she felt she had learned how to hide pain by following his example. The dialog she had with his presence created some headway in resolving her conflicts. She later said, "I felt anger at the losses and feelings of guilt at being angry—the inner conflict resulting in pain."

She returned the following week with no pain in her hip, yet continued to experience pain in the right mid-thoracic region and a mild pain in her left forearm. This time, my examination revealed a weakness in the erector spinae muscles of spinal extension and the muscles of hip extension, the gluteus maximus and hamstrings. She had done some gentle exercises I had suggested for her. I felt encouraged by her changes, so I asked her to practice Locust Pose to strengthen the hips and lower back. As her right sacroiliac appeared unstable, I had her do the Locust three times in varying widths, from legs together, to one foot apart, to two feet apart. Each lift was for a measured two breaths. She was stable for this amount of a hold. Beyond it, she trembled and began to twist her pelvis. So at this level of exertion, she was giving her musculo-skeletal structures stability. More than this would destabilize her body at this time.

We continued doing gentle Yoga Bodywork on the same forearm site as at the initial session. In the process of releasing this pain, she spoke of how her lover had left her with no words. He had simply left and stopped all communication. She felt abandoned, angry, and hurt. She asked, "What can I do to heal from this?" I encouraged her to use this phrase as a mantra and allow her intuition to reveal the answer she needed. Her self-reflections continued to deepen until a more formal meditation and prayer practice was set up two months later. Today she says she feels she has tools to effectively regulate the stress of her life.

Chapter 30

STRENGTHENING THE
IMMUNE SYSTEM

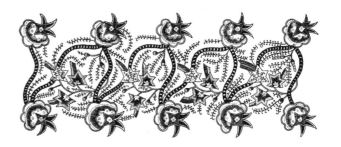

The immune system is made up of the spleen, bone marrow, lymph nodes, and various kinds of white blood cells, some of which circulate throughout the body, while others reside in the various tissues of the body, including the skin. Candace Pert tells us that its overall purpose is to defend the body against pathological invaders that threaten health and to repair any damage these invaders cause. "The immune system defines the boundaries of the organism, distinguishing between what is self and what is not self, determining what is part of the organism and what needs to be repaired and restored, versus what is part of a tumor and needs to be killed."[1]

Pert's definition is particularly intriguing when we look at the biological function of "distinguishing between what is self and what is not self." This is the prime directive of the Classical Yoga training of Patanjali in his *Yoga Sutras*, especially the cultivation of discriminative thinking, as espoused in chapter III, sutras 36–37 and 53–57. To know yourself is the first step of the yogic journey to life. Often, this journey is a return from secrecy and ignorance; on other occasions, it is a return from denial. A proverb about healing states

> *He who conceals his disease cannot be cured.*

This was particularly true for one of my clients facing the heart-wrenching challenge of fibromyalgia and chronic fatigue syndrome.

---

[1] Candace Pert, *Molecules of Emotion: Why You Feel the Way You Feel* (New York: Scribner, 1997), p. 181.

CASE STUDY—HELEN

Helen came to me on a referral from a caseworker at the Beth Israel Deaconess Hospital's Mind Body Medical Institute, where I offered classes to the staff and their patients. Helen is a single 46-year-old who had previously worked as a highly motivated career counselor for industrial workers. She was diagnosed with irritable bowel syndrome and had lost fifteen pounds from this condition. She had developed symptoms of chronic fatigue three years prior to being diagnosed with the condition. Her symptoms included trigger spots of intense muscle sensitivity (for which she was also given a diagnosis by a rheumatologist as fibromyalgia), extreme food sensitivity (there were only 20 items left on her diet that did not cause irritation), and low white blood cell count (indicative of lowered immune response). She managed to hide her symptoms for some time. Then one day she stopped trying to "control herself" and collapsed. Because of her extremely low energy, Helen lost her job. Her husband divorced her "to be with a woman who was more fun." She was forced to live with her parents, as she had no one else to take care of her daily needs. Like many of my clients, Helen had been exposed to yoga during her college days and had fond memories of its relaxation and peace-promoting benefits.

Because her energy levels fluctuated, we did a variety of yoga techniques. The major practice I emphasized was the development of breath awareness and sensitivity to how that affected her thoughts and feelings. On days when her energy level was higher, I gave her a gentle standing sequence for learning to have rhythmic motions in harmony with her breath. On days where fatigue was more acute, we did fewer yoga poses and more supportive, stationary or restorative poses, as developed by yoga master B. K. S. Iyengar.

We began with learning yoga breathing exercises consisting of resting in a supine position with the pelvis elevated. This position was for the purpose of increasing venous and lymphatic fluid return via the thoracic duct. She began by learning low abdominal breathing in this modified supported Bridge Pose. Iyengar has used this pose frequently for improving immune response in students with chronic stress. For Helen, at first her mind had difficulty focusing upon the breath, but this improved with the addition of having her press with her palms on the lower abdomen during exhalation. By developing a sensitivity to the changing shape of her lower abdomen, she learned to relax her pressure on inhalation to fill the lower abdomen, and increase the pressure to promote fuller exhalation.

As abdominal breathing has been shown to lower indicators of stress, it also began to increase her awareness of pent-up feelings. That which was hidden began to come to the surface. At first, she was extremely sensitive to touch, a symptom associated with irritable bowel syndrome. Then, as she learned to grade the pressure applied with breathing, the sensitivities revealed a whole host of emotions—anger, sadness, grief, memories of abandonment, loss of marriage and job. When the emotional content came up, I encouraged her to relax the structural tensions of her neck, shoulders, and face, which would increase as the emotional waves grew. There were times when the intensity of experiencing the buried feelings was too much for her, so I helped her to find alternate ways of breathing that would lessen the surfacing of her emotions.

Helen began to feel better and decided to take an eight-week yoga course, with the provision that she could do as much as she felt like and not be pushed by the group. When she first started, she was asked how much she felt she could do and replied that about 15 minutes was all she was up for. I suggested she do 7 minutes. Each time she returned, the same procedure was used, so that she began to have different values for her energy level. At the end of the eight-week course, she could do a full hour class without feeling fatigued.

I continued to see Helen for the next two years, though with less intensity, as she gradually improved in her vitality and energy level. While still struggling to fully regain her health, she is much more vocal about her emotions and no longer feels a need to hide her feelings. She found relaxation training working with Yoga Nidra and conscious breathing to be the most effective methods of healing herself. Yoga Nidra is a guided progressive relaxation method in which the physical body is consciously relaxed in a systematic manner. The full process lasts one hour. I created two tapes with variations to address Helen's particular needs for her to use.

Chapter 31

MEDITATION TRAINING TO DEVELOP A SPIRITUAL PRACTICE

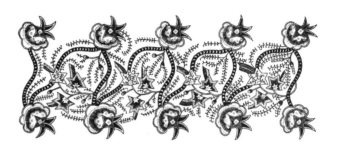

Once stress levels are under control, training in meditation and heightened awareness can proceed. Herbert Benson, M.D., was the first physician to study the physiological effects of Transcendental Meditation. In his groundbreaking book, *The Relaxation Response*, he described the factors that are necessary to induce the naturally occurring state of relaxation as a prelude to the experience of meditation.[1] While he did not practice yoga, Dr. Benson's research can be seen as a restatement of yoga's ancient doctrine. He found that four basic factors were all that was required to enter a state of meditation. These four factors are:

1. A quiet environment free of internal and external distractions;

2. A repeated mental device that reflects your deepest personal beliefs;

3. A passive attitude toward intrusive thoughts;

4. A comfortable position, consciously relaxing the body's muscles.

Note the similarity to the following aphorisms from Patanjali's *Yoga Sutras*, written two millennia earlier.

> 1. To eliminate obstacles to concentration, practice of a single technique should be made, the object may be any beloved object (I, 32).

---

[1] Herbert Benson, *The Relaxation Response* (New York: Avon Books, 2000).

2. Communion is gained through devotion to your chosen form of the inner Self (I, 23).

3. Consistent, earnest practice and dispassionate detachment can stop the vacillating waves of perception, which cloud realization of the Self (I, 12).

4. Yoga pose is comfortable and steady (II, 46).[2]

The practice of a regular prayer or mantra, or simply watching the regular rhythm of your breath, creates the relaxation reflex. To have regularity with practice requires interest and a desire sufficient to take the steps necessary to fulfill that desire. If you find that you're not committed, you may want to take another look at your goal. Does it fit in with your desired life-style?

Some people meditate easily with the help and camaraderie of a group. Others do best alone. If what you're doing isn't working—change. If you continue doing what you've always done, you'll keep getting what you've always gotten.

It has been said that we are not humans striving for a spiritual experience, but rather spiritual beings having a human experience. It doesn't matter to me which is true. In either event, regular meditation practice and the development of a spiritual practice support a harmonious life-style and contribute to the well-being of the entire planet.

We were all born, and, just as surely, we will all die. The beauty of birth, the mystery of death, and the magic of life are available to all equally. Meditate, not just for the benefits of health, or peace of mind, but also for the thrill of knowing yourself. There is such magnificence in us. There are inner worlds to explore. Sights, sounds, places we've never dreamed of are accessible only through meditation and heightened-awareness training. The blessing of a spiritual life doesn't just fall from the sky. It can be gained through the blessings of a teacher, a spiritual master or from God directly. Yet we can't hold what is given without training and self-discipline.

CASE STUDY—RACHAEL

Rachael, a retired 57-year-old registered nurse, came in early winter to request a personalized program of yoga to complement her training in Ayurveda. Her initial symptoms included chronic neck tension and acute pain in her right great toe. The pain in her toe was so debilitating that she was having trouble walking. She had been raised a religious Catholic and had been married for over thirty years to a dentist, who was also religious. Having this background allowed her to be open to the exchange of ideas between physical yoga and the energetic perspective of Ayurveda. She had been exposed to yoga prior to coming for private sessions. A right-hip injury four years prior, for which she had gotten help from osteopathic manipulation, had challenged her health. She had gone to an Ayurvedic physician for a more recent difficulty with chronic fatigue syndrome, which was attributed to candida yeast infection. This painful condi-

---

2 Stiles, *Yoga Sutras of Patanjali.*

tion was relieved by the Ayurvedic physician's use of random deep-tissue bodywork to release her "emotional armor." While the pattern of pain was broken, there was still recurrent pain in the middle and upper back, focused at the latissimus, trapezius, and sternocleidomastoid muscles. The chronic fatigue was treated with diet and herbal recommendations.

She had been doing an extensive yoga program consisting of 15 minutes of alternate-nostril breathing, 30 minutes of meditation, and 45 to 90 minutes of yogasanas beginning at 6 A.M. In Ayurvedic analysis, she was a vata/pitta type (air/fire), with an air imbalance.

In taking this training into consideration, I decided to recommend that she eliminate all other yoga exercises and had her practice only the Joint-Freeing Series. I asked her to do the series just as it is shown in this book, and to pay particular attention to maintaining rhythmic breathing. By so doing, she was also encouraged to feel the prana energy flowing directly to the joint in motion. Together, this concentration and physical exercise have been shown to relieve chronic pain.

The Joint-Freeing Series is particularly beneficial in relieving pain from vata conditions (which are the most common Ayurvedic imbalances). This is more likely to stabilize both the irregular occurrences of pain and the underlying energetic imbalance. Vata, or air type, is the most sensitive and has potentially the greatest intuition. One characteristic of this constitutional type is a tendency to instability that can come about by overdoing recommendations or by continually changing your routine based on the advice of several different practitioners. Often, with this quality, less is actually better, as doing less gives the energy field an opportunity to find a harmonious rhythm.

In our first session, I spent the majority of the time getting acquainted, as establishing rapport is critical to long-term success in working with this constitutional type. The evaluation noted a diminished external hip rotation of about 10 degrees from normal (35 degrees). The internal hip rotation motion was slightly above normal by approximately 3 to 6 degrees. Both internal and external hip rotators were found to be weak. Of these, the most marked weakness was in the left psoas. Her radial and navel pulse diagnosis revealed a displacement of the fire energy of digestion known as agni. This energy, which should be centered at the navel, had moved to the left of center. This can sometimes be correlated with weakened left psoas, which I found in her case.

At this session, she spoke of the challenges of maintaining her independent self while being deeply connected in her marriage. I then recommended she practice the Jesus Prayer, an ancient Christian mantra. In this practice, the phrase, "Lord Jesus, bless me with peace," is used.[3] By connecting the inhalation to the first half of the prayer and the exhalation to the second half, this practice can bring inner awareness to any activity. Since her husband was not interested in meditating with her, I recommended that she do this practice while having his psychic presence with her, the intention being to deepen the physical and psychic energy connection for the stability of their relationship. The

---

[3] Helen Bacovcin, *The Way of a Pilgrim* and *The Pilgrim Continues His Way* (Garden City, NY: Image Books, 1978). The description of a Russian pilgrim seeking advice on how to pray continuously using the Jesus prayer.

practice of rhythmic pranayama, accompanying prayer/meditation, is particularly beneficial for the relief of vata type of pain, which Rachael had been experiencing.

In successive programs, we emphasized the development of a meditative inner focus with her yoga exercise program. I began to explain many of her perceptions in terms of yogic anatomy, in order to deepen her connection to energy and prayer. We talked extensively about prana as an energy channel to access memory. By learning to feel the sensations of energy as they coursed through her body, she could also feel the directions in which that energy had continued, which, in turn, had created her postural distortions.

In the follow-up session a month later, Rachael was pleased to report the complete relief of the acute pain in her toe, and a complete return of mobility. Her fire energy, pitta, was found to have returned to the center of her abdomen, so that now a more normal recommendation could be given. I focused on giving her a sequence of poses to stabilize the fire energy and to tone the left psoas. The sequence consisted of doing the Half Boat Pose (Ardha Navasana), starting from a supine bent-knee position and exhaling up to the balanced position, then staying in the balanced position, keeping knees bent and together until stability was achieved and slowly curling the spine to the floor. After a few moments rest, this was repeated a total of six times. This motion balances the rectus abdominis muscle with the psoas. The second pose was to come to the Cobra Pose on inhaling and to lower the body on exhaling. Her capacity for this exercise was six repetitions. Doing full Locust in the same manner as the Cobra followed this. The final pose recommended was to catch hold of her ankles, as in Bow Pose, and remain, lifting nothing but her head and shoulders for as long as possible. The ideal duration was to be two minutes. The purpose of this sequence was to stimulate her vitality and produce a pleasant release of tension so that her body could naturally assume the relaxation reflex upon its completion. The sequence was created based upon reading her capacity to open and relax, a preliminary for the full procedure of relaxation training using the Joint-Freeing Series.

Four months after beginning sessions, Rachael began to come weekly. She now has a commitment to regular yoga practice and study, and is presently facing with courage her deeper psychological and spiritual issues. She has been a regular client, now, for six years.

CASE STUDY—JOE

Joe, a 45-year-old professor at a nearby university, came to me on referral from a physician for help with his body. In the initial interview, Joe said, "I hate my body. I use it to run away from myself. I want to learn how to get in harmony with myself and stop running away from myself." He had been an abused child, and had a difficult time being intimate with people to whom he felt attracted. He said he had an addictive personality and went to 12-step programs for substance abuse. His 12-step program had been a true saving grace. For him, it was a clearly defined spiritual path. He also claimed he ate, smoked, and drank too much. Joe described himself as spiritual, but not religious. He had been raised a fundamentalist. His current exercise program, which he had been doing for ten years, consisted of running three times a week and doing 80 to 100 push-ups in two sets of 40 to 50.

While I did give him a physical assessment in the follow-up interview, I focused the initial session on giving Joe the practice and the experience of meditation. I chanted the meditation mantra I had been given by my spiritual teacher, Swami Muktananda, for a few minutes; then we settled into a silent meditation for 20 minutes. The first sitting for him was profound and deeply stilling. I asked him if he wanted to read something about the science and practice of meditation. He declined, saying he just wanted to hold the experience.

In the second session, two weeks later, Joe talked about his concern over a growing hunchback (khyphosis) of the thoracic spine due to Schuermann's disease. This condition progressively increases the hunchback of the spine, making it rigid. He wanted help doing those yoga practices that might help lessen this spinal curvature. The physical examination revealed khyphosis that was accompanied by a sunken chest and rounded shoulder girdle. He appeared to have lost about two inches of height from the spinal compression. There was diminished scapular adduction and shoulder flexion on both sides. On the left, flexion was 70 degrees, on the right, 80 (normal is 90). The thoracic spine curvature could not be reversed when doing backbending poses. His hip flexion was limited to 100 degrees on both sides (normal is 135). The right internal hip rotation was diminished by 15 degrees, while the right hip external rotation was increased by the same amount. Essentially, his lying supine posture had a tendency to turn his feet to the right. In terms of muscular weakness, he showed a need for strength in the right psoas, right internal hip rotators, both hip flexors and hip extensors, and the posterior shoulder group—posterior deltoid, middle trapezius, and latissimus dorsi.

For the structural yoga portion of his program, I had Joe do modified push-ups from Cat Pose, to develop the posterior shoulder muscles, with the intention of progressing to opening his chest and elevating his standing posture. I also gave him muscle isolation and strengthening exercises for the individual components noted. During the next two weeks, Joe was quite faithful and did his program 12 of 14 days. As a result of doing the physical toning, and developing a trusting rapport, he began to unveil his inner issues. As a child, he had been overweight and had developed a panic-based fear of dying of a heart attack. This showed itself in his current restrained respiration. Even during mild exertion, he would become winded. We continued to end each session with a meditation session.

After the first month, Joe revealed that he had attempted to chant on his own and said, "I think the mantra's probably going to get me. For it's not lack of stimulation, but a lack of the true Self that I fear." I spoke of the teachings of the Classical Yoga text, *Yoga Sutras,* and its method of overcoming fear through understanding the nature of the mind and the True Self. At most sessions, these teachings were discussed as a way to understand the difficulties of his mind. Joe got a copy of my interpretation of the *Yoga Sutras.* He read from it frequently, and often came with questions about yoga philosophy and the veils of the mind (koshas).

After the second month of practice, Joe had made great progress in the strength and flexibility of his shoulders. I was pleased at his capacity to do 20 full push-ups with great form—not wavering from using what had formerly been weakened muscles. We arranged to meet monthly from this point on.

During the next month, Joe talked of his fear of the pattern of abused children growing up to become abusers, or being attracted to others who would keep them in a victim role. He spoke of his mother and wife as interchangeable. He might begin to tell me about his mother, and then say the word wife, and vice versa. I gave him a tape of my spiritual teacher chanting the meditation mantra. We sat in silent meditation for 20 minutes together. I explained that one meaning of the word mantra is "the sound that protects you."

Joe called me about three weeks later to tell me he had been in an auto accident. He said, "the mantra saved my life." A taxi driver who was taking Joe to work had panicked and lost control of the car due to a stuck accelerator pedal. Joe remained calm. He told the driver to turn off the ignition, but the driver, who didn't speak English, failed to understand him. Joe then relaxed into the yogic Fetal Pose and began to intently repeat his mantra. The meaning of his mantra is "I honor my inner Self." It implies that the inner Self is always with you, protecting, guiding—the One Presence worthy of being honored. The car crashed at high speed into a concrete divider separating the on-coming traffic, throwing the driver through the windshield and killing him. Joe came out of the crash with a mild injury to the right shoulder, a broken right ankle, and a pelvic displacement that created mild right sciatica. It took some time for him to recover from this event, so he waited until he was ready to come to me again.

I adjusted Joe's program to compensate for the injuries he had sustained and we went to a bi-monthly program to help him recover more quickly. Over the next summer, Joe made great progress in physically recovering his former strength, though he continued to lack full mobility in the right ankle. He discovered that chanting worked well for controlling his pain. He made good use of this finding.

Now, nearly nine years after his initial session, Joe continues to make appointments six times a year. Over this long period, he has also gotten relief from stomach acid by the practice of the yoga pranayamas Bastrika and Uddiyana Bandha. Yoga also seemed to empower him during an extremely difficult period of nearly two years, when he divorced his wife and gained equitable custody of his son. He has set aside an appointment for himself every day at 10 A.M. for an hour of practice. As a result, he looks and feels great. His stamina is much improved by his current regular practice of 35 to 50 minutes of Sun Salutations with variations that I gave him. Joe has been a remarkable client, in that he has made a commitment to doing his yoga practices, no matter what happens in his life.

The following is a quote from Joe about his experience with yoga therapy:

> More important than pain control, which was minor, was meditation's help with the nightmares of post traumatic stress disorder—two to three per night, falling (as in falling through space, accelerating in the cab), for about ten months. I found that, by meditating, I could get into a space that was not quite sleep, so not nightmarish, that left me refreshed in the morning. As I write this, I find it very interesting that, although I am loath to meditate routinely, when I really needed it, I embraced it gratefully.

I continue to encourage Joe to deepen his practice by incorporating a prayer to begin his meditation. I suggested that he pray for a higher power that loves him unconditionally.

Due to his long-standing involvement in 12-step programs, he found this compatible to his way of thinking.

Symptoms of Inner Peace*

Watch for the signs of peace, as they are the developing of stability in sattva guna. As you develop in the fullness of yoga life-style, there are signals that events are taking place that may be beyond your control. These symptoms are a wonderful ease (not dis-ease) that is contagious. You are cautioned to share them with everyone you meet.

1. A tendency to think and act spontaneously rather than from fear;

2. An unmistakable ability to enjoy each moment;

3. Loss of interest in judging others;

4. Loss of interest in judging yourself;

5. Loss of interest in interpreting the actions of others;

6. Loss of interest in conflict;

7. Loss of ability to worry (a very serious symptom);

8. Frequent, overwhelming episodes of appreciation;

9. Feeling connected with others and with nature;

10. Frequent attacks of smiling for no apparent reason at all;

11. Increased tendency to let things happen, rather than make them happen;

12. Increased susceptibility to giving and receiving love.

If you have more than three of the above symptoms, please be advised that your condition may be too advanced to return to your former self. If you become exposed to someone exhibiting these symptoms, remain exposed at your own risk.

*Excerpted and adapted from the poster SYMPTOMS OF INNER PEACE by Saskia Davis © 1984 all rights reserved. No transmittals or reproduction in any form is allowed without the written permission of Saskia Davis, LLC. www.symptomsofinnerpeace.net

Deepening Yoga Therapy

The yogic view of anatomy indicates that we are multidimensional beings. This translates to the perspective that what we feel may not always be in our physical body. Pain felt in the chest could be other than muscular, cardiovascular, neurological, or respiratory. It could be the pain of losing a dear friend. This emotionally based pain can lead to a shortening of muscle fibers and a resultant feeling of tension and stress. When we translate all feelings into physically caused reactions, we look to a medical specialist for the answer. When we translate feelings as something based in emotional psychology, we are more prone to consider a psychotherapist or psychoanalyst for help. When the pain or stress is of unknown origin, we may consider seeing both.

The yogic perspective is to consider all pain as having its source in a lack of understanding of our selves. When we know the body well, we can find the tools to be free of physical pain. In the same way, when we know our emotional nature thoroughly, we can direct our attention to the state of just being present to immediate feelings this can have a tendency to remove the pains of the past.

When changes to our body are due to nonphysical stress, the body will still react. Muscles tense, joint freedom diminishes, flexibility is lost, circulation is decreased, vitality is lost, and a depressing mood is generated. By changing any of these factors, however, the cycle can be reversed. This is where a constant and regular yoga practice can make a difference. If you make a commitment to stay in touch with your self and your body's messages, you will constantly be adapting to the stressors of life and lessening their impact. Swami Vivekananda, the man responsible for bringing yoga to America over 100 years ago, said:

> Every mental state creates a corresponding state in the body, and every action in the body has its corresponding effect on the mind.[4]

The perspective that Swami Vivekananda gives is that the body reveals the consciousness that made it. Through self-analysis of the body, you come to know the formative thought process. Hence, by changing your consciousness, you can change your body.

Candace Pert reflects this perspective at a molecular level in her research into the *Molecules of Emotion*:

> In summary, the point I am making is that your brain is extremely well integrated with the rest of your body at a molecular level, so much so that the term *mobile brain* is an apt description of the psychosomatic network through which intelligent information travels from one system to another. Every one of the zones . . . of the network—the neural, the hormonal, the gastrointestinal, and the immune—is set up to communicate with one another, via peptides and messenger-specific peptide receptors. Every second, a massive information exchange is occurring in your body. Imagine each of these messenger systems possessing a specific tone, humming a signature tune, rising and falling, waxing and waning, binding and unbinding, and if we could hear this body music with our ears, then the sum of these sounds would be the music that we call our emotions.[5]

Scientists no longer think of emotions as having less validity than material substance, and are beginning to see emotion as a cellular signal that is involved in translating information into physical reality. We are, literally, transforming mind into matter![6]

---

4 *The Complete Works of Swami Vivekananda* (Calcutta: Advaita Ashrama, 1989), p. 39.
5 Candace Pert, *Molecules of Emotion: Why You Feel the Way You Feel* (New York: Scribner, 1997), p. 188.
6 Pert, *Molecules of Emotion*, p. 189.

The Hatha Yoga perspective is that by making a difference in our physiology, we can make a difference in our consciousness. With yoga asanas, we change our posture dramatically in a positive manner. We know from subjective experience that we feel better following a good class. Physical therapists often parade about in a T-shirt that says "If it's physical, it's therapy." We can all relate to this.

Yet, there are pains and dis-ease that surgery, physiology, or physical therapy cannot touch. The stress of these pains seems inevitable. People hurt people. We disappoint ourselves. We carry this woundedness with us and it becomes us. Our postures change, our physiology changes, our behavior changes, in reaction to this nonphysical pain. What can we do?

One suggestion is to ask yourself three questions and reflect upon the one that produces the most reaction—physiological or psychological. Ask yourself:

What am I afraid of?
What am I angry about?
What am I holding onto?

The manner in which to ask the question is to repeat it over and over for a minimum of ten minutes and just listen to the response or, better yet, write it down. Watch carefully for your body's answers, as well as listening to your mental insights. If the pain is truly challenging, I suggest digging deeply with the questions and allowing yourself to open hidden doorways to your body's manner of answering you.

When faced with a situation that is beyond our experience, we need to challenge ourselves in a manner totally foreign to our past. The best we can do may be to meditate, reflect, and pray to a Higher Authority, however we understand that Being or Consciousness. Some guidelines for this are offered in chapter 6.

There may not always be a way to be free of pain and/or suffering from events of the past. But there is a way to be free of future pain, according to the teachings of Patanjali's Classical Yoga.

> The suffering from
> *pain* that has
> *not yet arisen*
> is
> *avoidable.*
>
> The *cause* of that *avoidable pain*
> is the close *association*
> of the *Seer* with the *seen,*
> so that one does not distinguish
> the True Self.[7]

---

[7] Stiles, *Yoga Sutras of Patanjali*, chap. II, sutras 16–17.

Patanjali recommends diving deeply into yourself and uncovering the True Self, the Self that has always been there. That Self is quite empathic. Its nature could be said to be of compassion, love, and peace.

Chapter 32

YOGA THERAPY

SECRETS

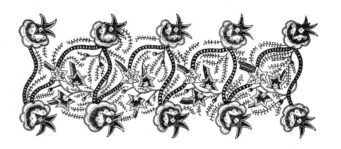

Many yoga students find that doing yoga is therapeutic for all levels of themselves—for everything from bad backs, mood swings, and the mid-life crisis of Where am I going? All can be dealt with through yoga. You are a multi-dimensional being. Doing yoga can be therapeutic for many areas of your life. This is true whether the issues are predominantly physical, psychological, or spiritual. Yoga therapy adapts its wide range of benefits to your uniqueness.

This is not to say that yogis and yoginis do not benefit from psychotherapy. Long-term practitioners know of difficulties of both students and teachers that might have been prevented with good therapy. I have personally benefited greatly from regular psychotherapy and twelve-step programs. While yoga can become a comprehensive discipline, I do recommend that you keep a perspective on its limitations and seek to know more of its benefits. The array of practices and philosophical viewpoints available can bring about a more glorious future than you might imagine.

> Yoga creates pathways in your consciousness through which the creative and healing forces can operate. Creativity, healing and wisdom are like your blood. Just as blood is a fact of your physical body, creativity is a fact of your spiritual body and nothing you must invent.[1]

---

[1] Julie Cameron, *The Artist's Way* (New York: J. P. Tarcher/Putnam, 1992), p. xiii.

The principal proponent of yoga therapy in this century was Professor T. Krishnamacharya. He was a lifelong student of yoga, Ayurveda, Sanskrit, and the healing arts. Krishnamacharya was the teacher of the world's most noted Hatha Yoga teachers, including his brother-in-law B. K. S. Iyengar, Pattabhi Jois, Indra Devi, and his son/successor T. K. V. Desikacharya. He was the heir of a family tradition of yoga teachers that can be traced back to Nathamuni, who lived during the 9th century. Krishnamacharya lived to the age of 100. This remarkable man often described yoga as "healing without surgery" and claimed that the "*Yoga Sutras* are for suturing the wounds of life."[2]

Krishnamacharya stated that the key Yoga Sutra for yoga therapy is the first aphorism of the second chapter on purification practices, or Kriya Yoga. This chapter contains the summation of practices that prepare the student for the deeper practices of meditation and ultimately result in Self-realization. The sutra is as follows:

> The *practical means (kriya yoga)*
> *for preparing the desired state*
> conducive to harmonious life
> consists of three components:
> *self discipline and purification (tapas),*
> *self observation*
> *stimulated by reflections on the scriptures (svadhyaya),*
> and *living your life*
> *as service*
> *to the inner Lord (Isvarapranidhana).*[3]

In Krishnamacharya's teachings, each of these three components plays an equal role in yoga therapy. The first of these principles, *tapas*, derives from the root word *tap* meaning "to burn." The practices of tapasya include leading a disciplined life-style (regularity of eating, sleeping, exercise), and practices to purify the body and mind (seasonal cleansing diets, longer yoga practices during times of difficulty, and selfless service to others without seeking recognition for your charitable acts).

The second quality, *svadhyaya*, means analysis of one's self. The root word *sva*, means "one's own," and *dhyaya* means "analysis." This quality of self-reflection is developed through philosophical study, the reading of works of self-analysis and scriptures on the nature of the True Self. By reading the texts of the timeless teachings known as the Sanatana Dharma, a personal experience can be gained from the visionary insights of master teachers. Svadhyaya also implies spending time with great beings, having the experience of living with an advanced teacher or a saintly person. It implies honoring your elders and the contribution that they have made to society.

The third quality, *Isvarapranidhana*, develops ethical qualities like humility and devotion to a Higher Power than your own self. The word's roots are *Isvara,* meaning

---

[2] Personal communication from Paul Copeland, student of Krishnamacharya, 1971–1973.
[3] Stiles, *Yoga Sutras of Patanjali*, chap. II, sutra 1.

"Lord of all, Supreme spiritual consciousness or God," *pra,* implying "fullness," *ni,* meaning "under," and *dhana,* which means "placement." Literally, it could be taken to mean "to place oneself under the fullness of the Lord." Classical Yoga is theistic, or more precisely, it offers belief in God as a valid way to serenity. There are many manifestations of this in practice. For some, it is the act of just doing yoga, no matter what, a surrender in faith to the tradition and practice of yoga. For others, it is a religious quality deepening their pre-existing religious beliefs and reaffirming the importance of prayer and rituals, and taking time for reflection. For others still, it is the profound Christian attitude of compassion to do unto others as you would have them do unto you. As the Dalai Lama has put it, "My religion is kindness."

The three principles feed each other. The practice of self-observation reveals a need for self-discipline, which in turn shows the limitations of self-effort, and the need for dependence upon a Higher Power. They can be summarized as right life-style, right thinking, and devotion to a God or to your personal conception of a power greater than yourself. When they are in place, your life-style becomes healthier, thoughts are more optimistic. Regular contact with a Higher Power elevates the intellect to its spiritual nature, bringing humility.

Ayurveda and Yoga Therapy

This first sutra of the second chapter of the *Yoga Sutras* can also be interpreted as a corollary to the sister science of yoga, Ayurveda, which emphasizes proper life-style, diet, and the application of yoga for personal therapy. Classical Yoga is renowned as a spiritual science emphasizing how to know yourself. In contrast, Ayurveda provides the necessary foundation for living in the world and the disciplines for longevity to support the lengthy spiritual practice necessary to make the most of life. According to Ayurveda, there are three unstable qualities or doshas that need regular attention to promote balance in life-style and in the mind. These qualities are vata (composed of the elements of air and ether), pitta (formed from fire and some water), and kapha (derived from earth and the remaining water). Kapha is the stabilizing force of the body. Pitta is the warmth of the mind and digestive strength. Vata is the rhythm of life and the connection to the life-force.

The practice of self-study promotes a balance of prana, the energy that is the root of Ayurveda's vata quality. When you observe yourself and inquire into the nature of life and your actions, prana is drawn inward to quiet your mind and produce deep restful sleep.

The process of self-discipline directs the pitta quality. When persisted in for some time, this elevates it from its bodily function as the source for digestive fire to the quality called tejas. This is the spiritual light that produces discriminative thinking and spiritual insights.

The practice of devotion to your chosen form of Higher Power, Goddess, or God leads to the goal of yoga as absorption into Spirit or samadhi. This experience produces a refinement of the quality of kapha into its essence known as ojas. Ojas is the closest substance to a spiritual material there is. It can be consumed as ghee made through the purification of butter from well-loved cows. It is also available to us from our loving mother's milk. Through the direct experience of a loving God's presence, ojas is produced, giving devotees a radiant aura and a peace-promoting countenance.

The Yogic View of Therapy

According to a dialogue between Rama and the sage Vasistha in the latter's *Yoga Vasistha*, there are three major causes of disease. The first is a wrong connection between the mind and the senses. The second is knowledge of good action present in the mind but overpowered by addictive or egoistic behavior. The third is external influences, such as a change in climate, cultural patterns of diet and life-style, and accidents.

The remedy given for the first cause of disease is the study and practice of Classical Yoga. To understand the mind and the senses, the view, or darshan, of Patanjali's *Yoga Sutras* and its related philosophical system, Samkhya, are most beneficial. To pursue this study, a good teacher of meditation practice is of the utmost importance. Seek and you will find.

The remedy for the second cause of disease is consistent earnest practice at being mindful in your life-style. To overcome this difficulty, you must not look to be free of present pain, but rather look deeper, to the root cause of the imbalances you are currently experiencing.

One of my most challenging teachers, an American who chooses to remain anonymous, used to talk about the cycle of life as being tests, lessons, and blessings. When difficulty arises, there is a test. If the mind is trained to look for the lesson and focuses intently enough, the present layer of the lesson can be learned. One can grow intellectually, intuitively, and spiritually from the lessons of life. Often, these lessons produce the blessings of health, happiness, or freedom from conflict.

The remedy for the third cause of disease is the process of learning from life. This is greatly helped by studying the "science of life" known as Ayurveda. Ayurveda and yoga are considered sister sciences, meant to be learned fully as branches of the same family tree. Ayurveda is an indigenous natural health system of India that has been in existence nearly as long as yoga. While yoga is considered to be the older and wiser sister, Ayurveda and yoga are both concerned with spiritual health. Ayurveda is more focused upon physical health. Yet together, their practices are highly renowned for their capacity to restore health and promote longevity.

The *Caraka Samhita* text of Ayurveda also cites the "causes to disease of both mind and body as being threefold—wrong utilization, non-utilization, and excessive utilization of time, mental faculties and objects of sense organs. The body and mind constitute the substrata of diseases and happiness and therefore positive health. Balanced utilization of time, mental faculties, and objects of sense organs is the cause of happiness."[4]

The spiritual goal of Ayurveda is succinctly stated in the *Caraka Samhita*, as, "salvation is detachment."[5] A similar sutra was written a thousand years earlier by Patanjali in

---

[4] Ram Karan Sharma and Vaidya Bhagwan Dash, *Agnivesa's Caraka Samhita*, "Quest for Longevity" (Varanasi, India: Chow Khamba Sanskrit Series Office, 1976), vol. I, sutras 54–55, pp. 39–40.
[5] Sharma and Dash, *Agnivesa's Caraka Samhita*, "Quest for Longevity," vol. II, sutra 142, p. 346.

his *Yoga Sutras.* In chapter one, sutra 12, he cites that the means to success in yoga is through "consistent earnest practice and dispassionate non-attachment."[6] These terms are elaborated in the following sutra:

Non-attachment
is the *consciousness*
of Self-*mastery,*
wherein one is *free from craving*
for sense *objects,*
whether they have been *experienced*
or imagined based on
promises in the scriptures.

That ultimate state of non-attachment
arises from *Self-realization*
in which there is even *freedom*
from the primordial forces of desire,
as everything
and everyone
is experienced as one's
own True Self.[7]

The Sanskrit word for health is *swastha,* which, literally translated, means "living in one's own self." Thus health and spirituality are interconnected for the yogic and Ayurvedic practitioner. The means to this goal is to become "freed from the primordial forces of desire," (in Sanskrit, the gunas). The gunas, like the Ayurvedic concept of the doshas, are three naturally arising forces. Unlike the doshas, which are based on biological qualities, the gunas are philosophical concepts of the nature of the mind.

Rajas — Sattva — Tamas
Activity — Balance — Inertia

The state of balance, or harmony, is called sattva. This is the goal of yoga therapy—to achieve a sattvic state of peace and tranquillity. For the yogi, it is a naturally arising state originating from being true to your inner teacher, guru or God. By purifying the body, senses, and mind, the yogi experiences his natural self.

At first, you identify with the actions you perform, the roles in life you lead, or the praise and criticism you receive from others. This state of activity and hyperactivity is called rajas. It is a state in which you identify yourself with your actions and seek to gain the rewards of a full life. In the rajasic state, the mind is identified with the concepts of karma. Whatever you sow, so you will reap. The concept of karma defines three attributes to its qualities. There is the karma that is presently being experienced as a result of

---

[6] Stiles, *Yoga Sutras of Patanjali,* chap. I, sutra 12.
[7] Stiles, *Yoga Sutras of Patanjali,* chap. I, sutras 15–16.

the past actions, heredity, and the social conditions we find ourselves in. There is the karma of that past that has yet to produce results in our life. There is also the present course of actions, which will produce a rather predictable future. Collectively, all three qualities are known as our karma. By having an active memory, we can see what has been the course of our life events and, to the extent that we have a clear mind, we can see how we have gotten into the grace or difficulty that we presently experience. Yoga therapy encourages us to have insights into this bundle of karmas and to gain a life-style that produces peace of mind.

The third quality of the gunas is called tamas. Tamas refers to darkness, ignorance, and the lazy nature of the mind. To give this up is to move toward the center of the cycle of the mind.

The methods recommended to achieve the sattvic, balanced state of body and mind are to watch the indicators of balance and carefully adjust our life-style, diet, physical and mental exercise for maintenance of harmony with the natural rhythms of life. Eat non-animal fresh foods that are seasonal and locally produced. Live a life-style in harmony with the seasons, so that sleeping, meals, and work are regulated daily events. In a balanced utilization of time, the ideal life-style will incorporate meditation and prayer as the first and last events of the day. Wake and rise before the Sun to capture the delight of the glorious sunrise. Exercise during the period before breakfast. The major meal of the day should be lunch, eaten between noon and 2 P.M. The evening meal should be light or moderate, eaten at the time of sunset. The hour prior to bedtime should be spent in restful pleasant activity, such as reading or walking in nature. An ideal bedtime is around 10 o'clock, and not later than 11 P.M.

Chapter 33

A COMPLETE
CLASSICAL YOGA PRACTICE

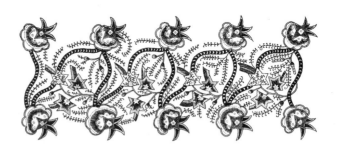

It is important to know your starting point in yoga. Without knowing this, it is at best difficult to evaluate your progress. By knowing yourself and making a regular commitment to re-evaluate yourself, you can know that you are making progress in the multitude of layers of your body/mind/Spirit that can express the natural harmony of your True Self. Continue to allow yourself to be re-appraised by colleagues, teachers, or even the yogini you meet on the street. By exercising self-study (svadhyaya), you can watch your freedom in yoga grow, being nurtured by your commitment to yourself.

I recognize three levels of students in yoga. These levels are not determined by flexibility, but rather by a number of factors that reveal a change to your personality. Table 7 (page 326) summarizes these phases of progress. You may find that, according to my summary, you are a beginner in some areas, a regular student in others, or even a committed student in one or two areas. These differences are natural. I encourage you to aim to stabilize all dimensions of your practice (sadhana), until it has become more fully integrated with the rest of your life.

In the same manner that the factors in Table 7 have levels, so I also find levels for the mastery of each of the techniques presented within this book. Following is a summation of all the practices for the Structural Yoga Therapy™ process that lead you more deeply into Classical Yoga.

1. Joint-Freeing Series is first done to evaluate joint freedom and learn anatomy. Regular practice maintains limber joints and improves circulation. Committed practice will shift attention to the energy level of pranayama practice to create a pranic flow through the pranamayakosha to awaken your intuition.

Table 7. Phases of Progress in Yoga Practice (Sadhana).

QUALITIES	BEGINNER	REGULAR	COMMITTED
Flexibility	Body moves in units, two joints at a time. Range of motion 80 percent.	Beginning to isolate joint motions and has full range of motion.	Can isolate strength or stretch to specific muscles.
Strength	Trembles on holding poses more than 3 breaths.	Steady in most poses for 6 breaths.	Steady in all poses for holds up to 12 breaths.
Alignment and Body Awareness	Feels awkward in balancing poses. Tight in forward bends, uncertain of anatomy.	"Adjusts" self frequently. Attempts to release specific tensions. Aware of fear.	Comfortable with body as it is. Watches for opportunities to open self.
Breath Awareness	Conscious for only few moments.	Irregularly breathing fully and rhythmically.	Comfortable at watching breath.
Diet	Irregularly eats "healthy foods."	Fascinated with "eating right."	Eats with a feeling of reverence and feels food becoming part of self.
Effort	Works hard at relaxing, toning, yet irregular.	Works fully, but relaxing with effort. Stays in touch with body.	Actively creates conditions for self-awareness. Paces self.
Desires	Wants to be relaxed, yet feels stressed.	Wants to meditate, beginning to relax consistently.	Wants to be in a continuous state of mindfulness.
Philosophy	Work hard and you'll get your reward.	Hard work isn't what its puffed up to be.	Take things as they come or go. Life is its own reward.

2. Strength exercises are first done to evaluate for potentially weakened muscles and analyze spinal freedom. Regular practice keeps the spine supple and will develop stamina in infrequently used muscles. Committed practice will eliminate weakened muscle tone and the spine will be free to comfortably hold many variations of the same asana.

3. Yoga asanas are practiced to increase sensitivity to stressed areas, distinguish stretching from strengthening, and tone overall body. Regular practice returns the body to improved posture by working to an aligned, stable base of support. Committed practice will focus on *Yoga Sutra* II, 47, to perfect the poses, gradually uncovering a feeling of connectedness within the natural currents of sensation that arise while the posture is held longer.

4. Pranayama is given to beginners to heighten their capacity to be self-observant. Regular practice enables students to remain ever-mindful of the wave of the breath, to be more open during daily activities. Committed practice reveals the omnipresent energy of prana and its ever-present mantra sound.

5. Mudras for the beginner are an extra challenge in self-observation. Regular practice expands the areas of the body of which one can be simultaneously aware. Committed practice connects the mind to the energy body and to one's immediate surroundings.

6. Bandhas for beginners develop the tone of the pelvic floor and the diaphragm, and freedom of the neck. Regular practice stimulates reflexes to lower heart rate and control elevated blood pressure, thus relieving physical stress. Committed practice heightens a smooth transition into meditation.

7. Meditation for beginners challenges their ability to stay centered and self-observant. Regular practice brings meditation insights into daily life. Committed practice develops into a personal spiritual practice to connect the student to themselves and to a Higher Power or Divine Presence.

Yoga Principles and Spiritual Guidelines

Underlying the Structural Yoga Therapy™ method is a commitment to practice within the guidelines established in the textbook of Classical Yoga, Patanjali's *Yoga Sutras*. From practicing in this manner, I have noticed certain basic principles that keep me focused while presenting this work.

1. The highest spiritual attainment is selfless service to others sharing your experiences with humor and joy.

2. Yoga postures can be perfected by the recollection of one's bodily experience during the grace-filled moments of Step 1. The teachings that come in this manner take precedence over the priority of perfecting the outward form of the poses.

3. The postures are perfected in a systematic manner—the first priority is to restore natural flexibility/range of motion; the second is to maintain symmetry in muscle strength; the third is to create an energy flow that leads to the experience of naturally arising spontaneous meditation.

4. Breath/pranayama training is for the purpose of facilitating steadiness during motion, release of suppressed emotions and thoughts, and to cultivate the state of "great respect and love."

The process of structural yoga is therefore presented as part of a larger scheme aimed at contentment through self-realization. It is very important, when practicing any type of physical or Hatha Yoga, that you remember Yoga. Don't get so caught up in the "determined effect" (the literal meaning of "hatha" yoga)—the struggle—that you lose awareness of harmony, union, and being at peace with your Self.

327

How, then, can we keep reminding ourselves that the process of Hatha is to serve the deeper process of Yoga? These guidelines have served me well:

1. *Remain a beginning student.*

By being open to learning and staying inquisitive, your mind remains alert and clear, free from trappings of idealism and preconceived views. One delightful story elaborates on this point.

Two monks had been walking in silence for many weeks on a pilgrimage to see their teacher. They came to a stream and discovered a young, quite beautiful woman stranded on their side wondering how to cross without being carried away by the current. The beginner monk offered to carry her across on his back. Together, the two of them succeeded in fording the stream. The woman left on a different path to visit her family.

The elder monk was getting distressed at how his student had broken his vow of brahmacharya—avoiding the company of women. His mind became heated as he struggled with whether to tell their teacher and if so how to explain the novice's failure. Finally, he felt compelled to scold the novice. He said, "How could you break your vows of celibacy? Have you no mindfulness? What got into your head that you thought you could touch that lovely woman and hold her so tightly?"

After the elder's indignation was spent, the novice replied, "I put her down on the side of the stream, why are you still carrying her so tightly?" The elder couldn't hear this and told the novice to leave his company because he was impure.

The two monks arrived separately at the teacher's abbey, and the story was told to the master. The master sent the elder monk to clean the kitchen, while he spoke in private to the novice. Touching the novice sweetly and tenderly, the master bestowed upon him, through a secret touch, his blessings, and told him he was ready to be on his own. He said the novice would only be hindered by such companionship at the abbey. The novice was sent to a foreign land to establish his own way—the way of the novice.

2. *Seek out the presence of a living master.*

The word "Buddha" comes from the Sanskrit root *buddh*, which means "to reveal," "to understand." As we remain beginners, we can see how life reveals its secrets. Until a master teacher comes to us, the beginner's attitude provides the means of revealing secrets even from the mouths of fools. The process of seeking implies a reaching for the light of knowledge. As we reach beyond Hatha, Raja Yoga is revealed. *Raja* also means, "to shine," "to illumine," in the same way that *buddh* means "to clarify." Raja Yoga comes as an illumination of the mind—not only from practice, but also from openness to what pre-exists before, during, and after training.

The process of meditation prepares you for meeting your master. Patanjali says that one of the easiest "ways to meditation is to let your mind rest on a Self-realized being who has transcended human passions and attachments."[1] In keeping the company of such a mentor, the mind becomes calm and serene, and the teacher's experience and knowledge become yours.

---

[1] Stiles, *Yoga Sutras of Patanjali*, chap. I, sutra 37.

3. *Contemplate writings that uplift you.*

I entered yoga practice from reading a yoga book. I have much regard for how the message, the search for one's esssential self, can be conveyed through an excellent teacher's clear communication of his or her experience. There are many writings, not necessarily scriptures, that can keep you focused on your process. I recommend reading an inspirational chapter or sutra every night just before bed. This is the ideal time to absorb lofty impressions into your deep consciousness. Some of my personal favorites are cited in the recommended readings at the end of this book.

4. *Keep good company.*

By following the first three guidelines, you will be brought to "good company"—people who seek to be loving, aware, and at peace with themselves. The Sanskrit term for good company is *satsang*, literally, "in the company of Truth." Joining a satsang of like-minded seekers is beneficial to spiritual development. Best of all is to keep the satsang of your own inner Teacher. Sometimes self-observation brings you closer to people along the path, sometimes your spiritual seeking (sadhana) leaves you alone. Be true to yourself and, in so doing, sadhana will manifest of its own nature. *Sadhana* means literally "keeping the Truth." If you can keep good company inwardly, then, outwardly, good company will be attracted to you and come of its own accord.

Above all else, stay happy and practice smiling.

Bibliography

Arbogast, Donna. "Massage, Yoga and Aromatherapy—Can They Help GI Conditions?" *Digestive Health and Nutrition*. Bethesda, MD: American Gastroenterological Association, January/February 2000.

Baba Hari Das. *Ashtanga Yoga Primer*. Santa Cruz, CA: Sri Rama Publishing/Hanuman Fellowship, 1981.

Bacovcin, Helen. *The Way of a Pilgrim* and *The Pilgrim Continues His Way*. Garden City, NY: Image Books, 1978.

Batmanghelidj, F. *Your Body's Many Cries for Water*. Falls Church, VA: Global Health Solutions, 1995.

Baxter, Christopher. *Kripalu Hatha Yoga*. Lenox, MA: Kripalu Center for Yoga and Health, 1998.

Bell, R. D. and T. B. Hoshizaki, "Relationship of Age and Sex with Range of Motion of Seventeen Joint Actions in Humans." *Canadian Journal of Applied Sports Science*, 6 (4).

Benson, Herbert with Miriam Klipper. *The Relaxation Response*. New York: Avon Books, 1975.

Brofeldt, B. Thomas. "Rebel with a Cause." *Sacramento Magazine*, June, 1997.

Cameron, Julie. *The Artist's Way*. New York: J. P. Tarcher/Putnam, 1992.

Christensen, Alice. *American Yoga Association Beginner's Manual*. New York: Simon & Schuster, 1987.

Couch, Jean. *The Runner's Yoga Book*. Berkeley CA: Rodnell Press, 1991.

———. "Balance." *Yoga International*. Honesdale, PA: Himalayan International Institute, August/September 1998.

———. "In Defense of Stretching." *Yoga Journal*. Berkeley, CA: California Yoga Teachers Association, July/August 1983.

Daniels, Lucille and Catherine Worthingham. *Muscle Testing—Techniques of Manual Examination*. Philadelphia: W. B. Saunders, 1980.

Datey, D. K., et. al. "Shavasana: A Yogic Exercise in the Management of Hypertension." *Angiology*, 1969, vol. 20.

Desikachar, T. K. V. with R. H. Cravens. *Health, Healing & Beyond: Yoga and the Living Tradition of Krishnamacharya*. New York: Aperture, 1998.

Douillard, John. *Body, Mind, and Sport*. New York: Crown, 1994.

Evjenth, Olaf and Jern Hamberg. *Auto Stretching*. Alfta, Sweden: Alfta Rehab Forlag, 1997.

Foster, Titus. *Agaram Bagaram Baba: Life, Teachings, and Parables—A Spiritual Biography of Swami Prakashananda*. Berkeley, CA: North Atlantic Books; and Patagonia, AZ: Essene Vision Books, 1999.

Funderburk, James. *Science Studies Yoga: A Review of Physiological Data*. Honesdale, PA: Himalayan International Institute, 1977.

Griner, Thomas with Maxine Nunes. *What's Really Wrong with You?—A Revolutionary Look at How Muscles Affect Your Health*. Garden City, NY: Avery, 1996.

Ghosh, Shyam, ed. and trans. *The Original Yoga as Expounded in Siva-Samhita, Gheranda-Samhita and Patanjali Yoga-Sutra*. New Delhi: Munshiram Manoharlal, 1980.

Harrigan, Joan (Arpita). "Physiological and Psychological Effects of Hatha Yoga: A Review of the Literature." *Research Bulletin*. Honesdale, PA.: Himalayan Institute, vol. 5, nos. 1 and 2, 1983.

Hay, Louise. *You Can Heal Your Life*. Carlsbad, CA: Hay House, 1987.

Hoppenfeld, Stanley. *Physical Examination of the Spine and Extremities*. New York: Appleton-Century-Crofts, 1976.

Hymes, Alan and Phil Nuernberger. "Breathing Patterns Found in Heart Attack Patients." *Research Bulletin*. Honesdale, PA: Himalayan International Institute, vol. 2, no. 2, 1980.

Iyengar, B. K. S. *Body the Shrine, Yoga Thy Light*. Bombay: B. I. Taraporevala, 1978.

——————. *Light on Yoga*. New York: Schocken Books, 1979.

Jacobs, Susan with Jason Serinus. "Living with AIDS." *Yoga Journal*. Berkeley, CA: California Yoga Teachers Association, July, 1987.

Jung, C. G. *Psychology and the East*. R. F. C. Hull, trans. Princeton, N.J.: Princeton University Press, 1978.

Keeffe, Emmett. *Know Your Body: The Atlas of Anatomy*. Berkeley, CA: Ulysses Press, 1999.

Keim, Hugo and Robert Hensinger. *Spinal Deformities: Scoliosis and Khyphosis*. Summit, NJ: CIBA-GEIGY Corporation, vol. 41, no. 4, 1989.

Kraftsow, Gary. *Yoga for Wellness: Healing with the Timeless Teachings of Viniyoga*. New York: Penguin/Arkana, 1999.

Kurtz, Ron. *The Body Reveals*. San Francisco: Harper and Row, 1984.

Kuvalayananda, Swami. *Pranayama*. Philadelphia: The SKY Foundation, 1978.

Lannoy, Richard. *Anandamayi: Her Life and Wisdom*. Boston: Element Books, 1996.

Leonard, George and Michael Murphy. *The Life We Are Given*. New York: J. P. Tarcher/Putnam Books, 1995.

Lowen, Alexander. *The Language of the Body*. Old Tappan, NJ: Macmillan Company, 1971.

Lucas, George. *The Empire Strikes Back*. London: Lucasfilm, Ltd., 1980.

Lugaresi, E., G. Coccagna, and F. Cirignotta. "Snoring and Its Clinical Implications," cited in C. Guillemainault and W. C. Dement, eds. *The Sleep Apnea Syndromes*. New York: Alan R. Liss, vol. II, 1978.

Muktananda, Swami Paramahansa. *Meditate*. South Fallsburg, NY: S.Y.D.A. Foundation, 1980.

——————. *The Nectar of Chanting*. Oakland, CA: S.Y.D.A. Foundation, 1975.

Nikhilananda, Swami. *The Upanishads*. New York: Ramakrishna-Vivekananda Center, 1978.

O'Shea, Michael. "Fitness." *Parade Magazine*. September 5, 1993.

Paramahansa Yogananda. *Autobiography of a Yogi*. Los Angeles, CA: Self-Realization Fellowship, 1998.

Pert, Candace. *Molecules of Emotion: Why You Feel the Way You Feel*. New York: Scribner, 1997.

Pratinidhi, Bhanawanvo Pant (Raja of Aundh). *Surya Namaskara: An Ancient Indian Exercise*. Hyderabad, India: Orient Longman, 1989.

Saraswati, Swami Muktibodhananda. *Hatha Yoga Pradipika*. Munger, India: Bihar School of Yoga, 1985.

Satchidananda, Swami. *Integral Yoga Hatha*. New York: Henry Holt, 1970.

Satyananda, Swami. *Surya Namaskara (A Technique of Solar Vitalization)*. Munger, India: Bihar School of Yoga, 1983.

Sharrard. W. J. W. "Muscle Recovery in Poliomyelitis." *Journal of Bone Joint Surgery*, vol. 37B, 1955.

Singh, Jaideva. *Siva Sutras: The Yoga of Supreme Identity*. Delhi: Motilal Banarsidass, 1979.

Singh, Kirpal. *The Crown of Life*. Delhi: Ruhani Satsang, 1971.

Sivananda Yoga Center. *The Sivananda Companion to Yoga*. New York: Fireside, 2000.

Sri Aurobindo. *The Synthesis of Yoga*. Pondicherry, India: Sri Aurobindo Ashram, 1984.

Sri Chinmoy. *The Body: Humanity's Fortress*. New York: Aum Publications, 1978.

Stiles, Mukunda. *The Yoga Poet*. Brookline, MA: Patanjali Press, 1999.

————. *The Yoga Sutras of Patanjali*. York Beach, ME: Samuel Weiser, 2001.

Stutley, Margaret. *The Illustrated Dictionary of Hindu Iconography*. Boston: Routledge & Kegan Paul, 1985.

Venkataram, T. N., ed. *Maharshi's Gospel: Books I and II*. Tiruvannamalai, India: Sri Ramanashram, 1994.

Vishnu-Devananda, Swami. *The Complete Illustrated Book of Yoga*. New York: Three Rivers Press, 1988.

Vivekananda, Swami. *The Complete Works of Swami Vivekananda*, 8 vols. Calcutta: Advaita Ashrama, 1989.

Warren, C. G., J. F. Lehmann, and J. N. Koblanski. "Elongation of Rat Tails Tendons: Effect of Load and Temperature." *Archives of Physical Medicine and Rehabilitation*, 52(3), 1971.

—————. "Heat Stretch Procedure: An Evaluation Using Rat Tail Tendon." *Archives of Physical Medicine and Rehabilitation*, 57(3), 1976.

Recommended Reading

ANATOMY, KINESIOLOGY, AND WELL-BEING

Calais-Germain, Blandine. *Anatomy of Movement*. Seattle, WA: Eastland Press, 1993. A most helpful manual of functional anatomy written by a dancer.

Clemente, Carmine D. *Anatomy: A Regional Atlas of the Human Body*. Baltimore, MD: Urban & Schwarzenberg, 1987. My favorite detailed reference to human anatomy.

Daniels, Lucille and Catherine Worthingham. *Therapeutic Exercise for Body Alignment and Function*. Philadelphia: W. B. Saunders, 1977. Evaluation and exercise planning for gradual improvement in postural alignment.

Hoppenfeld, Stanley. *Physical Examination of the Spine and Extremities*. New York: Appleton-Century-Crofts, 1976. How to locate structures and pathology.

Kendall, Henry, Florence Kendall, and Gladys Wadsworth. *Muscle Testing and Function*. Baltimore: Williams & Wilkins. 1971. Manual of physical examination.

Jerome, John. *Staying Supple*. New York: Bantam Books, 1987. Lay language to understand how the body works, the physiology of suppleness, with commonsense practical advice.

Netter, Frank H. *Atlas of Human Anatomy*. Summit, NJ: CIBA-GEIGY Corporation, 1989. A modern classic, artistic rendering, with some anomalies cited.

Northrup, Christiane. *Women's Bodies, Women's Wisdom*. New York: Bantam Books, 1998. A modern classic on listening to your wisdom body and nurturing yourself.

Olsen, Andrea. *BodyStories: A Guide to Experiential Anatomy*. Barrytown, NY: Station Hill Press, 1991. The title says it all, a delightful book to learn about yourself.

Palmer, M. Lynn and Marcia E. Epler. *Fundamentals of Musculoskeletal Assessment Techniques*. Philadelphia: Lippincott, 1997. Comprehensive evaluation methods for body reading from a perspective of physical therapy.

Pearsall, Paul. *The Heart's Code*. New York: Broadway Books, 1999. Fascinating account of cellular memory confirming yogi's secret Heart as the true seat of consciousness.

Pert, Candace. *Molecules of Emotion: Why You Feel the Way You Feel*. New York: Scribner, 1997. A modern classic by a neuroendocrineimmunologist scientist/Sherlock Holmes.

Sieg, Kay and Sandra Adams. *Illustrated Essentials of Musculoskeletal Anatomy*. Gainesville, FL: Megabooks, 1996. A great student's guide with large drawings.

Thompson, Clem. *Manual of Structural Kinesiology*. St. Louis: Times Mirror/Mosby, 1989. A college textbook of functional musculo-skeletal anatomy.

Todd, Mabel. *The Thinking Body: A Study of the Balancing Forces of Dynamic Man*. Brooklyn: Dance Horizons, 1939. A classic source of inspiration to all who love the body.

THEORY AND PRACTICE OF CLASSICAL YOGA

Bernard, Theos. *Hatha Yoga*. Thesis. New York: Columbia University Press, 1945; reprinted New York: Samuel Weiser, 1974. A thorough overview of Classical Yoga, citing Hatha Yoga medieval texts.

————. *Heaven Lies Within Us*. New York: Charles Scribner's Sons, 1939. A fascinating account of Classical Yoga training in India to master poses to a 3-hour duration by the first American scholar/sadhu.

Desikacharya, T. K. V. *The Heart of Yoga*, Rochester, VT: Inner Traditions, 1995. Contains many photos of the great master Krishnamacharya, by his son, with an overview of his life and teachings, and commentary on the *Yoga Sutras*.

Feuerstein, Georg. *The Yoga Tradition: Its History, Literature, Philosophy and Practice*. Prescott: AZ: Hohm Press, 1998. A scholarly, in-depth view of the development of yoga teachings.

Frawley, David. *Yoga and Ayurveda: Self-Healing and Self-Realization*. Twin Lakes, WI: Lotus Press, 1999. A comprehensive view of Classical Yoga practices in an Ayurvedic framework.

Iyengar, B. K. S. *Light on Yoga*. New York: Schocken Books, 1979. The yogi's reference on asanas—names, how to do them "properly," source for Structural Yoga poses, with an excellent introduction to Classical Yoga.

Kingsland, Kevin and Venika. *Complete Hatha Yoga*. New York: Arco, 1983. A thorough overview of Classical Hatha Yoga practices, well balanced with discussions of philosophy, relaxation, meditation, and diet.

Mohan, A. G. *Yoga for Body, Breath, and Mind*. Portland, OR: Rudra Press; and Los Angeles: International Association of Yoga Therapists, 1993. An excellent book surveying basic teachings of Krishnamachar and Desikachar. It covers 20 poses, fundamentals of practice with yoga therapy.

Saraswati, Swami Satyananda. *Asana Pranayama Mudra Bandha*. Munger, India: Bihar School of Yoga, 1983. An excellent, thorough commentary on all aspects of Hatha Yoga.

Shyam, Swami. *Patanjali Yog Darshan*. Montreal, Canada: Be All Publications, 1980. My favorite commentary to Patanjali's *Yoga Sutras,* filled with insights from a delightful master.

Stiles, Mukunda. *Yoga Sutras of Patanjali—With Great Respect and Love*. York Beach, ME: Samuel Weiser, 2001. A poetic rendering of the textbook of Classical Yoga.

CONTEMPORARY YOGA AND STRETCHING EXERCISE

Alter, Michael J. *Sport Stretch*. Champaign, IL: Leisure Press, 1990. Three hundred stretching positions arranged by muscle groups, with recommendations for 28 sports.

Blakey, W. Paul. *Stretching without Pain*. Stafford, England: Bibliotek Books, 1994. A guide by an osteopath on tissue, physiology, and mental-emotional aspects of stretch.

Douillard, John. *Body, Mind, and Sport*. New York: Crown, 1994. A fitness guide with comments from top athletes, based on Ayurvedic and yoga principles.

Evjenth, Olaf and Jern Hamberg. *Auto Stretching: The Complete Manual of Specific Stretching*. Alfta, Sweden: Alfta Rehab Forlag, 1997. A beautifully presented book of stretches, with specific muscles detailed for each motion.

Laird, Joan. *Ageless Exercise: A Gentle Approach for the Inactive or Physically Limited*. Williamsburg, MI: Anglewood Press, 1994. A manual for those confined to chairs or with limited mobility. Well done with variations to mobilize even the most challenged.

Ohlig, Adelheid. *Luna Yoga: Vital Fertility & Sexuality*. Woodstock, NY: Ash Tree, 1995. An important book on women's issues and yoga.

YOGA THERAPY AND RESEARCH IN YOGA

Funderburk, James. *Science Studies Yoga: A Review of Physiological Data*. Honesdale, PA: Himalayan International Institute, 1977. An overview of all research data on Hatha Yoga.

Harrigan, Joan (Arpita). "Physiological and Psychological Effects of Hatha Yoga: A Review of the Literature." *Research Bulletin*. Honesdale, PA.: Himalayan Institute, vol. 5, nos. 1 and 2, 1983. Reprinted in *The Journal of the International Association of Yoga Therapists*. Lower Lake, CA: IAYT, vol. 1, 1990. An overview of all research on Hatha Yoga with an excellent summary.

Jarrell, Howard. *International Yoga Bibliography, 1950 to 1980*. Metuchen, NJ: Scarecrow Press, 1981. An exhaustive report of 1700 listings of research studies and journals.

Monro, Robin, R. Nagarathna and H. R. Nagendra. *Yoga for Common Ailments*. New York: Gaia Books, 1990. Yoga therapy as used in the world's finest clinic and research center—Vivekananda Yoga Kendra in Bangalore, India.

Nagendra, H. R., ed. *New Horizons in Modern Medicine*. Bangalore, India: Vivekananda Kendra, 1990. Articles of recent research in yoga therapy from several Indian centers.

Satyananda, Swami. *Yogic Management of Common Diseases*. Munger, India: Bihar School of Yoga, 1983. Comprehensive overview of diseases treated by Australian physicians trained in Sivananda style yoga. See also separate titles including *Yoga & Cardiovascular Management* (1984); *Asthma and Diabetes* (1984).

Vivekananda Kendra Yoga Research Foundation. *Yoga Research Contributions (1983–1998)*. Bangalore, India: Vivekananda Kendra Yoga Prakashana, 1999. A bibliography of over 100 international research papers and dissertations they have sponsored.

MEDITATION

Dayananda, Swami with Janaki Vunderink. *Hatha Yoga for Meditators*. South Fallsburg, NY: SYDA Foundation, 1981. A guidebook of practices that facilitate entry into meditation practice and experience.

Osborne, Arthur, ed. *The Collected Works of Ramana Maharshi*. York Beach, ME: Samuel Weiser, 1997. Ramana was the first Indian spiritual teacher introduced to Western seekers. His method of contemplative inquiry into the eternal question "Who am I?" is most profound.

Muktananda, Swami. *Meditate*. South Fallsburg, NY: S.Y.D.A. Foundation, 1980. A powerful voice on the innate drive for spirituality, and an excellent guide for all methods of meditation.

————. *Play of Consciousness.* South Fallburg, NY: SYDA Foundation, 1978. A spiritual autobiography detailing awakening of kundalini, piercing of the chakras, and the journey to self-realization.

Ram Dass. *Journey of Awakening: A Meditator's Guidebook.* New York: Bantam Books, 1978. From Harvard professor to spiritual mentor, Ram Dass has helped raise America's spirits.

Ravi Dass, Narendra Dass and Anand Dass, eds. *Between Pleasure and Pain: The Way of Conscious Living.* Sumas, WA: Dharma Sara Publications, 1976. More than a guide to yoga and meditation, Baba Hari Dass's students provide insights into the Yoga of Life.

Singh, Kirpal. *The Crown of Life.* Delhi: Ruhani Satsang, 1971. A superb introduction to the varieties of yoga by a meditation master of the Sikh lineage.

Index

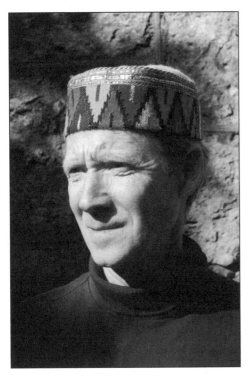

About the Author

Mukunda was first exposed to yoga while a cadet candidate for West Point Military Academy in 1969. In this unlikely setting he had a spiritual awakening, which transformed his curiosity into a lifelong passion. Subsequently, he has received extensive training in Classical Yoga and meditation under the guidance of the world's finest teachers. Most of his yoga teachers, including B. K. S. Iyengar and Indra Devi, are students in the lineage of Professor Krishnamacharya.

Another transformation occurred from receiving the gift of Shaktipat ("the descent of Grace") in 1974. From this devotional process, a continuous purification of body, mind, and Spirit were set in motion guided by the lineage of Nityananda of Ganeshpuri. Over the next eight years, he was yoga instructor at four of his spiritual teachers' residential ashrams and studied in India with both renowned and hidden teachers. His academic training includes a degree in religious studies from the University of California, Davis, and a year of graduate study in physical therapy at the California State University in Sacramento. He created Structural Yoga Therapy™ in 1976 after training at America's first professional yoga school, the Institute for Yoga Teacher Education (renamed the Iyengar Yoga Institute).

Since 1978, he has given certification courses in Structural and Ayurvedic Yoga for teachers and therapists. Mukunda is the author of a poetic rendering of *The Yoga Sutras of Patanjali* (soon to be published by Samuel Weiser), *The Yoga Poet*, American Yoga College asana course manuals, and is editor of the International Ayurvedic Institute's course manuals. He has taught and given workshops on four continents.

Mukunda welcomes inquiries and feedback at:

Yoga Therapy Center
3585 19th Street
Boulder, CO 80304
303-442-7004
yogimukunda@comcast.net
www.yogatherapycenter.org